BREAST CANCER

BREAST CANCER
A Family Survival Guide

Lucille M. Pederson
and
Janet M. Trigg

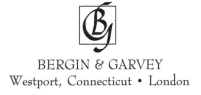

BERGIN & GARVEY
Westport, Connecticut • London

Library of Congress Cataloging-in-Publication Data

Pederson, Lucille M.
    Breast cancer : a family survival guide / Lucille M. Pederson and
Janet M. Trigg.
        p.   cm.
    Includes bibliographical references and index.
    ISBN 0–89789–293–3 (alk. paper)—ISBN 0–89789–438–3 (pbk.)
    1. Breast—Cancer—Popular works.   I. Trigg, Janet M.   II. Title.
    [DNLM: 1. Breast Neoplasms—therapy.   2. Breast Neoplasms—
psychology.   3. Family—psychology.   4. Social Support.
    5. Adaptation, Psychological.   WP 870 P3716 1995]
    RC280.B8P34   1995
    616.99'449—dc20
    DNLM/DLC
    for Library of Congress   94–37836

British Library Cataloguing in Publication Data is available.

Library of Congress Catalog Card Number: 94–37836
ISBN: 0–89789–293–3
        0–89789–438–3 (pbk.)

First published in 1995

Bergin & Garvey, 88 Post Road West, Westport, CT 06881
An imprint of Greenwood Publishing Group, Inc.

Printed in the United States of America

The paper used in this book complies with the
Permanent Paper Standard issued by the National
Information Standards Organization (Z39.48–1984).

10 9 8 7 6 5 4 3 2 1

To the women and their family members
who have generously shared their private feelings and
experiences so that they can help others
coping with breast cancer.

Contents

Acknowledgments   ix

Introduction   xi

1   Finding and Reacting To a Lump   1

2   Physical, Emotional, and Psychosocial Effects of Breast
    Cancer   13

3   Types of Breast Cancer and Treatments   27

4   Breast Reconstruction   43

5   Holistic and Alternative/Complementary Treatments   55

6   Effects of Breast Cancer on Couple Relationships   71

7   Effects of Breast Cancer on Children and Other Family
    Members   83

8   Relationships with Health Care Professionals   93

9   Communicating about Breast Cancer   103

10 Coping with the Breast Cancer Experience   117

11 Supportiveness of Family, Friends, and Community   131

12 Coping by Looking and Feeling Attractive   141

13 Coping with Medical Forms and Insurance   145

14 Coping with Recovery   149

15 Opportunity for Growth   157

16 Coping with Death   163

17 Survival Guidelines for the Woman with Breast Cancer   175

18 Survival Guidelines for Spouse/Partner, Children, and Other
    Family Members   183

19 Guidelines for Friends   189

Epilogue   193

Appendix A   *Suggested Readings*   197

Appendix B   *Resources*   201

Appendix C   *Questions to Ask Doctors*   207

Appendix D   *Procedures for Detecting Breast Cancer*   211

Appendix E   *Precautions for Avoiding Lymphedema*   213

Appendix F   *Bill of Rights for Cancer Patients and Family
               Members*   215

Appendix G   *Twenty-five Practical Tips You Can Use to Help
               Those Facing Serious Illness*   217

Notes   219

Glossary   237

Bibliography   243

Index   267

Acknowledgments

We are deeply indebted to all those who participated in our study and others who volunteered to share their experiences. We have been honored by their candidness and graciousness as well as their belief in this project.

To the Graduate Research Council at the University of Cincinnati for a grant to undertake a pilot study, we are grateful. We also express our appreciation to the College of Nursing and Health for the Herbert S. Rabinowitz Nursing Research Fund Award to begin our main investigation. We wish to thank Barbara Valanis, who got this project started.

Without the assistance of physicians who recommended to patients that they might wish to participate in the study, we could not have proceeded. We thank Drs. K. A. Keichert, W. J. Cormier, R. L. Coith, M. B. Popp, John Bismayer, Donna Stahl, and others. We are especially grateful to Dr. Michael G. Leadbetter and to Dr. Henry W. Neale for their support and referrals. We give special credit to their surgical assistants, Jeri Murray and Zae Roderer, for their help and encouragement. Others to whom we are grateful are Joy Webb, former director of nurses, and Mary Ann Joslin in the cancer division of Our Lady of Mercy Hospital, as well as the American Cancer Society and Reach to Recovery. We appreciate Nina Weber's generosity in lending us a tape of the show on breast cancer that was aired on Lifetime Television. The late Roger Stuebing, who analyzed the data in our study, deserves our deepest respect and gratitude.

We are also indebted to editors Sophie Craze for believing in our book and Lynn Flint for her patience and encouragement. We appreciate the efforts of Karen Davis and Alice Vigliani at Greenwood Publishing Group for their help in bringing this to completion.

To our husbands and family members and the friends who have given us their time and support, we express our gratitude.

Introduction

We remember well the first persons close to us who had cancer. Mine was a very dear friend with whom I spent many hours watching over our children as they learned to swim in her outdoor pool. When our children were in school we sometimes snatched time for ourselves to dabble in watercolor painting or to play golf. I'll never forget the day she made a hole-in-one.

Then Lois got breast cancer. She was one of the bravest women I've known. She took the loss of her breast with a smile and said, "Well, if I were 16, it would matter. I have my children; it's not important now." A former prisoner of war in the Philippines, Lois had learned what was really important. Just when it seemed she had recovered, the cancer recurred and the treatment was failing. At that time we didn't know nearly as much about treatment as we do now; chemotherapy was in its infancy.

I saw her, but not as much as before because I gotten busy in a part-time job. Our conversations became rather superficial—not like they had been. I know Lois was terribly lonely, and I'm embarrassed to say that I didn't know what to say to her and didn't make as much effort to be with her as I should have. I've always had regrets about that dear friend because I think she might have wanted to talk about her life, and I didn't give her the opportunity. I guess neither of us knew how to approach the subject of her impending death.

Since then, I have had many friends and a family member with breast cancer, some of whom, like Lois, did not overcome it. Others have, and all those who have coped with it have been an inspiration. For me, the person who has made the most remarkable recovery and adjustment is my sister-in-law. About two years after she had had a mastectomy another tumor appeared in her arm, but it was a different type from that found in her breast. This cancer, in the arm opposite from her mastectomy, required extensive excision of the tumor and lymph nodes as well as radiotherapy. Through all this she has gone on with her life, handling traumas and personal losses in a way that sets an admirable example of courage for all of us. Now she is experiencing the returning effects of polio (post polio syndrome) that she had after the birth of her second child. Wearing a brace and using a cane when she has considerable walking to do, she carries on an active life without complaint.

Janet, too, has experienced the cancer of someone very close to her. She tells you her story: "Just as we all remember what we were doing the day John F. Kennedy was shot, I recall vividly where I was the day my brother Bill called me long distance to tell me he had colon cancer. 'I've had cancer in the back of my mind since the polyps were found two years ago,' he said. His words came as a shock, but Bill was so faithful about having his six-month check-ups and sigmoidoscopies that I felt confident this was an early malignancy that could be cured with surgery.

"I went to stay with him during his first surgery at a cancer center 200 miles away from his home and family. All reports were positive for a successful removal of all cancer. However, within a year, a recurrence required another surgery. When the physician found that the cancer had spread to the liver and spine, I lost hope for his survival.

"The quality of Bill's life for the next year was poor. He endured a great deal of pain that was never relieved. He had no appetite and lost weight.

"Traveling 400 miles every two months, I tried to be a support to him and his family, even though my own grieving made me numb. I listened to Bill's concerns and his wife's. When I cried, he would console me. During these two years I wept in solace as he and his wife suffered. I witnessed the many frustrations my sister-in-law felt as she became solely responsible for every facet of their lives.

"After Bill died, I reflected on this experience with ambivalence. Had I supported each of them as well as I should have? How could I live with the sadness of my loss? From his death I learned the devastation for those who are left, but I also gained strength from Bill. The courage and dignity with which he had handled his illness and death provided me with an admirable model.

Although both of us have undergone the pain of losing someone close to us with cancer, neither of us had breast cancer. However, both of us have experienced the anxiety of lumps in our daughters and in our own breasts. So far they have tested negative. This book has not been written out of our personal anguish with breast cancer but from the experience we have gleaned from the many close friends, relatives, women, and their family members who have generously shared with us.

Our book has evolved from a study that we have worked on together for at least eight years at the University of Cincinnati. A colleague in epidemiology (the study of specific causes of outbreaks of infection or disease) asked me to assist her in a study of the effects of breast cancer on the family. My communication background encompassed the teaching of family communication, and she wanted the family's as well as the patient's perspective. I had also been interested in how families cope with chronic illness and had done some research on the topic. Janet, who teaches courses on breast cancer in the College of Nursing and Health, soon joined us. We had just completed our pilot study when our colleague Barbara, who initiated the study, was lured away from our university to another position.

Although breast cancer has been studied extensively, Janet and I were convinced from what we have learned in our pilot study of nine women and their families that we had a need to fulfill. We have continued the project, following a group of women and their families through a year of adjustment to breast cancer.

In addition to the nine in our pilot study, another forty-five women and their families (except for three who live alone) answered questionnaires and shared their experiences in interviews. Our endeavor was to enlist a greater number of women and their families, but we needed to be sure that their physicians felt they were emotionally ready. Indeed, we found that some women did not want to talk about it and that a number of their spouses would not consider discussing it. We are fully aware of the personal and private nature of breast cancer, and we respect their right to privacy. However, many women and men who were not a part of our structured study have volunteered to add to our information.

Since we began our investigation, the disease has increased and is now affecting one in nine women, according to the latest figures from the American Cancer Society. Shirley Temple Black, Betty Ford, Betty Rollins, and other prominent women who went public with their stories have made breast cancer less stigmatizing, and now people are more open to the discussion of it.

Breast cancer can have profound effects, both negative and positive, on a woman and on her spousal and parental relationships. Since the breasts are a part of a woman's nurturing and sexual image, some women and spouses may view breast cancer as the worst thing that could happen to them. As we have found, it can indeed be devastating—but it also can have positive outcomes.

Past studies have documented the trauma and adjustment women undergo and, to some extent, the problems that spouses experience. Recently, researchers have begun to look at the effects on children. As those of us who have experienced the illness of a family member are aware, the illness affects every member in some way. Children are particularly sensitive to a parent's illness.

The families who have shared their feelings and experiences with us have done so out of their desire to help others. Through sharing, some of them have found that it has been personally helpful. They have expressed gratitude in being able to talk about their problems and feelings.

We have witnessed the bonds of marital partnership grow stronger, and in several cases, break apart. For those couples whose marriages could not withstand the strains, the illness was perhaps the final straw in the emotional gap that had grown between them and the build-up of unresolved problems.

Today, the advances that have been made in detection, surgical procedures, treatments, and reconstructive surgery have given women more options and more hope for recovery. The factors that are crucial to this recovery are awareness, early detection, and early treatment.

In these chapters we share with you our findings and the experiences of families who have faced breast cancer. Not all of them have overcome the disease, but even those whose prognosis for recovery was poor accepted the reality of the disease and endeavored to live as fully as possible to the end. A number of women and their spouses have said that cancer has given them an acute realization of the value of life.

Our task has been gratifying and inspiring. Both of us have a deeper understanding of what it means to be devastated, depressed, courageous, tenacious, compassionate, positive, and spiritual. We want to impart some of the things we have learned to you.

One young mother said to us, "Breast cancer definitely changes your life but does so in a different way for each woman. When I had my first mastectomy [she has now had the second] I looked for a book about someone who had the same feelings and problems I was having—someone with whom I could identify. I didn't find anyone in my reading, but I did finally get acquainted with a woman in my neighborhood who has been understanding and helpful."

The women who participated in our study, as well as their spouses and other family members, have signed consent forms for the publication of their experiences. Except for well-known women, several deceased friends, and living relatives whose cancers have been made public, names and details have been changed so that the persons remain anonymous. Among them we hope there is someone with whom you can identify.

BREAST CANCER

Chapter 1

Finding and Reacting To a Lump

Peggy Thompson was taking her shower one morning when she felt a lump in the lower part of her right breast. She called her husband Dave, who kidded her and said, "Ah, the usual tease. This is the best invitation I've had all day." Then he felt the lump and she knew . . . his facial expression told her.

"I knew right away there was something there," Dave interjected.

After their initial panic, Peggy explained, they immediately called the gynecologist, who told her to have a mammogram. "I called the Breast Center [located in a large city near their town] and they said they could schedule me in seven weeks."

"We couldn't wait that long!" Dave exclaimed.

Peggy continued, "So we went to a doctor here who said that there was something in my system that didn't belong there, and that bothered him. 'Let's take it out,' he said."

"When he took out the tumor, it was negative but behind the tumor there were malignant cells. We've been told that we were very lucky that this doctor looked beyond the tumor," Peggy explained.

She worked for a physician at the time, so she was very knowledgeable: "The cancer cells were in situ (confined to the site of origin) and had not invaded neighboring tissues. The tissue in both breasts had severe dysplasia (the cells were altered in size, shape, and organization)."

"My mother had died of breast cancer when I was 16 years old," Peggy continued, "and an aunt had had a mastectomy. The doctors told us that because I was young and the dysplasia was so severe something should be done. They were very frank."

"We panicked and feared the worst but we didn't fool around with it,"

Dave said. "Many people wait and let it go; then, when they do see the doctor, the cancer may be advanced."

THE WAYS OF DETECTING BREAST CANCER

The case of Peggy and Dave illustrates the way that some women find a lump—when bathing or showering. Peggy's story also demonstrates the importance of seeing a physician immediately and having one who is thorough in looking beyond the apparent lump, particularly if the woman senses that something is wrong.

Another woman with whom we talked, Jane Adams, found her lump quite by accident when playing baseball with her family. Jane related her experience: "I was in the outfield. My husband Larry hit the ball and it struck me. I was sweating and rubbed my hand over the area [she demonstrated her hand movement] and I felt a lump there. I tried to ignore it, thinking it would go away. Then I talked with a friend who urged me to have it checked. I found a doctor who was highly recommended and made an appointment. I worried about it because I just had a feeling that it was serious. I don't know if I felt that way because of what my friend told me or if I just sensed it. I had been feeling tired all the time, and that told me something was wrong."

Jane's story explains why the American Cancer Society advocates examining your breasts during a bath or shower as a first step in self-examination. Hands glide more easily over wet skin. Because her skin was wet with perspiration, Jane's hand movement happened to glide over the lump— which she might not have noticed for some time unless she inspected her breasts regularly and carefully.

Breast self-examination (BSE) can aid in detection of breast cancer, but a mammogram may disclose suspicious calcification or lumps in their earlier stages. It can show tiny areas that cannot be felt by hand. For example, in the case of Doris Stanton, her breast cancer was discovered in its early stage because of a very cautious physician who urged his young patients at age 39–40 to have mammograms. Doris explained, "I was so fortunate to have had a good doctor. When I was 39 years old, he told me he wanted me to have a mammogram to use as a baseline." Several years later Doris went for her regular check-up and a mammogram. "That was how they found my breast cancer—by comparing mammograms. The doctor detected a change in the tissue from my baseline mammogram. He told me that it would have been another two years before I would have felt a lump." By that time the tumor would have been much more advanced. Although Doris did have a mastectomy, she did not have lymph node involvement and she feels confident that the cancer is gone. She is grateful for having a cautious physician.

Although the mammogram is the best detection tool at this time, it does not always reveal changes in the breast tissue. Some tumors are so hidden or fast growing that they are not detected even with sophisticated methods.[1] Such was the case with Eloise Crowell, who told us about her experience: "I had been having problems with soreness and discomfort in my breast for several months. I was getting ready for our youngest son's graduation from college and was having everyone here for a big party. In preparation I was doing some landscaping, wallpapering—things that I don't do every day. When I felt the soreness I thought I had pulled a muscle and strained myself, so I just sloughed it off. Two weeks after the party I decided something was wrong and I called my gynecologist. I had two mammograms and nothing showed. That was when I told the gynecologist that I was having problems with my breast. I was still uneasy about the soreness, so I had another mammogram. Still they could find nothing and the doctor suggested it might be a hormonal problem. I accepted that."

Two weeks later Eloise discovered a lump when doing a breast self-exam (BSE). "I called the doctor immediately and he told me to come in. 'That was not there before,' he said." He tried to reassure her and told her he thought she had nothing to worry about because it was on the chest wall, not the breast. He reminded her that pain doesn't occur with breast cancer. "But," he said, "we'll take it out because it's bothering you."

Eloise's lump was malignant. In her case mammography did not help in the detection of cancer, but her body and her persistence did. She knows now that although it is rare, you can have pain with breast cancer; and she warns her sisters and friends to check out any discomfort they feel.

Although some pain, or discomfort, is a common breast symptom, it is not usually associated with breast cancer. However, according to Preece and associates, 15 percent of the cases of operable breast cancer have pain. In very rare instances, pain that is referred to as noncyclical, or "target-zone" pain (it stays in one specific area), can be a sign of breast carcinoma. Whatever the cause of breast pain, it arouses the fear of cancer and should be investigated.[2]

Jean Doerger's experience was similar to that of Eloise. She said, "I was scheduled to have a hysterectomy and shortly before my admission to the hospital I found a lump in my breast. I have had fibrocystic disease with lots of lumps, but this lump felt different. After examining it, the doctor thought it was just a fibrocystic mass that should be left alone. When I went back after the hysterectomy, I wanted him to check it again and he said, 'Maybe we should take it out.' The excised lump had all the signs of being benign, but it was malignant." Jean underwent a simple mastectomy that disclosed that the cancer had invaded the tissue throughout her breast.

In another instance, Mindy Bishop was advised that the lump she had found could "be watched." Mindy, in her early thirties, mother of a toddler, said "I just wasn't comfortable with that, so I went for another opinion and cancer was found." Mindy had a mastectomy, underwent chemotherapy, and has had two "scares" since then. Fortunately, on both occasions the tissue was clear, but Mindy checks immediately when any disturbing symptom appears. "If I had taken the first doctor's advice of waiting and watching," she said, "I might not even be here now." When we last saw Mindy she had just had a check-up and was relieved to know she has no signs of recurrence.

There are other instances in which a woman's feeling that something is wrong and her persistence have led to the detection of breast cancer. Judy White had an uneasy sense about the results of a mammogram. Her concern led to finding her cancer. When Judy had her yearly mammogram the doctor thought there was something questionable but did not send her to the Breast Center for a further check, so she called the Center herself. She recalls that the receptionists constantly put off making an appointment for her. "It took me three months to get in because I didn't have a definite lump. If there had been one, they said they could get me in right away. Because there wasn't, I was put on a waiting list. All the people I had contacted up to that point were treating it very lightly. I have had a past history of breast problems and I felt as though they thought I had become neurotic about it." Judy continued to be persistent; breast cancer was found and she underwent a mastectomy.

Breast cancer may be detected by noticing changes in one's body. Willa Morrison, who had been widowed for over eighteen years and has no family nearby, lives alone. She described the circumstances of discovering a lump in her breast: "I was bending over to make my bed and I noticed a change in the shape of my breast. There was a large lump." The lump was so large (one and a half inches) that Willa immediately sensed it was probably malignant, so she was somewhat prepared for the diagnosis. She had a mastectomy and chemotherapy and has had no recurrence.

Sometimes breast cancer is found when a patient sees a physician for a condition that is unrelated to cancer, as in the case of Esther Seifert. "I had gone to the eye doctor with headaches," she explained. "He wanted me to have a CAT scan, but in order for our insurance to cover it, I had to see my family doctor who would then send me to the hospital. In reviewing my medical history, my family doctor asked me if I had ever had a mammogram. I told him I hadn't. He recommended I have one because I'm over forty." Esther took his advice and had the mammogram along with the CAT scan.

"After the tests," she explained, "the hospital personnel told me to contact my doctor the next day. I made an appointment and my husband went with me. I was worried that something had shown up in my CAT scan, that I might have a brain tumor. The doctor said, 'I have some bad news about your mammogram. You have a tumor in your breast.' Stunned, I just sat there and looked at him. 'I thought there was something wrong with my head,' I muttered. 'No,' he replied, 'there is nothing wrong with your head. We need to do a biopsy to determine if your tumor is malignant.'

"When it sank in I looked at my husband and he was sitting there crying.

I went to pieces then, too. After I got home and settled down, I thought, 'I have so much to be thankful for. It's not a tumor in my brain, where they might not be able to operate.' " The biopsy revealed cancer cells, and she had a mastectomy.

Esther had felt no lump or soreness. The doctor told her that by the time she would have felt a lump the cancer may have spread. She realized she was very fortunate that her headaches had prompted her to see a doctor.

In another case, Shirley Ottenheimer's doctor had found calcification in her right breast, which he wanted to watch. A year later a palpable mass (one that could be felt) was biopsied and the doctor advised her to have either a lumpectomy with radiation or a mastectomy. However, because Shirley's husband George needed surgery, she waited a few months to make a decision. The surgeon told her he couldn't understand how she could have waited. "Most women can't tolerate the anxiety of a long wait," he commented. Shirley confessed to him that she was afraid she might have waited too long. His reply: "No, you gambled and fortunately won."

Cancers grow at different rates. Most grow slowly but some are fast-growing, and some grow in spurts. When the cancer grows slowly, waiting may not be disastrous. However, if the cancer is fast-growing, the type that Fran Humphrey found, immediate treatment is necessary. Because her large breasts were contributing to problems with her back, Fran, who was working as a family counselor, was preparing herself to undergo surgery for breast reduction. "One Friday I noticed a kind of tightness or pinching in my breast," Fran recalled, "and that weekend I began to get sharp pains. As you know, the assumption is that if you have pain, it is not malignant. On Monday I felt a mass and immediately went to my family doctor, who referred me to a surgeon. I think he knew at once, but I was sure it was a cyst that was just going to go away."

Fran had bilateral surgery because the cancer had spread into the lymph nodes and the physicians thought it would soon be in the other breast. She had just completed chemotherapy when she had a recurrence and had to begin treatments again. She was fortunate that pain had alerted her to the cancer and that she could get to her doctor immediately. Laughing and calling it "a crap-shoot," Fran continued to counsel troubled families and finished her master's thesis. She had a third recurrence and each time was determined to fight it. Her optimism and "will to live" has been an inspiration.

Another woman, Ellen Barckley, is an example of how breast cancer can be found when other symptoms lead a woman to consult her doctor. Both Ellen and her husband Bob were retired, so they spent several winter months in Florida playing golf and tennis. For some time before they went to Florida, Ellen had not been well. First she had a viral infection, then shingles. "While in Florida," she said, "I began to lose weight and I didn't know what was wrong because my problem had always been keeping weight off.

My tennis game was terrible. I couldn't hit the ball; everything seemed too much for me."

She resolved to see her doctor when she got home and some weeks later made an appointment. After listening to her rather vague symptoms, the doctor diagnosed her problem as depression and prescribed a tranquilizer. She said to him, "I could be depressed, but I don't want to let it go with that. I'd really like to go into this more and have a thorough physical exam." He agreed to do a complete blood count, and at the same time he did a breast examination. "While he was examining me," she said, "I remembered that I had felt a lump when we were in Florida. I had completely forgotten that. I think it may have been denial or something, but I just completely forgot that I had felt a lump. I didn't really think about cancer."

Ellen went on with her story: "After the doctor told me I had a lump as well as the diabetes he had just discovered, he sent me for a mammogram and then to a surgeon, who did a biopsy. When the surgeon told me the lump was malignant, I was so shocked that I couldn't tell him anything about my health. I couldn't tell him why I was taking medication; I couldn't remember anything. I had never really felt so upset before."

Ellen's vivid description of her physical condition prior to going to her physician and her reaction to the diagnosis reveals the stress that she was undergoing. It may be that Ellen has lumpy breasts and that what she felt wasn't that unusual for her. On the other hand, her story may demonstrate an unconscious denial or a preoccupation with "feeling awful" and having low energy, which made her forget the lump she had felt. Fortunately, her other symptoms prompted her to see her physician and she was assertive enough to express her uneasiness with his first diagnosis.

THE IMPORTANCE OF EARLY DETECTION

The stories these women have told us illustrate some of the various ways by which they or their physicians discovered breast cancer. Their experiences emphasize the importance of awareness, vigilance, and assertiveness in taking responsibility for our health. If we pay attention to body changes and follow the American Cancer Society's guidelines for early detection, breast cancer can be detected and successfully treated. The most effective methods are breast self-examination, clinical breast examinations by a doctor, and mammograms.[3]

The changes that are constantly occurring in a woman's breasts make the identification of a lump that might be cause for concern very confusing for women. During menstruation the breast tissue swells, becoming tender and sometimes painful. An early sign of pregnancy is tenderness, and throughout pregnancy and breastfeeding lumps can develop. Sometimes milk cysts form.

Other changes may be a cyst, a fibroadenoma (a lump that forms during early years of menstruation), or a pseudolump (which sometimes appears during pregnancy and lactation). Some women have lumpiness that is normal breast tissue; this may cause considerable anxiety unless a woman is familiar with her breasts.[4]

The lump that causes real concern will be clearly distinct from other lumpiness. Dr. Love explains that when you are examining your breasts, "you are looking for one lump (or possibly two or three—rarely more) that's at least a half-inch in size, stands out, and is persistent and unchanging." This lump remains in the same place and does not disappear after menstrual cycles, whereas noncancerous lumps may go away after several menstrual cycles. A cancerous lump will not be felt until it is large enough for tissue to have formed around it. Any prominent tissue thickening that does not disappear should be checked.[5]

METHODS OF DETECTION

The foremost method of detection is the mammogram, which uses a low level of radiation. Mammography is an effective screening device whereby findings indicate the possibility of cancer. It can reveal abnormal areas of density or cancerous tissue, clusters of calcified spots, and cancers too small to be felt, even by an experienced physician. The American Cancer Society makes the following recommendation:

1. A screening mammogram should be done for women age 39–40; women between ages 40 and 49 should have a mammogram every one to two years. Women age 50 and over who have no symptoms should have a yearly mammogram.

2. "A clinical physical examination of the breast by a physician every three years for women ages 20 to 40, and every year for those over 40."[6]

3. A breast self-examination by women ages 20 and over once a month.

Unless a woman has a high risk of developing breast cancer, mammograms are not recommended if she is under age 35. The most important reason is that even though the amount of radiation has been reduced significantly in recent years, a young person has greater risk of developing cancer from radiation exposure. By age 35 the radiation risk becomes insignificant or nonexistent. Also, because of the density of breast tissue in a young woman, Dr. Love states that the mammogram can be ineffective as a detection device in young women.[7]

The mammogram must be done with an accredited dedicated mammography machine, which means the equipment is only used for mammographs. Two views should be taken by a skilled technician. It is also important to have a skilled radiologist to study the X ray. When you call to inquire about having a mammogram, you can ask about the equipment and the number of mammograms performed by the technicians operating it.

Mammograms involve some additional exposure to radiation. However, the National Cancer Institute and the American Cancer Society have recommended safe radiation levels and it has been established that the procedure is safe. The possible risk from mammograms is one additional cancer per million per year.[8] This is an extremely small risk in exchange for an early diagnosis.

The second method of detection recommended by the American Cancer Society is a regular physical or clinical breast examination. The physician palpates, or feels, the breast for consistence of parts beneath the surface. Any irregularities can be checked with a mammogram or ultrasound.

The third method, breast self-examination (BSE), is recommended by the American Cancer Society because many breast cancers are found by women themselves. The monthly breast self-examination is recommended "as a routine good health habit for women 20 years or older."[9] Through this procedure some women find lumps that have developed during the time between mammograms and regular physical examinations.

How does one do BSE? As the *first step* the procedure should include a check of the breasts while showering. Using flat fingers, feel for lumps as you glide your hand over every part of your breasts. The *second step* is a visual examination before a mirror with both arms raised overhead and then with hands lowered to the hips while you flex the chest muscles. The *third step* involves looking for any changes in coloration, contour, dimpling, nipple inversion, or sudden prominence of veins. The *fourth step* involves palpating or feeling the breasts while lying on your back with one arm behind your head and a pillow tucked under the shoulder of the side being examined. With the other hand press the breast gently in a clockwise circular motion—or, as Dr. Love suggests, you can invent your own pattern. Some breast centers demonstrate how to examine one's breasts when you get a mammogram. The important thing is to feel the entire breast and be aware of changes that may occur. The *last step* is to squeeze the nipple gently. If there is any discharge, it should be checked with a doctor.[10] Women who have certain risk factors should be especially conscientious about using the three methods of detection. (See Appendix D for procedures).

Ultrasound

This technique uses high-frequency sound waves that are projected toward the breast. An image of the interior of the breast is produced by converting the patterns of echoes from the sound waves. It is not good for screening but can be used for examining a specific area or a lump that has been detected. Rather than doing a mammogram on a very young person,

Dr. Susan Love uses ultrasound, which does not involve radiation, to determine if a lump she has detected by physical examination is solid or fluid-filled (a cyst).[11]

CAT Scan and MRI

The CAT scan (computerized axial tomography) and MRI (magnetic resonance imaging) are methods of examining the body in cross-sectional slices. Because they use higher amounts of radiation than mammography and are costly, they are not routinely used for screening and early detection. They are used for further evaluation of diagnosed breast cancer, for detecting metastases, and for evaluating responses to therapy. As researchers Kim et al. predict, in the next decade MRI will "play a significant role in the detection of breast cancer."[12] Scans are also referred to as CT scans followed by the part of the body being scanned, i.e. CT scan of the liver.

RISK FACTORS

There are certain factors that can increase the risk of developing breast cancer. Because of their family history, some women may be unduly concerned about their risk.[13] Before we discuss what makes some people more susceptible to a disease than others, it is important to note that Dr. Love suggests you should not become overly anxious if you have one or more risk factors. At the same time, you should not have a false sense of security if you have none. Cancer has many causes and interacts with other factors in ways we don't understand, so it is best to follow the guidelines for detection even though you may be low-risk.[14]

What are the risk factors? The major ones are as follows:

1. *A person's sex.* Although men can develop breast cancer, it is predominantly a disease of women.

2. *Age.* Breast cancer risk increases progressively as women age. Two-thirds of breast cancer cases occur in women over the age 50, after menopause. It does not occur often in women under the age of 30, but it increases sharply in the early forties. It levels off after age 45 and increases again after age 55. The yearly incidence in 70-year-old women is three times greater than in 50-year-olds.[15]

3. *Family history.* This may be the most important factor, especially in women who have a history of immediate relatives who have breast cancer.[16] The number of American women who have inherited a susceptibility to the disease is as many as one in two hundred.[17] Women whose mothers or sisters have had breast cancer are two to three times more likely to develop it. If it has occurred

in both breasts of these relatives and before menopause, the risk is increased. A family history of breast cancer need not indicate a genetic cause.

4. *Previous cancer.* If a woman has had cancer in one breast, the risk of her developing it in the other breast in the twenty years following the initial diagnosis is between 10 and 15 percent.[18]

Among the factors that have been associated with cancer risk are diet, obesity, national origin, and economic status. High-fat diets and obesity appear to increase the likelihood of breast cancer. Women of North American or northern European origin have a much higher incidence of breast cancer than do Asian and African women. The lowest incidence occurs in Japanese women who remain in their native land, where they subsist on a diet low in animal fats. This indicates that risk may be related more to diet than to race. There is also a higher frequency of breast cancer among women of higher social and economic classes.

Other risk factors are pregnancy, menstrual history, and hormones. Women who have not borne a child or whose pregnancy occurred after age 30 have a higher risk. Early onset of the menstrual period along with late menopause also seems to increase the risk, whereas early menopause lessens it. Finally, the relationship of hormones is not well established. Some breast cancers are clearly related to estrogen; others are not. Although the effects of birth control pills and estrogen supplements have been very controversial, conclusive evidence has not been found to establish them as a cause of breast cancer. The risk of cancer for long-term users of the pill and hormone replacement therapy (which is now being taken to retard osteoporosis) will be under investigation for some time. Results thus far are somewhat contradictory.[19] It is wise for any woman taking these pills or supplements to have frequent check-ups with her physician.

FAILURE TO UTILIZE METHODS OF EARLY DETECTION

Despite the recommendations of the American Cancer Society and the National Cancer Institute, many women still fail to take the precautions of regular breast self-examination (BSE), mammography, and breast examinations by physicians. Studies that have assessed the competency of women who practice BSE have reported that it is often done improperly. Instruction by a nurse or physician improves a woman's confidence and, therefore, the value and (it is hoped) the practice of self-examination.

Women avoid taking these precautions of early detection for several reasons.[20] The cancer screening process engenders fears of death, mutilation, and loss of desirability and feminine identity in them. Because people often respond to a woman on the basis of her appearance, much of her self-esteem and psychic energy is invested in being physically attractive.[21] Women are afraid they may find cancer and lose a breast.

An additional reason for failure to have mammograms is the pain associated with them. Some women with fibrocystic disease have breast tenderness and report that having the mammogram causes discomfort. Some women who experience severe discomfort believe that mammograms are harmful because the breast tissue is squeezed so tightly, causing pain. After such an experience one woman vowed she would never have another mammogram. Another woman said she was bruised for weeks and questioned the value of a test that would have a damaging effect.

Each person has a different tolerance for pain, and for some women that tolerance may be low. A recent study of the discomfort reported by women who have mammograms found that only 1.1 percent were "very uncomfortable" and only 0.2 percent were "intolerable." The study concluded that the pain caused by the high degree of compression necessary in a mammogram can be tolerated. It is important that a trained, experienced technician conduct the mammogram in a sensitive, caring manner.[22] In cases where women experience great discomfort they should discuss this with their technicians and physicians. We recently asked a radiologist about the extreme pain some women have; she assured us there is no damage from the process. Nonetheless, it is difficult to convince a woman who has suffered an unpleasant experience to have regular mammograms. However, the benefits of early detection outweigh the short duration of pain and discomfort.

Other reasons for neglecting to have mammograms include fear of radiation and biopsies, and the high cost of a mammogram. Some insurance companies are now paying for the mammogram; but for women with limited incomes and no insurance, a mammogram can be unaffordable. Cancer centers in some hospitals employ financial counselors who help women with limited resources.

When a woman finds a lump or other symptoms of cancer, the first inclination is often to deny it. Others take a "wait and see" attitude. Still other women see their doctors immediately. If a woman has become familiar with her breasts and their hormonal changes during the menstral cycle, she will be better able to judge the urgency of seeking medical advice. In Chapter 3 you will learn more about the breast, types of lumps, and treatment options.

PREDICTIONS FOR NEW CASES OF BREAST CANCER

The predictions for new cases of breast cancer in the United States in 1994, as published in *CA—A Cancer Journal for Clinicians* (1994), was estimated as 182,000 new cases among women, or approximately one in every nine women. Although breast cancer rarely occurs in males, an estimated 1,000 new cases and 300 deaths were predicted for men, the same as predicted for 1993. Since the early 1970s to 1990, breast cancer mortality rates increased about 2 percent a year, but they have decreased about 3 percent a year in women under age 65. There are an estimated 46,300 deaths from breast cancer predicted for women in 1994. The increased incidence of localized cases, especially where lesions were under 2 cm, have accounted for most of the earlier increase in rates. Because of early detection and improved treatment, mortality rates have remained the same or have decreased for patients diagnosed with regional spread or with distant metastases. Breast cancer is the second major cause of cancer death in women.[23]

With the methods now used in treating early detected breast cancer, the survival rate had improved in 1993. For localized breast cancer the five-year survival rate has risen from 78 percent in the 1940s to 93 percent in the 1990s. The survival rate approaches 100 percent when the cancer is not invasive (in situ). When it has spread regionally to surrounding tissues and lymph nodes at the time of diagnosis, the 5-year survival rate is 72 percent. If the cancer cells have spread to other organs in the body (distant metastases), the survival rate is 18 percent.[24]

To summarize this chapter, we have enumerated some of the various ways in which women have found breast cancer. Their messages have emphasized the need to take advantage of screening and early detection methods and to be aware of body changes. The improved techniques for early detection and methods for treatment have greatly enhanced the chances for a full and longer life. What makes a difference in terms of survival is that both detection and treatment should occur early in the development of breast cancer. We have also reported 1994 predictions for new cases and survival rates.

Historically women's breasts have had great significance in feminine psychology and have become the foremost symbol of femininity and sexual desirability in our culture. This idealization has made breast cancer and the subsequent loss of breasts a very traumatic experience for women.

In the following chapter we will consider the physical, emotional, and psychosocial problems that may result from breast cancer. We will examine some common, or self-protective, methods of coping with the initial shock of diagnosis and the difficulties of making critical decisions. We will also discuss emotional reactions and some of the more disturbing effects of breast cancer, as well as the problems that require practical solutions.

Chapter 2

Physical, Emotional, and Psychosocial Effects of Breast Cancer

Joy Martin, a university professor who lost both breasts and feels very lucky to have caught her cancer early, described her experience in this way: "Having breast cancer is like being on a roller coaster when you haven't even signed up for the amusement park." Joy was describing how she felt as she reacted to and dealt with the ups and down caused by an event over which she had no choice or control. Not only did she have to deal with the initial shock of being on this turbulent course, but she also had to make immediate critical decisions. The decisions involved physicians and treatment, her family, her job, and other disruptions in her life. In addition, the disease created short-term as well as ongoing physical, emotional, and psychosocial problems.

One researcher noted that people cope psychologically not "with the disease of cancer, but with the *impact of cancer*."[1] The impact is the combined force of all the distressing and disrupting problems caused by the disease that make a woman and her family feel as though they've been "hit by a ton of bricks." It can change family relationships, strain friendships, and cost a patient her job. Dr. Jan van Eys of M. D. Anderson Hospital and Tumor Institute said that in some ways "the physical cure is not as important as the psychosocial cure."[2]

With the increase in treatment options and women's desire to participate in making decisions about their treatment, the subject of breast cancer is more openly discussed. Also, the quality of life is receiving more emphasis. As we know, women react very differently to the diagnosis of breast cancer. Adjustment is more difficult for women who are young, single, pregnant, or nursing. It is also more difficult for those who lack a good support system, who have suffered from mood disorders such as depression, or who have engaged in substance abuse.[3]

A number of circumstances can affect a woman's reactions and ability to cope with the shock. Her psychological makeup, her resources and coping abilities, as well as her stage in the life cycle will determine how she handles the disease. Additional factors are the unexpectedness of the diagnosis, the stage of the cancer, other stresses in her life, and her normal response to stress. Because the disease can be life-threatening as well as damaging to a woman's body image, her self-esteem, and her sexual life, the impact on her and those she loves can be profound.

The diagnosis of cancer becomes a crisis event for a woman and her family when their usual methods of coping with unpredictable events are inflexible or inadequate. Marked changes in behavior may occur. Feeling helpless, they may act in unconstructive and ineffective ways. They may undergo changes in body functions and experience insomnia, loss of appetite, memory lapses, difficulty in concentration, and decreased tolerance for frustration and additional stress.[4] The acute state may last for only a brief time or it may continue for an extended period. In any case, the woman and each family member will begin immediately to manage the shock in his or her own way.

A THEORY OF COPING

One way to understand the efforts we make to manage a crisis situation is to view coping as a "process" that we move through. This theoretical explanation of coping explains behavioral changes that we may notice in others who are experiencing a crisis. They may not act as they usually do in an upsetting situation. Moreover, their methods of coping may change as the stress increases or diminishes. Also, some coping efforts appear to be largely emotional, whereas others are more rational and focused on solving the problems created by the disease.[5] Because the diagnosis of cancer is usually a great shock, our first coping behaviors are efforts to withstand the shock and ease the emotional distress. They are self-protective forms of coping that help us tolerate the emotional turmoil we are experiencing.

SELF-PROTECTIVE RESPONSES TO STRESS

A common method of protecting oneself is to deny the seriousness of the diagnosis, saying that it is a mistake. Denial is an effective short-term means of coping with great stress because it allows time for the body and mind to adjust to the shock.[6] This first phase of adjustment usually lasts only a short time. However, by continuing to deny the diagnosis, some women may delay seeking medical treatment, thus giving a malignant tumor time to become more advanced. A woman should move on to accept and face the realities of the disease.

Another self-protective device is stoicism-fatalism. The stoic fatalist takes the attitude that "this is the fate I must bear," or "we all have to die sometime; this is the way I'm supposed to go." Possibly the stigma or fear of the disease, which are reasons for avoiding mammograms and physical examinations, may account for a stoical-fatalistic defense that some women take.

Projection, displacement, faith, and prayer are other forms of self-protection. A woman who blames the physician for the advanced stage of her cancer when she has delayed for many months before making an appointment is projecting her negligence onto the doctor. That same woman might displace her feeling of guilt for her procrastination in getting medical help by becoming angry with her husband or yelling at her children. Other women depend on their faith and prayers to heal them rather than seeking or following the advice of a physician. An example was Shirley Ottenheimer, whose doctor had told her she had a mass that needed surgical treatment. Relying on her faith in God to protect her, she displaced her anxiety to her ill husband until she was afraid that she had delayed her own surgery too long.

Physical illness almost always results in an upset in one's emotional balance, particularly when there is an unpredictable outcome such as changes in body appearance or functions, and threats to self-esteem and self-image.[7] In seeking treatment some women would prefer to find a competent physician and trust him or her to do what is best. However, more and more women want to be involved in the decisions concerning their treatment and recovery. A problem is that at a time when she is emotionally upset, a woman must often make these critical decisions without sufficient information.

MAKING IMMEDIATE CRITICAL DECISIONS WHEN IN SHOCK

Recently, at a luncheon I was seated beside a young woman who had been a student in one of my classes several years ago. We had much "catching up" to do, of course, and the subject of breast cancer was mentioned. Julie said, "I've had it," and added that she had chosen to have a lumpectomy. When I asked her what the experience was like for her, she told me the shock was indescribable. Even though she is a nurse, decisions about her treatment had been especially difficult to make. Fortunately, having a good network of medical professionals, she had great confidence in the surgeon she chose. Being a nurse, she said there were disadvantages in knowing too much; she had not wanted to do a lot of reading on the subject, but preferred to rely on the information her surgeon gave her. After he had outlined her treatment options, she posed this question to him: "If it were you or your wife, what would you do?" His reply was, "I'd choose a mas-

tectomy; but then, I'm not a woman." Julie went through a period of agonizing uncertainty before she elected to have a lumpectomy, which has
proven to be a good decision in view of recent research.

My conversation with Julie reinforced what we have learned about some
of the most difficult moments that a woman with breast cancer endures.
She must find a surgeon in whom she has confidence as well as an oncologist
and/or oncology radiologist, if further treatment is recommended. Then,
providing the cancer has been found early, the second major decision is the
surgical procedure; whether to have a mastectomy or a lumpectomy.

Treatment options have been very controversial. For early stage invasive
breast cancer the surgical options are (1) modified radical mastectomy, (2)
breast conservation (lumpectomy) with radiation, and (3) modified radical
mastectomy with either immediate or delayed breast reconstruction. As with
Julie's doctor, many physicians recommend the mastectomy as the best way
of removing all the cancer. However, recent research indicates that there is
little difference in recurrence rates between the mastectomy and the lumpectomy with radiation therapy, which leaves most of the breast intact. In
the event that both breasts are diseased, the decision may be more difficult.

When breast cancer has been found, a woman needs a good deal of information in order to make decisions. She needs to know what her choices
are, and what she can expect. Certain criteria should be used in making her
selection: (1) *Her age*—She may undergo breast conservation therapy at any
age. (2) *Her family history*—A strong family history does not hinder her
from breast conservation, but she should be counseled regarding her individual risk. (3) *Size of her breasts*—They should be of adequate size for
tumor excision and radiotherapy. Complications can occur when breasts are
too small or too large. (4) *Presence of collagen vascular diseases*—If she has
discoid or systemic lupus erythematosus or scleroderma, she should avoid
breast conservation because of possible acute and late side effects from radiotherapy. (5) *Her motivation*—She should have a strong desire to preserve
her breasts and a willingness to have daily radiotherapy as well as continuous,
periodic check-ups. Any fear of radiotherapy and relapse should be con-
fronted. (6) *Stage and size of her tumor*—It should be early stage and the
size should be less than 4 cm, with no metastases and no node involvement.
With the exception of two small lesions or microcalcifications within a sphere
of less than 4 cm in diameter, a lumpectomy may not be done if there are
multiple tumors.[8]

A woman who elects to have breast conservation should know the advantages and disadvantages of her decisions. Because gathering information and
asking the right questions occur at a time of high emotional distress, a
woman can benefit from assistance in learning what her choices are. No
matter what decision she makes, she will be less likely to become anxious
or depressed if she has had a choice.[9]

OBTAINING AND ABSORBING INFORMATION

A problem for women and their families who are undergoing the breast cancer experience is obtaining and absorbing information. Some may feel they are not given adequate information. Many are hesitant to ask questions. However, those who are upset about their health may encounter the difficulty that Ann Schneider experienced when she was first diagnosed—the inability to listen attentively. Ann admitted, "One of my problems was that even though I asked questions, I just wasn't absorbing all of the answers the first time the doctor told me. It took at least the second time of explanation to comprehend what he was saying. I was too emotional the first time."

Ann realized that she was responding as most people do when they are emotionally upset: their ability to listen and absorb information becomes extremely limited. As we related earlier, Ellen Barckley vividly described the paralyzing shock that she experienced when she went to the surgeon. Her thought processes were so disrupted that she couldn't even remember why she was taking medication or that she had suffered a heart attack several years prior to this diagnosis.

One surgeon, who has done the surgery on several women in our study, helps his patients to understand and recall what he has told them by taping his conversation with them. He records his diagnosis, his explanation of the options that are open to the patient for her treatment, her prognosis, and any instructions he has for her. He then gives her the cassette tape to take home, where she and her family can listen to it as often as they like before making any decisions about her treatment. This surgeon also has an assistant who has had breast cancer herself, and who will talk with the patient whenever she has questions or feels the need to talk.

A female physician told the story of her inability to hear what was said to her when she was told she had breast cancer. During the days while she was waiting for the surgery she confessed that it was as though she were deaf. She heard almost none of the information given her and was unable to comprehend the meaning of what she did hear.

EMOTIONAL KINDS OF COPING

Women often react to the diagnosis of breast cancer with anger. In fact, almost every woman with whom we talked has mentioned the intense anger that she felt at some point in the experience. For example, as Kathryn Lathrop was sharing her feelings she said, "When the doctor told me I had breast cancer in my other breast, I became angry. I thought, 'I have done everything right; what has gone wrong? What did I do?' I was very angry because I had behaved myself for twelve years from the time of my first mastectomy and somehow or other believed that if I did all the right things, it would not happen again. But it did."

Kathryn explained that at first she was so upset she nearly went out of her mind, but then she said, "I decided this was not going to help me at all and I realized the best thing to do was to break everything down to very small pieces. I thought if I could just live from today until tomorrow, I could handle it. I don't take medications, but the last two days before going in for surgery I finally gave in and took the Valium the doctor had given me. I moved from being angry and upset to the point of accepting, where I am now. A large part of my acceptance has come about because I feel fine now and I am active. I am doing everything that I was doing before."

Anger can be a positive reaction if one can step back, think through the situation, and decide to take positive action. Kathryn decided to take her treatment one step at a time. She also decided to have reconstructive surgery to make her feel better about herself. As soon as she had recovered from her surgery, she resumed her activities.

Dottie Corman, who was undergoing chemotherapy, was feeling intense anger. Before her breast cancer was found she had broken an engagement because marriage meant moving to another country and culture. It was a difficult decision in midlife. To compound that loss, a long-standing close friend was moving abroad to live there permanently. The cancer reinforced the anger that Dottie had been feeling for a long time and intensified her grief over the separation from the man she loved, a close friend, and her breast. Persistent dreams about dying prompted her to find a psychotherapist, who was helpful.

The expense and limited insurance coverage prohibited Dottie from getting the continued help she needed. In fact, the action she took to help relieve her anger added to her financial problems and to deeper frustration. After the treatments and reconstruction were completed, Dottie had worked through much of her anger. She was coping in a more positive way even though she had little power to change most of the circumstances troubling her. She was moving toward an accepting attitude.

Kay Sherwood, a minister's wife with grown children, also admitted that part of her immediate reaction to the breast cancer diagnosis was anger. "Why me?" she thought. Then, being an optimistic person, a few minutes later she said to herself, "Why not me? It happens to people in all walks of life."

Kay's anger flared briefly before she changed her view of the breast cancer and accepted it as a challenge. That is not to say that she did not use emotional coping again, but she was soon able to act in positive ways. After her recovery from surgery, one of her first steps was to volunteer for Reach to Recovery, where she has been able to help other women as well as herself.

FEAR OF PAIN

The major fears, termed the "five D's," that are associated with cancer are death, disfigurement, disability, dependence, and disruption of relationships. Another fear, perhaps the most frightening, is the fear of severe pain that often accompanies cancer. Some of our fears stem from myths and lack of information. Justified fear of pain often results from experiences with friends and family members who have had cancer.

The frequency of pain varies with the stage and side effects associated with treatment, whether it is surgery, radiation therapy, chemotherapy, or bone marrow rescue. Whatever the cause, there are ways of controlling pain through the use of analgesic or narcotic drugs.

The brain creates substances or "natural opiates," called endorphins and enkephalins, that reduce the patient's perception of pain in a manner similar to narcotic drugs. In addition, analgesic (pain-relieving) drugs are available to help manage the pain. Among these are the nonprescription drugs (aspirin; acetaminophen, or Tylenol; and ibuprofen) for mild to moderate pain. Also, a number of nonsteroidal anti-inflammatory drugs are sold only by prescription and are felt to be more potent and less irritating, if taken as prescribed. Finally, an important method of pain control is the use of narcotic drugs, "controlled substances," which must be prescribed and carefully administered. Some patients choose to endure the pain rather than take a narcotic drug.

A common breast pain, mastalgia, causes many women discomfort and concern about cancer. The pain can be cyclical, noncyclical (also known as target-zone breast pain), or pain in the chest area that is not really breast pain. Cyclical pain is related to the menstrual cycle, whereas noncyclical or target-zone pain occurs in a specific place and is more or less constant. Target-zone pain may be difficult to diagnose. Nonbreast pain may be caused by an arthritic condition. Hormonal treatment is used for cyclical pain, but little is known about treatment of these breast pains.

Some studies have shown that nondrug methods, such as meditation and visualization, can be effective in managing pain.[10] Physical therapy, biofeedback, hypnosis, local stimulation of the skin, and exercise may be used in combination with analgesic drug therapy, giving the patient a sense of control over her pain. Simonton and others advocate relaxation, meditation, imagery, and hypnosis. A study conducted by a pain management center confirmed Simonton's observation that "the more kinds of treatment that a patient participates in, the more his pain decreases."[11] From Dr. Love's experience, some of these techniques may stimulate the body's immune system and give a woman a role in her own care.[12] How widely these nondrug treatments are used is not known.

GUILT

Physicians Holland and Cullen have pointed out that some approaches for coping with cancer, specifically the Simonton technique, have "a potential for arousing guilt in those patients who are prone to self-blame and who already worry that 'they waited too long to go to the doctor.' "[13] A woman may feel responsible for her illness because she has been careless about her health. Or a woman who tends to blame herself may feel the disease is punishment for past actions—as in the case of Millie Davis, who blamed her breast cancer on her early use of the pill. (Although more studies are being undertaken on effects of the pill, evidence of its relationship to breast cancer has not been established.)

In their book *Guilt: Letting Go*, Freeman and Strean state that women have admitted feeling guilty when they show dependency, vulnerability, or physical weakness.[14] According to psychologist Harriet Lerner, "women are encouraged to feel guilty and, therefore, often have difficulty sorting out when guilt is justified."[15]

Sometimes we have good reason for feelings of guilt for a wrongdoing, but as Felder reminds us, this kind of guilt serves to teach us that we should be kinder, more sensitive, and more thoughtful of others. However, the kind of guilt we feel for imagined mistakes and inadequacies can be harmful. Self-criticism can be detrimental to health when it drains our physical and emotional strength.[16]

The spouse or partner of a woman with breast cancer may feel guilty because he is healthy when she is ill. He may blame himself for her illness because of something he did or did not do. She may increase his guilt by criticizing him. Most of all, young children who do not fully understand how illness is caused may suffer guilt.[17] They have a natural tendency to feel that anything bad that happens to the family is somehow their fault. The guilt that adolescents experience may take the form of resentment and anger as demands made upon them by the illness occur just when they are struggling to pull away from the family.

Felder suggests that we take steps against our guilt by identifying regrets, feelings, and things that upset us. Once we have listed these guilt feelings we can sort them into those that we can change and those that are inaccurate or impossible to change. By determining a constructive action that will correct guilt-causing actions, we can alleviate the guilt feeling. For wrongs that are past or imagined, we can forgive ourselves for being human, learn to laugh at our imperfections, and give up the idea that the cancer is a form of punishment.[18]

If you are suffering from guilt, we recommend that you read Felder's book, *When a Loved One Is Ill*. His chapter entitled "Conquering the Nasty G-Word (Guilt!)" is insightful. See the Bibliography for the publisher.

MOOD DISTURBANCE, LOW SELF-ESTEEM, AND NEGATIVE BODY IMAGE

Mood swings, lowered self-esteem, and negative body image are often effects of breast cancer. Shirley Ottenheimer found that her moods went from high to low and she was not able to handle upsetting events as well as she had before her mastectomy. She had sought the help of two different psychologists and thought she should probably continue to see one of them. "I've always had a low self-image and inferiority complex," she confessed, "and I think it is accentuated more since my surgery."

Part of Shirley's lowered self-esteem resulted from losing her breast. She found that looking at her scar increased her feelings of inadequacy. Her supportive husband was sensitive to her needs and encouraged her to socialize, but she resisted, even avoided family gatherings. That troubled him and he seemed grateful that she felt comfortable in sharing her feelings with us.

Although not all women have mood disturbances, clinicians often cite them as a problem experienced by their breast cancer patients. Lynn Robbins disclosed the wide range of intense emotions she felt that began with her anger at having to lose both breasts. She confessed that after her surgery she was so angry that she told an acquaintance, "There are ten other people who deserve this more than I do. It's not fair. I am a single parent trying and struggling to make it. I'm working, going to school, taking care of my kids, and now I have to suffer through this. Why wasn't it somebody who sits around and does nothing all day long? It just seems I do get more than my share."

Things certainly weren't easy for Lynn. As a single mother she earned a minimal salary, and with the child support her children's father gave her, she was barely managing. She admitted that she often indulged in self-pity, especially during her recovery from surgery. When she began to feel sorry for herself the man she was dating, a very supportive, compassionate man, allowed her so many minutes to vent her feelings. When the time was up he stopped her and pointed out the bright side of her life. He explained that she has always had low self-esteem and tends to dwell on her imperfections. He viewed himself as a stabilizer for her, a role he carried out by giving her encouragement and making her laugh at herself.

The support Lynn received, her own sense of humor, and her efforts to change her situation were coping resources that resulted in personal growth for Lynn, despite the poor body image she continued to have. At the end of a year she was pleased with her progress, especially her weight loss. However, she still could not look at her body in a mirror. Lynn illustrates another reaction to breast cancer—negative body image along with the low self-esteem she already had.

It took the sensitivity of Shelley Young's husband Jack to understand why

she, at age 27, a new mother, was having such difficulty accepting the loss
of her breast. Shelley was still coping on the emotional level not too long
after her reconstructive surgery. Her tone conveyed a mixture of anger and
dejection. "I guess I feel this way because I'm so young," she revealed; "I
didn't feel that the cancer had spread and that I was going to die or anything."

Jack expressed his view of Shelley's feelings to her. "You had a self-image
problem. Also, the cancer took us by surprise." Turning to me he continued, "What I felt for her was not so much anger as concern; I was worried
about her." A year later Shelley was a much happier woman. She had returned to her job, she and Jack had resumed the outdoor sports they share,
and they were enjoying life again.

Body image changes upset many women who have lost a breast or both
breasts. Reconstructive surgery and prostheses help them feel and look better in their clothing. Several women were ecstatic about their reconstructed
breasts. In fact, Joy M., who lost both breasts and underwent reconstruction, proudly claims to have "a 16-year-old bust in a 45-year-old body."

Chemotherapy, which will be discussed in the next chapter, also has negative effects on the body image of some women. Loss of hair and weight
gain can be demoralizing. Women are grateful for wigs and have been sur-
prised and delighted to have their hair grow back thicker and sometimes
curly. A few drugs used in chemotherapy can cause weight gain, which has
a disheartening effect on body image. Three women told us that gaining
weight upset them more than any other aspect of the entire experience.

Eloise Crowell gained weight with her chemotherapy treatment, but, she
confessed, "I did overdo. I might as well admit it. I was feeling sorry for
myself and people brought goodies and I felt good to be eating. I can't say
the 30 pounds I've gained is all the medication. The doctor told me she
would rather have me tell her I want to eat rather than that I can't eat."

Physicians emphasize the need to maintain a nutritious, sensible diet when
undergoing chemotherapy to help the body's defense system. However, especially when a woman suffers with nausea, being able to enjoy food again
when the nausea has passed can lead to overeating.

FEARS OF DYING AND RECURRENCE

Women who have breast cancer must also cope with fears of dying and
recurrence. With several exceptions, many women in our study admitted
that fear of dying was their first thought, as it was for Carol McNeil. She
said, "I had a real fear of dying because there was a possibility that the
cancer had spread."

As time goes on the fear of dying recedes. However, most women continue to harbor a fear of recurrence that surfaces before each physical check-
up, causing great anxiety. Even those who say they never think about their

cancer, when asked directly, will confess that they are "nervous wrecks" before they see their doctors for a check-up.

As an example, Millie Davis expressed her feelings about recurrence. "I am back to normal again as though nothing has ever happened except for worrying about the cancer coming back. I am always going to worry about it, I think." Another woman, Mary Lynn Gordon, feels strongly about the prevalence of this fear. She said emphatically, "I know that it's on the mind of every woman who has had a mastectomy. It becomes almost an obsession, not that she admits it or talks about it. Every time she thinks something in her body feels different, she becomes frightened and worried." Shari Lovell, who had made an excellent adjustment, agreed; "I'm not as confident about being 'okay' as I was earlier. Every time I hear of a friend having a recurrence or dying, I think 'Am I next?' I probably won't ever get over it."

DEPRESSION

Periodic feelings of being low, or having the "blues," can occur to breast cancer patients and can become severe for some. Esther Seifert's experience is an example of depression that developed after she had made what appeared to be a good adjustment. As soon as she realized that having breast cancer was much better than the inoperable brain tumor she had feared, she became very accepting and grateful for her good fortune. Soon after the surgery, her outlook was remarkably optimistic.

One year later Esther was seeing a therapist for depression. "It seemed that I had been coping very well," she reflected. "Maybe I was just laughing it off and was not accepting things as well as I thought I was. Every time I get sick or something goes wrong, I worry that there is more cancer. I keep thinking about being here to see both my boys graduate from school."

Esther may have partially explained her delayed depression. Her ability to "laugh it off" initially suggested emotional control, which researchers Watson et al. found to be associated with depression.[19]

SEXUAL RELATIONS AND CHILD-BEARING

Two other aspects of breast cancer that disturb women and their spouses is the effect on their sexual relationship. After Carol McNeil's pathology report confirmed that the cancer had not spread, her fear of dying was replaced with other fears. "I wondered," she said, "how this would affect my energy with all that was going on in my life. How would it affect my sexual relations with my husband? There was no one to talk with about that. Then I called Cancer Share and asked to speak to someone near my age. That is how I met Sandy, who is the first person I could ask about what this would do to my sex life."

Carol raised a subject that few couples talk about—the effect of the loss of a breast or breasts on their sexual life. In the questionnaires that were given to thirty couples in our study, 40 percent of the women and 75 percent of the men reported that the breast cancer had had no effect on their sexual lives. The remainder disclosed adjustment problems; and over the course of a year, some men and women indicated changes, either for the better or worse, in satisfaction with their sexual life. However, because this was a small sampling of couples, the results cannot be considered to be typical. This subject will be discussed at more length in a later chapter on relationships.

Breast loss is also a great concern for unmarried women, particularly the effect it will have on dating and marriage. Judy White and Rachel Dunne each had grown children and were divorced, both hoping to meet someone. They expressed their concern about a man's reaction to their having lost a breast. Fortunately, Judy, who had had reconstructive surgery, did not have to wait long to find out. Six months after disclosing her apprehension to us, she was dating a man who proposed marriage. When asked how she had approached the subject of her breast cancer, she confessed she was very nervous about it. She had not said anything to him until the relationship began to get serious, then decided she had to tell him. As it happened, he already knew through a mutual acquaintance, even before he began dating her. It obviously made no difference to him.

Mindy Bishop, whose breast cancer resulted in the termination of her marriage, felt extremely pessimistic about dating. She said, "I would not feel it fair to a man. I'd feel he was being cheated." Mindy's reactions were affected by her former husband's lack of compassion, which had given her a negative body image, as well as the fact that childbearing would be very risky for her. She had asked her doctor about having more children (she had a toddler at the time of her surgery). The doctor's answer had been, "I'm not telling you not to have more children because it might not be a problem, but we advise women to wait five years."

Mindy's response to the doctor was, "I'm going to be 35 and I need to know when I'm dating what kind of a future I can give another man." The doctor was frank: "It's like adding logs to a fire. If there are stray cancer cells, pregnancy could make them grow faster." He was sympathetic: "One of the tragedies for young women with breast cancer is that is affects childbearing."

Mindy no longer feels that she has little to offer in a marriage. As her energy returned and her check-ups continue to be good, her outlook has become very positive. In fact, she has now married a man she has known since high school.

The message to Kathy and Alan Mayer and Shelley and Jack Young was the same as Mindy had been given. Having additional children would be risky. Fortunately, all three of these couples have had one child, but all of them would like more. It's a very difficult decision that only they can make.

In the case of Ann Jillian, who took the risk, bearing a child may have no ill effects on the health of a woman who has breast cancer.

The decision to become pregnant after breast cancer is a personal one that depends upon a woman's values. Dr. Love states that pregnancy will not cause cancer to spread.[20] However, if a woman has any cells in her body from a previous hormone-sensitive tumor, the pregnancy hormones will possibly stimulate cancer cells to develop more rapidly than if she were not pregnant.

Chemotherapy may stop menstrual periods temporarily, and if the woman is close to menopause, permanently. If a woman is young, the chemotherapy will not affect the ovaries because the eggs are not made up of dividing cells; she can become pregnant. It is important that women obtain accurate information from their physicians and then make their own decisions.

PROBLEMS REQUIRING PRACTICAL SOLUTIONS

Other adjustments that must be made because of the illness encompass financial matters, insurance claims, childcare and housekeeping tasks, personal care, and transportation for treatments. A number of women cited insurance forms, delayed payments, and the confusing statements from billing departments as problems that were worse than the treatment of breast cancer. In other instances, the high cost of psychotherapy and the refusal of some insurance companies to pay for reconstructive surgery may frustrate women who need or want these treatments. Others have lost income by having to cut back their hours of employment or by having to resign from jobs because of treatment regimens and fatigue. These problems will be discussed at greater length in another chapter.

Housekeeping tasks and childcare make great demands on women with babies and young children. When these women are undergoing surgery and treatment, the burden of care often falls upon the spouse. Several spouses admitted that they found this additional responsibility very tiring, but it has given them a greater appreciation of what their wives do. The added work load is stressful for husbands who must continue with their jobs as well as make hospital visits, oversee the children, and manage housekeeping details. One overworked spouse said he felt neglected when all the support from friends was directed toward his wife.

Additional and ongoing strains such as an ill parent, a job crisis, the death of a parent, and problems with children can further tax both the woman's and her spouse's energy and coping skills. One woman said that watching what her illness did to her husband and family was more distressing for her than what she was experiencing herself.

These problems require actions that bring about practical solutions. Often the two forms of coping, emotional and problem-focused, work together to help in managing the problem. As an illustration, Ann Schneider explained how she handled her anxiety when she found her last two lumps (she has undergone surgery and treatments three times and is doing fine now). "Since I'd been through it before, I knew what to expect. I'm always a nervous wreck until I get to the doctor. First I called for an appointment. I knew there would be a delay—I never get in the first day. In the meantime, I mentally prepared myself by reviewing the steps I knew I'd go through. After the last diagnosis I questioned the doctor: 'This means I will have radiation?' When he said 'yes,' it did not come as a big surprise; but the first time it was a great shock."

In this situation Ann's emotional coping mechanism (anxiety) prompted her to call for an appointment (a problem-directed action) to help ease her anxiety. Then, to prepare herself, she mentally rehearsed the steps and the possible diagnosis (an analytic process). In this way each of the two forms of coping worked to facilitate the other; Ann was able to relieve her anxiety somewhat by taking the steps necessary for getting a diagnosis of the lump she had found. Had she continued to rely on emotional methods of coping, they would have blocked her rational, problem-solving approach to her recurrence.

Gagnon and fellow researchers concluded that overall, the adjustment following early stage breast cancer is good, especially if women were "well adjusted" prior to their mastectomy. They will have "a good quality of life."[21] However, the recent practice of giving chemotherapy or radiotherapy to all women with early breast cancer has increased the stress that they undergo. Side effects, such as nausea and fatigue, and disappointment in outcome of the surgery may result in emotional trauma.

In conclusion, in this chapter we have discussed the emotional and psychosocial effects and other problems that women may experience with breast cancer. We have also discussed their initial coping efforts. When the usual methods of managing an unexpected event are inadequate, the event becomes a crisis. Customary behavior for dealing with crisis situations may be different; it may undergo changes and may be both emotional and rational. The initial emotional responses will help to handle the shock. Then rational or problem-solving efforts facilitate effective management of problems. These two kinds of coping efforts may either hinder or work together to accomplish recovery.

In the next chapter we review the behavior of cells, how tumors develop, kinds of lumps, and cancer types. The surgical treatments, radiation, chemotherapy, hormonal therapy, and autologous bone marrow rescue—or transplant—along with possible side effects and complications, are explained. As in the case of each chapter, women's accounts of their experiences illustrate the treatment methods and effects. The brief explanations will provide you will some understanding of choices and, we hope, motivate further reading before you make decisions about treatment.

Chapter 3

Types of Breast Cancer and Treatments

How do cancer cells grow and spread? Before we begin to discuss cancer types, breast lumps, and treatment options, let us summarize what is known about the behavior of cancer cells. This will help in understanding how treatments are use in the attempt to hinder or stop their growth, some of their side effects, and why they succeed or fail in destroying the cancerous cells.

BASIC CELL STRUCTURE AND FUNCTIONS

In the nucleus of each cell that makes up the body tissue there are strands of DNA (deoxyribonucleic acid) that are organized in twenty-three pairs of chromosomes. Twenty-two contain "look-alike" chromosomes; the twenty third set contains X and Y chromosomes, which determine sex. Genes are the tiny molecular units of DNA that are strung on each chromosome. They carry and send messages to the various parts of the body, telling them how they should function. Most of the time the genes send the right messages, but with the incredible number of genes and messages, sometimes alterations can occur in the process of cell division. For example, environmental factors—such as X ray and ultraviolet rays from the sun, or food toxins—can alter the DNA. Most of the damage is repaired, but if it occurs at certain points near regulator genes, the cell's ability to control important genes is disrupted.

There are two types of genes. Growth-supporting protooncogenes (normal genes) can be transformed into oncogenes (tumor genes); tumor-suppressor genes, or antioncogenes, act as the "brakes" for undesirable cell growth. When these suppressor genes are altered, cells' growth is unchecked. An important tumor-suppressor gene p53, which has the function of suppressing growth of normal cells, is most commonly associated with breast cancer. When both of the two copies of the p53 genes are mutated or altered, cancer can occur.

Some oncogenes (cancer genes) may be turned on spontaneously; others may be triggered by exposure to a carcinogen, such as a virus, which puts the cell in a receptive condition for cancer development. The cell will remain harmless unless some other agent or condition, a promoter such as a chemical or element in the diet, comes along to trigger what the initiator has set up.

Normal cells perform their function as they should, to maintain the body's well-being. However, cancerous cells have no regard for the body's welfare. They grow uncontrollably, forming masses of tissue called tumors from which cells break away and spread, or metastasize. When trapped by the lymph nodes, cells remain at their original site; but if untreated, they will invade neighboring or distant tissue. They disrupt, damage, and generally harm the organs and body functions.[1]

Among the new approaches that researchers are exploring is genetic alteration of a cell that is aimed at improving the outcome of bone marrow transplantation.[2] Researchers have been able to pinpoint a breast cancer protein that combines with a receptor in the cancer cell membrane and stimulates growth of the cancer cell. This kind of research provides clues for developing anti-cancer drugs that will be able to interfere with the process and halt the growth of cancer cells. Researchers are also trying to identify a gene or oncogene that may be responsible for the cancer that occurs in generations of a family.

How rapidly do cancer cells grow? Love reported the growth rate calculated by Bernard Fisher, who found that the average doubling time of a cancer cell is 100 days. At that rate it takes about eight years for cells to multiply to the size of a centimeter, when they can be detected by mammogram. In about ten years the normal cancerous growth would be the size of a lump that could be felt. However, this rate is not characteristic of all malignant tumors because some grow at faster or slower rates and others grow in spurts. These calculations in growth rate have led to changes in the treatment of breast cancer.[3]

CANCER TYPES AND DOMINANT KINDS OF LUMPS

There are different cancer types. The lumps or tumors that appear in the breast and other organs are classified as carcinomas, the most common category of cancer. Lymphomas appear in the lymph system and spleen and may cause tumors to grow in other parts of the body. The types that occur least often are the leukemias and sarcomas. Leukemias occur in bone marrow, resulting in the production of white blood cells; sarcomas develop in connective tissue.

Four kinds of dominant lumps may occur in the breast. Three of these (fibroadenomas, cysts, and pseudolumps), related in some way to hormonal changes, are considered noncancerous and may go away after several menstrual cycles. Fibroadenomas often, but not always, appear near the nipple; they are hard, smooth and easily movable within the breast tissue. They frequently form during the early years of menstruation and in young women in their early twenties. At that age they do not need to be removed if there is no doubt that they are benign. Cells in fibroadenomas are usually removed to be sure they are not malignant.

Cysts form toward the onset of menopause. They contain fluid that can be aspirated (removed by suction through a needle) to relieve the pain they sometimes cause. Cysts are seldom malignant; in fact, the occurrence of cancer in cysts is only 1 percent.[4]

The third type, a pseudolump, is exaggerated lumpiness that results from the pressure of a rib, scar tissue, or extra breast tissue. This exaggerated lumpiness has been referred to as fibrocystic disease. The pseudolumps are biopsied or aspirated to make sure they are benign.

The fourth kind of lump (discussed earlier in Chapter 1) is distinctly different from other kinds of lumpiness. Dr. Love explains that a troublesome lump, which may or may not be cancerous, will be at least one-half inch (a centimeter or two) in size, will stand out, and will remain in the same location.[5] Its borders may be irregular or it may have a spindle shape or a poorly defined shape, whereas benign tumors are usually well defined.

An X ray (mammogram) may not show an actual lump but can reveal tiny calcified deposits that might be malignant. Other clues can be seen in a mammogram. If the pattern of calcified spots is irregular and clustered, this may be an indication of malignancy. In addition, ducts in an area may seem to be pushed aside or distorted. Also, the breast's architectural features may be different from the pattern shown in an earlier mammogram. It is for detecting these changes that baseline mammograms should be taken at an age (39–40) when the breasts are believed to be normal.[6]

Breast cancer is also classified by cell type:

1. *Invasive or infiltrating ductal carcinoma (sometimes called adeno-carcinomas).* These cancers are hard to the touch and tend to spread rapidly to the lymph nodes, even when quite small. They may cause retraction of the nipple or visible skin dimpling. About 70 percent of breast cancers are of this type, and their prognosis is poorer than for some other types.[7]

2. *Medullary carinoma.* This cancer, which looks like brain tissue, seems to grow within the duct in a capsule form. It may become

quite large but has a better prognosis because it does not metastasize as often as the more common ductal cancer discussed above.
About 5 percent to 7 percent of breast cancers are of this type.

3. *Infiltrating comedocarcinomas.* Beginning in the lining of a duct,
   this cancer grows into the duct and causes it to dilate. Although it
   can become quite large, it is not as likely to spread beyond the
   breast, so the prognosis is fairly good. This type accounts for about
   5 percent of breast cancers.

4. *Mucinous carcinoma.* This is a form of ductal cancer that is char-
   acterized by the production of mucous. It, too, may grow quite
   large without metastasizing. The prognosis tends to be good; about
   3 percent of breast cancers are mucinous carcimomas.

5. *Tubular ductal carcinoma.* So named because the structure of this
   tumor is tube-shaped, this rare form occurs in only 1 percent to 2
   percent of breast cancers and has a better outlook than the invasive
   ductal cancer.

6. *Invasive or infiltrating lobular carcinoma.* Starting in the breast
   globules, which branch off the lobes, this type accounts for 5 percent to 10 percent of breast cancers. The prognosis is generally
   poor.

7. *Noninvasive or preinvasive breast carcinoma in situ (also referred to
   as lobular and ductal carcinomas in situ).* These cancers are too
   small to be felt and may appear on a mammogram as tiny areas of
   calcifications. They are found in premenopausal younger women,
   whereas ductal carinoma in situ is more often found in women who
   average 55 years of age. Until recently these carcinomas were found
   in only 1 percent to 2 percent of all breast biopsies, but they are
   now found in almost 10 percent of the biopsies of nonpalpable
   lesions detected in mammograms and 45 percent of all nonpalpable
   breast malignancies.[8] Because of difficulty in predicting which will
   be become invasive, physicians disagree on treatment. Some advocate a wait-and-see approach, whereas others believe a mastectomy is advisable. When a woman has other risk factors to consider,
   she may elect to have the breast removed.[9]

8. *Paget's disease.* Following a long history of changes in the nipple,
   tumor cells appear in the nipple epidermis. This type is accompanied by itching, oozing, burning, and bleeding; it occurs in only 1
   percent of patients with breast cancer.

9. *Inflammatory breast carcinoma.* Symptoms are skin edema (accu-
   mulation of fluid), redness, warmth, and a hardening of underlying
   tissue. This carcinoma has a poor prognosis.[10] The percentage of
   occurrence was not reported.

STAGES OF BREAST CANCER

The stage, or progression of a tumor's growth, is classified according to an elaborate scale. A tumor in Stage I is less than 2 cm or .78 inches and has no detectable metastases, and lymph nodes are negative. In State II the tumor is larger than 2 cm but less than 5 cm. Lymph nodes are positive but no distant metastases are detectable. In Stage III the tumor is greater than 5 cm, or it may have invaded the skin or chest wall, or there is positive lymph node involvement in the collarbone area. Still no distant metastases are detectable in Stage III. The more advanced cancer is Stage IV wherein the tumor has metastasized to other areas of the body.[11] Breast cancer cells most often travel, or metastasize, to the lungs, liver, brain, and bones. Staging helps the physician to determine what treatment will be more helpful for a patient.

Medical professionals refer to abnormal growths as "lesions," "neoplasms," and "dysplasia." Dysplasia describes a precancerous condition of abnormal cell development in which the cells are altered in size, shape, and organization. Cancer that is "in situ," "noninvasive," or "preinvasive" is localized, and in its earliest stage.

TREATMENT FOR CANCER

When cancer is untreated, its continuous growth crowds and destroys healthy cells around it. Cells that break away begin to spread, or metastasize, and invade the lymphatic system and blood stream where they can travel to other vital organs. This is why it is important to find cancer early before cells have been able to metastasize.

The body's immune system works to control the cancerous cells but, for various reasons, may be unsuccessful. In this case, some kind of outside treatment must be used. Treatment is considered to be local when the breast itself is treated; it is systemic when the rest of the body is treated.

SURGICAL TREATMENT

In order to find out whether or not a lump is malignant, or cancerous, a biopsy procedure may be done. A woman should understand the types of biopsy so that she knows what to expect when her doctor says this procedure should be done.

Types of Biopsies

In the simplest type of biopsy, called a fine needle biopsy, only a few cells are removed from a lump with a fine needle.[12] More extensive biopsies are called incisional and excisional. Both are done with either local or general anesthesia but usually local. The incisional biopsy involves the removal of a portion of the lump, and an excisional biopsy removes the entire lump with a small amount of surrounding tissue.

According to Dr. Love, in any type of biopsy the excised cells or tissue samples are analyzed by a pathologist. In early days of breast cancer, surgeons used to wait for the pathologist's report and, if malignancy was found, the mastectomy was performed immediately. That is rarely done at present, as most women want to discuss their options before consenting to further surgery or treatment.[13]

A recent technological breakthrough in the diagnosis of breast cancer can eliminate the need for a surgical biopsy. This is called a stereotactic breast biopsy, or a mammotest.

The mammotest is a simple, two-step procedure. First, the woman lies face down on a mammotest table that has an opening through which her breast is positioned naturally and comfortably. A technologist takes two stereo X rays of the breast using a computerized mammography machine. This procedure helps locate the lumps and calculate where the radiologist should place the biopsy needle.

Second, the doctor injects a local anesthetic into the area where the needle will be placed. Several cores of tissue are taken with the biopsy needle and are sent to the pathology laboratory.

Women have reported that they experience very little discomfort with the mammotest. There is a slight sting from the local anesthetic injection. Some women say they feel a slight pressure at the moment the biopsy is taken.

After the procedure, a small bandaid and a pressure dressing is put on the breast. An ice pack may be applied for a short time. Most women return to work immediately unless their activity is strenuous.

The entire procedure takes about one hour. The woman experiences no general anesthesia, no surgery, no incision or stitches, and no scarring. Tests have proven that the stereotactic needle-core biopsy technique, or mammotest, is 98 percent accurate, which is the same rate of accuracy as a surgical biopsy. Moreover, it is less invasive, less expensive, and requires less time from work; but not all hospitals have the equipment to perform this procedure.[14]

Partial Mastectomy

The surgery with which most woman are familiar is the mastectomy. In its simplist form, the partial mastectomy, the lump and a part of the breast tissue surrounding it are removed. A partial mastectomy may also be referred to as a lumpectomy, a wide excision, a segmental mastectomy, or a quadrantectomy. The labels do not describe the amount of tissue to be removed except in a quadrantectomy; it may be more or less than a quarter of the breast. Otherwise the size of the lump and the surgeon's preference determine the extent of the excision. The surgeon may remove some of the lymph nodes from the armpit in a procedure called axillary dissection. The tissue is sent to the pathologist for analysis.

In 1989, the National Institutes of Health issued a statement based on scientific research that the lumpectomy treatment regime is an equally effective alternative to the mastectomy for selected cases. However, depending on the size of the tumor, the size of the woman's breasts, the location of the tumor, or the type of cancer cells, the physician may recommend a mastectomy instead of a lumpectomy.

Because of the wide differences in surgical practice and understanding of what constitutes a partial mastectomy, a woman should get specific information from her surgeon before having this surgery. She should be informed about the amount of tissue that will be removed and how the results will look. She will then be prepared should more of her breast be removed than she had anticipated. For current information on breast cancer, call the National Cancer Institute (1-800-4-Cancer).

Five women we know who have had partial mastectomies, or lumpectomies with radiation therapy, have reacted positively to the surgical treatment. For example, prior to her breast cancer Karen Miller had undergone surgery for a melanoma in her leg, which had left an ugly disfigurement. When she learned that she had breast cancer, a mastectomy was recommended with no other options. Karen was devastated; she could not face another deformity. She sought another opinion and learned that her cancer could be treated with a lumpectomy. Karen was able to cope with the removal of only a section of her breast. "The treatment," she said, "makes a big difference in how you deal with the shock."

Modified Radical Mastectomy

The breast and some of the axillary lymph nodes in the armpit area are removed in a modified radical mastectomy. The removal of breast tissue begins at the collarbone and extends down to the rib and around from the breast bone to the muscles behind the armpit. Some of the lymph nodes are removed as in the partial mastectomy. Unless a woman has chosen to have immediate breast reconstruction, which is done by the plastic surgeon following the removal of the breast and lymph nodes, the flaps of skin will be sewn together, resulting in a flat area. Drain tubes are inserted to siphon off tissue fluid while the skin is healing.

A majority of the women who have contributed to our study have had modified radical mastectomies with adjuvant chemotherapy (drugs used as an auxilary remedy with surgery) and/or radiation. Many of these women chose to have reconstructive surgery.

Radical Mastectomy

The surgical procedure for management of breast cancer has changed dramatically in the last thirty-five years. Prior to 1960, a radical mastectomy called the Halstead procedure was performed in an effort to remove all possible cancer cells in the breast area. This type of mastectomy is much more extensive than the modified radical mastectomy and is rarely done now unless the tumor is very large or has spread into the muscle. The radical mastectomy involves removal of chest wall muscles and lymph nodes in surrounding and axillary areas. Sometimes it is necessary to take a skin graft from another part of the body, usually the thigh. Cosmetically, this surgery results in more deformity. It may decrease arm mobility and result in swelling because lymph nodes have been removed.

The extended radical procedure is rarely done anymore because it does not seem to be significantly more effective than radiation to prevent recurrence. Some medical experts have credited the late Rose Kushner, who campaigned against immediate and radical surgery, with changing the thinking about surgical alternatives. Kushner wrote several comprehensive books on the subject of breast cancer.

Only two women in our study had had radical mastectomies. One of them, Kathryn Lathrop, had radical surgery on her right breast twelve years before cancer was found in her left side. Kathryn had reconstruction of the left breast but not the right. The remarkable thing about Kathryn's radical surgery is that she regained the range of motion in her arm and continued as the organist of her church soon after her recovery from surgery.

Preventive Surgery

A small percentage of women who think they may have a serious risk of developing breast cancer are electing to have their breasts removed before cancer develops. Where there is a history of breast cancer in families, some women believe that with preventive or prophylactic surgery, they can avoid getting the disease.[15] However, there is no consistent data concerning the degree to which prophylactic surgery reduces the risk. Nor has the effectiveness of preventive strategies been studied. Moreover, there are possible complications with this surgery. Women who consider it should become well informed and weigh the benefits and risks carefully before undertaking preventive surgery.[16] According to Vogel and Yeomans, it should be done only if evidence of an autosomal dominant syndrome (a syndrome related to paired chromosomes) is found or if there is evidence of premalignant changes in the breast. In cases in which a patient's fear of breast cancer is psychologically incapacitating, it may be advisable to have preventive surgery.[17]

Mastectomy Results and Possible Complications

With all forms of mastectomy the most common result will be the difference in the size and shape of a woman's breasts. If she has had both breasts removed (bilateral surgery) and undergone reconstruction, her breasts are more likely to be symmetrical. Where nerves have been severed or damaged in surgery, she will have numbness. This loss of sensation may diminish, but if it does not, it can be worrisome.

Several complications can result from removal of the lymph nodes. Fluid may form under the armpit and may need to be aspirated if the swelling becomes large and uncomfortable. A form of phlebitis, or an inflammation of the vein in the arm, can also occur with mastectomies. This may cause a feeling of tightness and pain, which will subside in a few days. An infrequent complication that occurs when fluid does not drain properly from tissue is lymphedema, or swelling of the arm.

The removal of lymph glands makes a woman more prone to infection, which increases chances of lymphedema. Because treatment of lymphedema is difficult, reasonable precautions—such as avoiding cuts and burns—should be taken to prevent infections. Also, lifting and carrying heavy objects with the arm down may cause swelling.

Although rare, another hazard of breast cancer surgery is possible injury to one or both of the motor nerves. This injury may cause arm fatigue or difficulty with the muscle that keeps the shoulder blade (scapula) flat against the back.

A woman whose treatment requires any one of these forms of mastectomy, particularly when lymph nodes are to be removed, should discuss the risks and possible complications with her physician prior to the surgery. She should also receive explicit instructions about exercises that are necessary for maintaining mobility in her arm and shoulder. See Appendix E for precautions to take in avoiding infection and lymphedema.

RADIATION

Radiation, a local treatment, has been used in conjunction with surgery to help cure or control an original cancer. It is frequently used to attack cells that may remain after surgery, and it can lessen pain or slow down the growth of a tumor by shrinking it. Radioisotopes can also be injected directly into the breast tissue. The rays halt the reproductive process of cancer cells, as well as the next generation of cells, by making the cancerous cells or tumor unable to multiply.

Radiation therapy is used in breast cancer treatment for the following:

1. For local control after lumpectomy or quadrantectomy when breast cancer is in Stage I or Stage II. Radiation therapy is typically used

with women who have health problems, such as heart disease, that
make them poor candidates for surgery.

2. When the chest wall is involved, or for control after a mastectomy
    with positive margins.

3. When a patient is a poor surgical candidate for axillary dissection
    and is at high risk for axillary metastases or, when gross disease is
    left behind, the axilla is irradiated.

4. If there are positive axillary nodes, radiation is used.

5. For management of metastatic disease of the brain, bone, or skin,
    additional areas are irradiated.[18]

In cases where diagnosis of breast cancer has been made early enough to
warrant conservative treatment, the lumpectomy with radiation therapy is
the preferred treatment. Several recent, reliable studies have changed surgeons' methods of treatment. Findings have shown that primary radiation
therapy, lumpectomy, and mastectomy with radiation for women having
Stage I and Stage II cancers may be equally effective.[19]

Possible Side Effects and Complications

The possible side effects of radiation for breast cancer vary greatly among
women. Even with advanced technology, damage occurs to some normal
tissue. The most common effect is seen in the skin, which has a sunburned
appearance. Some people break out in a rash or have redness, itchiness,
dryness. When radiation is applied to the breast, several changes may occur
in the breast tissue. The tissue may thicken and appear darker in color. The
breast may become sore. Occasionally, there may be permanent swelling.

Another possible side effect is fatigue, which may worsen toward the end
of the treatment and linger after the treatment is completed. Tiredness has
been cited by several women in our study as a reason for taking a leave from
outside employment.

Radiation may affect the soft rib bones and, in turn, cause rib fractures
to occur. Although symptoms may not be apparent, the fractures can be
detected by X ray.

Delayed complications may appear as muscle soreness and a form of ar-
thritis. Occasionally, sharp pains will occur. Before electing to have radiation, any woman should consult with her surgeon and oncology radiologist
to understand any discomfort and other side effects that are sometimes
caused by radiation. She should also receive guidelines for skin care during
treatment.

Personal Accounts of Radiation Treatment

Kathy Mayer was nursing her baby when the lump she had felt a few weeks before giving birth was diagnosed as breast cancer. A lumpectomy was performed, she underwent radiation treatments, and she had to give up nursing. These events, compounded by her new responsibility and her career as a lawyer, drained Kathy's energy. Pale and thin, her major complaint was exhaustion.

A dramatic improvement took place over the next six months, and at the end of a year Kathy looked fully recovered. However, she was concerned about the breast that had been radiated. She shared her misgivings; "I am so heavy on the side where I had surgery and radiation that it is always aggravating and often painful. Some women's breasts shrink with radiation, but mine is bigger and heavier." The third time I saw her, Kathy's breast was feeling almost normal. She still has some periodic soreness and pain, but most of the time she doesn't even think about it.

The experience of having radiotherapy was more challenging than the side effects Fran Humphrey experienced with chemotherapy. She described it this way: "Getting the treatment was a little scary because they put me in a room encased in styrofoam, made everyone leave, and closed a heavy steel door. I was alone with this big machine, which kicked into action with a screaming noise. I focused on this big machine as being a healing power, a positive thing. I really had to work on my focusing technique." Fran used visualization, which will be discussed in a later chapter, to help her cope and fight the cancer. Her energy held up well for about four weeks before she suddenly became very weak. It took several months to regain her energy, before she felt it was fully recovered.

Like Fran, Ann Schneider had radiation daily for five weeks, along with chemotherapy. She did not know what to expect of the radiotherapy and did not find it too unpleasant. "Actually, nothing was happening," she told us. "I looked the same. Finally, my skin started to turn pink and after the treatments stopped I felt that I had been microwaved and was still cooking. Then my skin began to slough off; there were blisters and oozing. It took eight weeks for it to heal. With the radiation and chemo together I was really fatigued and had to quit my job. I couldn't keep up with it."

CHEMOTHERAPY

Chemotherapy involves the use of chemicals, either ingested or injected, that circulate throughout the body and kill the cancer cells. Adjuvant chemotherapy is given after surgical removal of cancer to suppress, control, and extend the "disease-free survival" and improve the quality of life.[20] For many women with operable breast cancer it can reduce the risk of recurrence significantly and improve survival.[21] To treat locally advanced breast cancer

(Stage III) neoadjuvant chemotherapy is given before surgical removal of the cancer. "The goal is to shrink the local disease and reduce the risk of systemic spread.[22] Systemic therapy is used when the cancer has spread outside the breast.

Chemotherapy drugs work by interfering with the reproduction of cells, very much as the radioactive particles in radiation do. The drugs used in chemotherapy alter the DNA and kill cells by preventing them from making nucleic acids and proteins, which are essential to their survival and reproduction. In order to inhibit a cell's reproduction, anti-cancer drugs must attack the cell at a particular time in its reproductive phase.

To enhance the chances of destroying cancer cells, two kinds of drugs are used. "Cell-specific" drugs can harm the cells only at a specific time in the reproductive phase; "cell-cycle nonspecific" drugs can damage the cells during any phase.[23]

The practice of using chemotherapy soon after detection in combination with surgery and/or radiation has increased. There are a number of reasons why chemotherapy may not be used alone. First, when anti-cancer drugs are given, only a fraction of the cancer cells are destroyed. Meanwhile, other cells that are in a resting phase escape the effect of the drugs. Second, drugs become diluted in the bloodstream and may be too weak to affect cells. Moreover, their stay in the bloodstream is of short duration before they are excreted. Another explanation is that cancer cells react as people do to drugs; they become resistant or immune to them.

Chemotherapy has been found to work best when there are fewer cells to attack—which means that the earlier it is used, the more effective it can be. For this reason, early adjuvant chemotherapy (auxillary substances given to assist or aid another treatment) is now being recommended, particularly for premenopausal women.

Before the administration of chemotherapy, the blood count is taken to establish a baseline. During treatment the blood count is taken to monitor dosage levels, white cells, and platelets, which, if low, increase the risk of infection and bleeding. Although treatments are usually scheduled in three-week cycles, this will vary with the patient and oncologist.

Possible Side Effects and Complications

A common side effect with some drugs is nausea, vomiting, and loss of appetite.[24] The nausea associated with chemotherapy may last for a short time or continue throughout the treatments. The problem of nausea differs with each individual and with the kind and amount of chemicals being used. Some women have no difficulty with nausea at all; others are very ill for several days after treatment. In extreme cases, particularly when the injected drugs can be tasted, a patient may develop anticipatory reactions even before the drugs would produce such effects. Stimuli in the setting, such as needles and odors, and other reminders may trigger the nausea.[25] Medications for nausea, tranquilizers, and techniques such as visualization and relaxation may be helpful in controlling it. Along with nausea may be a loss of appetite or an aversion to certain foods. The release of new anti-nausea drugs is helping to reduce or eliminate side effects of chemotherapy.[26]

Another side effect is loss of hair (alopecia). This, too, depends on the particular drugs being used. For example, some drugs always cause the hair to fall out, whereas other drugs may sometimes or rarely cause hair loss.[27] Wearing a wig can alleviate some of the negative effect on body image until the hair grows back.

A number of other side effects may occur. Women report hot flashes, mood swings, cessation of menstruation, vaginal dryness, mouth sores, diarrhea, constipation, and other complications. A woman receiving chemotherapy should discuss with her oncologist the side effects that may occur with the particular drugs she will be receiving. For some women, knowing what to anticipate may have a negative power of suggestion. However, it is more important for a person to know what to report to the physician if side effects do occur. Furthermore, women can learn techniques, or alternative treatments such as imaging, that will help them to cope with stressful side effects.

Personal Accounts of Chemotherapy

When Mary Lynn Gordon's surgeon sent her to an oncologist who advocated chemotheraphy because of the advanced stage of her lesions, she said, "No." She didn't want to lose her hair. The oncologist called her several times urging her to take this additional treatment, and she finally decided to so. Although she lost her hair, Mary Lynn did not suffer with nausea so she was able to continue working.

It wasn't her hair that upset Ruth Thayer, it was the nausea. As her husband Mel expressed it, "The chemo turned her upside down. About the third or fourth day after a treatment the turmoil in her stomach would hit her. I would come home to see how she was feeling and she would be on the couch shaking. Every treatment made her feel horrible."

Chemotherapy also made Mindy Bishop nauseated for several days. A single mother, Mindy was the breadwinner; and chemotherapy affected her job. She told us, "I had a lot of time off from work and it lowered my job productivity as well as my personnel reviews. They said I was doing an 'adequate' job, but what they expected of me I could not do because of my health. I was draggy, tired, depressed. Now my co-workers see a big difference in me since the treatments ended. It's been a difficult time, but I think how lucky I am compared to other people."

Fran Humphrey's experience with chemotherapy illustrates the importance of having frequent blood counts and other tests during the treatments.

Her case also describes the anxiety resulting from side effects. Fran had just completed the radiation and chemotherapy treatments for a breast tumor, and she and her husband George were all set to get on with their lives. Then she found another mass. Chemotherapy had made Fran nauseated the first time, but, being a positive person, she had endured it. However, four days after the second round of treatments began, she had severe pain. She not only had pneumonia but her blood count was low, so low that treatments had to be discontinued.

Fran's husband George was upset with the decision. "The trouble I'm having," he related, "is that chemotherapy is supposed to be the last word here. Now, all of a sudden the doctors are saying, 'Maybe not.' What does this mean? I follow their reasoning but, emotionally, I feel we are bailing out, conceding some territory, in the middle of the fight."

The outcome of Fran's difficulty with chemotherapy was that other treatments were used. She underwent the bone marrow rescue treatment and radiation. The radiation, her own fighting spirit, and a strong support system kept her cancer in remission for some time.

HORMONE THERAPY

Another type of systemic treatment is hormone therapy. The growth rate of breast cancers can be altered by the presence or absence of estrogen and progesterone in a significant number of cases. These breast cancers are "hormone-responsive." The menopausal status and the effect of hormones on the cancer are key factors in the use of hormone therapy. Unlike chemotherapy, hormone therapy does not kill cancer cells directly. Hormones are naturally produced by the body and are not cytotoxic. In other words, they do not have a specific toxic action upon cells of special organs. Because hormones stimulate some breast cancer, manipulation of hormones involves elimination of estrogen and other female sex hormones. The objective is to reduce the estrogen that cancer cells depend upon for growth. In the past, removal of the ovaries (oophorectomy) was done by surgery or radiation to stop the production of hormones. Now, the use of the hormone is the common treatment.[28] However, as each case differs, before hormone therapy is given, a test can determine if it will be helpful.

The estrogen-receptor test, sometimes called the estrogen-receptor assay test, is used to determine a tumor's sensitivity to hormones. The cancerous tissue from the biopsy is examined in the lab to determine if cells are estrogen positive or negative. If the test indicates that a cell in a particular cancer is sensitive to estrogen, it is estrogen-receptor-positive. This means that there is a receptor in the cell that allows the estrogen molecule to enter the cell. It also means that the cancer cell is slower growing and will be responsive to hormone treatments. In other words, hormone therapy may be effective. If the test is negative (estrogen-receptor-negative), hormone treatments may not be effective.

A number of potential treatments—such as estrogen, androgens, progesterone, and others—can be used. Tamoxifen is an example of an anti-estrogen commonly prescribed to prevent recurrence or to treat metastasis to the bone, skin, lymph nodes, remaining breast tissue, and lung. Where a tumor growth is believed to be speeded by the production of hormones, this prevents the estrogen from entering the malignant cell to promote its growth. Tamoxifen has some side effects, most of which seem to be well tolerated by most women.[29] The side effects may be not flashes, vaginal dryness, nausea, vomiting, hypercalcemia (an excess of calcium in the blood), or a transient flare of breast cancer symptoms. These often decrease in a few weeks.[30]

Before making a decision to take any treatment, a woman should discuss the possible side effects with her physician. Newer hormones, which may be even more effective than what is now available, are being developed.

BONE MARROW RESCUE, OR TRANSPLANTATION

Before beginning this treatment, the patient undergoes a medical and psychological assessment and must sign an explicit consent form. Also, the family members have a meeting with the health care team during which their needs are considered. The consent form has a detailed description of the transplant process.

An autologous (products of the same individual organ) bone marrow transplant (BMT) is the most common type of transplant for breast cancer. It is also called a rescue. The woman's bone marrow is harvested during remission, frozen, and stored in a blood bank. At the time of transplant the patient first has high doses of chemotherapy to kill any malignant cells. During this preparatory or conditioning phase the patient's immune system is suppressed and susceptible to infection. Forty-eight to seventy-two hours after the chemotherapy is completed, the patient's harvested bone marrow is infused intravenously to rescue her bone marrow.

The period during which the graft-taking or rejection takes place can last from approximately six to thirty-five days. It is a difficult wait for the patient. She should be encouraged to express her concerns and to take "one day at a time." Family and friends can help her through this by planning surprises that relate to her interests. In addition to the long process that this treatment requires, there are both temporary and long-range effects.

Bone marrow rescue is used when other forms of treatment have failed to stop the growth of cancer. The woman who chooses to undergo it must prepare herself for a series of critical times. It has worked for Christy Duval, who has enjoyed almost two years of recovery since she underwent this treatment.[31]

During the last thirty years the approach to the diagnosis and treatment of breast cancer has undergone dramatic changes that have increased survival and the quality of life. Adjuvant chemotherapy and adjuvant hormone therapy reduce the risk of metastases and recurrence. Mammography, which is used routinely for early detection and screening, has resulted in earlier diagnosis of breast cancer and a 30 percent lower mortality rate in women who undergo screening. Breast conservation with radiotherapy and the availability of reconstruction options are other important developments. Another change is in the administration of neoadjuvant systemic therapy for primary breast cancer before other treatment. The use of autologous bone marrow transplant is increasing and prolonging the length of survival. Even with all these changes, however, treatment for metastatic cancer needs much improvement. Technological advances and clinical and genetic research are promising. Moreover, greater awareness of the social, emotional, and spiritual needs of patients and families, and the emphasis on preventive medicine, are important changes.[32]

In summary, the body's immune system may be able to fight off a few cancerous cells, but as the cells increase and become more aggressive, it may be unable to kill all the cancer cells without help. At some point the cells escape from their main source into the blood stream or lymph system to find other locations. Surgery, chemotherapy, radiation, and bone marrow transplantation, the major treatments that are being used to control cancer, have greater success when administered early in the life of the cancer cells. Meanwhile, the immune system itself must be stimulated.

Breast reconstruction, the topic of the following chapter, is another option for women who undergo the removal of a breast. A history of reconstructive surgery, current procedures, the positive effects, and the risks are reviewed. Also included are answers to questions for women who have problems with implants or think they may have an immune disease associated with a silicone implant. The chapter concludes with a discussion of women's reactions to breast reconstruction.

Chapter 4

Breast Reconstruction

Kathryn Lathrop's husband had discouraged her from having reconstructive surgery because he thought she had gone through enough suffering. "You don't need that, too," he said. "I don't care what you look like." Kathryn's retort was, "I do."

Without her husband's support, Kathryn had her breast reconstructed because her appearance is important to her. She expressed one of the foremost reasons why women want reconstructive surgery; it not only improves their appearance but it can also make a remarkable improvement in their psychological outlook.

Beginning with a brief history, in these next pages we will acquaint you with the alternative procedures, timing, benefits, possible complications, and controversial issues of breast reconstruction. Questions that you will need to ask if you consider this surgery are specified in Appendix C. Finally, we present attitudes of women and their spouses toward reconstruction and the testimonies of women who have undergone the surgical procedure.

HISTORY OF BREAST RECONSTRUCTION

Breast reconstruction was first reported in 1895, when a surgeon removed a fatty tumor (a tumor, usually benign, composed of mature fat cells) from another part of a woman's body and transplanted it to her previous mastectomy site. Not until twenty-two years later did another surgeon try to use a woman's own fatty tissue for transplantation after a simple mastectomy. The results were unsuccessful because of infection and reabsorption of the tissue. In 1963, silicone gel–filled breast implants became available. For the following eight years these implants were used in cosmetic surgery for enlarging the breasts. By 1971, surgeons were beginning to implant the silicone gel for breast reconstruction following a mastectomy.[1]

Alternative reconstructive procedures were described in the 1970 medical journals. They involved two major flap procedures, using a woman's own skin, tissue, muscle, and blood vessels from another area of her body for breast reconstruction.

Capsular contracture due to the formation of a fibrous membrane around silicone gel implants has been a concern since their inception in the late 1950s. In the 1960s polyurethane coating was added to the standard gel-filled implants to aid in the fixation of the implant. One major benefit was found to be the lessening of the fibrous membrane.

However, in 1991, charges were made that polyurethane had a potential for creating a toxic substance. This prompted an advisory panel of the Food and Drug Administration (FDA) to request reports of data from manufacturers of silicone gel implants. Because of adverse media exposure, companies that manufactured the implants voluntarily began to withdraw or discontinue availability of their products. The panel recommended that, while research was being done, implants remain available. Then, in January 1992, the panel called for a 45-day moratorium on the sale and use of silicone gel-filled implants.

Several months later, in April 1992, the FDA panel recommended that the use of implants for cosmetic reasons be "limited," but "broader" access be made for patients having immediate reconstruction (this constituted "urgent need" for implants).

Urgent need can be defined as those women who require permanent implants after the removal of temporary tissue expanders used for breast reconstruction. It also applies to replacement of ruptured silicone implants previously placed, and for situations where saline implants are unacceptable. All women receiving silicone implants must be recorded in a registry and must participate in ongoing research studies.

CURRENT BREAST RECONSTRUCTIVE PROCEDURES

Two kinds of reconstructive surgery following a mastectomy are currently practiced. They are the artificial saline-filled implant or a procedure using the woman's own muscle, tissue, skin, and blood vessels.[2]

Saline-Filled Implant

The saline-filled implant is placed under the pectoralis muscle in the chest. The muscle is pushed forward and the skin is closed over the top. At times it is necessary to stretch the muscle and skin prior to the insertion of the saline implant by means of a procedure called tissue expansion.

The tissue expander is a plastic bag that has a tube with a valve. The expander, from which the valve or tube extends to the surface of the skin, is placed behind the pectoralis muscle and is sutured closed. The woman must visit the doctor's office each week for a saline injection of about 100 ml (less than 1/2 cup) through the valve. It may take four to six months to stretch the skin to the desired size. When the size is achieved, the expander bag may be removed. The most current procedure is to use the same saline device for both the expander and the permanent implant.

Problems associated with the tissue expander may include discomfort, such as severe back pain, when the expansion presses on nerves. Also, there is always the possibility of infection when foreign material is introduced into a person's body. One woman reported that infection occurred where the expander was placed, necessitating its removal. Another woman stated that muscle spasms became more intense with each injection.

Myocutaneous and TRAM Flap

A procedure using a woman's own muscle and tissue is called the myocutaneous flap or the TRAM flap. A wedge of skin, muscle, and fat is removed from either the back muscle—called the latissimus muscle (LDMF procedure)—or the abdomen—called the rectus muscle (TRAM procedure). This wedge is tunneled under the skin into the removed breast area. The feeding artery and vein are not cut in this technique, so the blood supply remains intact. The site from which the muscle and fat is taken is sutured closed, leaving a scar in the area.

Some physicians believe this type of reconstruction has advantages over the artificial saline implants because there is extra skin that can be used to make a larger breast and it provides a more natural droop. Women have reported that they feel normal externally but that they still have reduced sensation. This type of surgery requires a short hospital stay, but a woman can be fully active in about six months.

Any of these procedures can be done immediately at the time of the mastectomy or at a later time. The most important point to be made is that you should be thoroughly informed of all the possibilities. You need to be sure you want the reconstruction when you agree to have it done immediately after removal of your breast. Another point to remember is that there are no time limits on reconstruction; it may be done at any time or at any age.

Nipple and Areola Reconstruction

Nipple and areola reconstruction usually requires a later surgery after the reconstruction. Reconstruction of the areola, the brown or darker pink area surrounding the nipple, can be done on an outpatient basis without anesthesia. One method is to tattoo a circle that matches the opposite breast in size and color. Another is to take skin from another part of the body, such as the lower abdomen, and graft it onto the circular areola.

There are several procedures to reconstruct the nipple. One method is nipple sharing, which looks most natural. Part of the opposite nipple is moved to the reconstruction side. Another procedure involves constructing a nipple from tissue taken from another part of the body to use as a graft. After the transplant the graft will take on a darker color to make a fairly close match with the original nipple. Nipple saving at the time of the cancer operation is not recommended by most physicians because of the possibility of retaining and transplanting cancer cells that may be present in the nipple.

Some women who have breast reconstruction decide against a nipple for various reasons. As in the case of Jean Doerger, some women do not want to go through more surgery. Others, on the other hand, feel that a nipple is necessary for them to look their best in their clothes. One patient said she wanted to look exactly as she had before surgery. Some women have the other breast reduced or augmented in order to have both breasts equal in size.

It is important to emphasize that each woman is unique and that, as Dr. Love points out, decisions need to be based on what is best for her.[3] A woman who has experienced breast cancer should not concern herself with guilt or whether her vanity is motivating her to have reconstruction. Dr. Love believes that each woman is entitled to do what she can to make the time after cancer surgery as comfortable as possible for herself.[4]

HAVING IMMEDIATE OR DELAYED RECONSTRUCTION

The dilemma of immediate versus delayed reconstructive surgery involves several issues. The first is personal choice. Although a woman may think she is not interested, she needs to be well informed prior to the mastectomy in order to make an intelligent decision. Second, there may be medical reasons that delayed reconstructive surgery will have the best outcome. For example, some surgeons may recommend a delay of several months to allow for healing before more complex reconstruction procedures, such as a TRAM, can be performed. Another reason may be that prolonged anesthesia could increase operative risks.[5] The medical team may agree that reconstruction should not be done until after radiation therapy is completed.

Reconstructive surgery should be delayed if the woman is too overwhelmed with the diagnosis and future treatment to make an immediate decision. This was the case with Martha Sherman, who felt ambiguous about reconstruction. At times she felt her surgery was "too drastic to consider the ordeal" of reconstruction. At the same time she wanted to have both breasts. Martha advises that a woman must weigh the matter carefully and make her own decision. She may change her mind later on if she isn't sure that she wants reconstructive surgery initially.

Although research studies have shown no statistical difference between immediate versus delayed breast reconstruction in regard to complications, recurrence, or survival, physicians have not reached a consensus regarding its timing. However, some take a strong stand on the matter. For example, Norman Hugo, chairman of plastic and reconstructive surgery at New York City's Columbia Presbyterian Medical Center, states his department's philosophy: a woman doesn't leave the hospital without a breast.

Among the research that has analyzed the psychological effects of immediate versus delayed reconstruction is a study by Stevens and associates.[6] They examined two groups of women (those who had immediate surgery and those who had delayed surgery) at three time periods and found that psychological reactions were significantly better for the group who had chosen immediate reconstruction. Only 23 percent of them reported that they suffered depression, whereas 83 percent of those who had delayed reconstruction were depressed.

Other positive effects for those who had immediate reconstruction are related to body image, sexuality, and femininity. Women had no feelings of deformity after the reconstruction and returned to their premastectomy style of clothing and activity. With the exception of three women, sexual functioning was not affected.

In contrast, the delayed group described feelings of deformity, disfigurement, imbalance, and mutilation after the mastectomy. Half of them wore loose clothing to decrease attention to their breasts. As to their sexuality, around 60 percent reported a decline in sexual functioning, which improved after they underwent breast reconstruction. An important finding of studies that compare immediate and delayed reconstruction is that women who decided upon immediate reconstruction were more informed about alternatives of breast cancer treatment. Most women who had delayed reconstruction did not know that immediate reconstruction was even available.

In summary, the research findings have shown a definite psychological benefit to those women who have had breast reconstruction at the time of the mastectomy. Many of the psychological problems they experience with the loss of a breast are lessened. An important advantage of immediate breast reconstruction is that there is only one anesthesia risk when both procedures are done at once. The saline implant/tissue expander is inserted easily and quickly after the surgeon removes the breast tissue. Surgeons have found less postoperative fibrosis and better cosmetic results because of the preservation and use of the uninvolved breast skin.[7]

An example of the positive psychological effect that breast reconstruction can have is given by Millie Davis, who told us how she felt about the surgeries she had undergone. "It was worth it because every time I had surgery, I looked better," Millie said. "It helped my self-image a great deal. Some people would ask me why I went through all this. They think I'm vain. I'd tell them, 'I would rather go through the surgery and look like everyone else than live without breasts.' "

If you choose to have reconstruction, you may hear insensitive remarks and jibes about your vanity. Learn not to react to others but make decisions for yourself. Remember that a woman's breasts have always been a part of her. If she wishes to restore her body to a feeling of wholeness with reconstructive surgery, that is her desire and need for a full recovery. It is not for everyone; whatever you do, you have made a valid decision.

THE RISKS OF RECONSTRUCTIVE SURGERY

Risks in the Surgical Procedure

The surgical procedure of inserting an implant can be performed under local or general anesthesia. It is usually an outpatient procedure. If the implant is not placed at the time of the mastectomy but is done months to years later, the existing incision is generally used.

As with any elective surgery that includes anesthesia, there are risks. Infection or bleeding may occur at a frequency comparable to any clean surgery. However, the course of the patient's cancer is not affected by implants, nor does it change a woman's survival expectancy.

Risk of Capsular Contracture

The most common problem of breast implants is capsular contracture. At the time of surgery the surgeon makes a pocket in which the implant rests. In a normal process, fibrous membrane, called a capsule, forms around the implant. Sometimes the capsule may shrink and squeeze the implant, which results in various degrees of hardness. This contraction may occur soon after the reconstruction or years later. It is not usually a health risk but is cosmetically distressful to the woman and may cause pain. The scar tissue around the implant can be surgically relieved or removed; the contraction can recur.

Risk of Implant Rupture

The trauma of an accident or breast compression may break an implant shell. The saline in the implant, which is not a foreign product, will be absorbed by the body. In case of rupture of a silicone gel implant, the contents are usually contained within the scar tissue and could, therefore, go undetected. Symptoms of a rupture include a change in the feel and shape of the breast or a persistent burning. New scar tissue will form around the ruptured contents within two to six weeks. Most plastic surgeons recommend that the implants be removed and replaced if a rupture occurs.

Risk of Cancer Detection

Women have expressed a fear that breast implants interfere with the detection of breast cancer by hiding a lesion lying beneath it. In regard to this fear, the Food and Drug Administration has issued a statement that "there is no evidence that women with breast implants are at an increased risk."[8]

Two studies have found that implants do not interfere with breast cancer detection, nor is there evidence that silicone gel implants increase the risk of cancer in humans. A study of more than 3,000 women in Los Angeles County showed no difference in the incidence of breast cancer between women who had implants for over eleven years and those who did not have implants. A Canadian study of more than 11,000 women who have had implants actually showed a decrease in the expected incidence of breast cancer.[9] This very important finding of the study indicates that implants are not carcinogenic.

The American College of Radiology, the American Cancer Society, and the American Society of Plastic and Reconstructive Surgeons agree that a woman with breast implants should have routine mammograms under the same American Cancer Society guidelines (see Appendix D) as a woman without implants. These organizations recommend that a woman with an implant should not receive a mammogram at a screening clinic where only two routine views of the breast are taken. She should be referred to a facility accredited by the American College of Radiology where the special "Eckland" four views are done to fully evaluate an implanted breast. It is important to ask whether the technician is experienced in performing mammography with breast implants. A woman should always inform the technician of her implant before the mammography so that special care is taken when compressing the breast to prevent rupturing of the implant. This is called the Modified Compression Technique.

The cost of this special mammogram is higher and the amount of radiation exposure is also somewhat greater with additional views. Information about accredited facilities can be obtained by calling the National Cancer Institute (1–800–4–Cancer) or a local chapter of the American Cancer Society (see Resources in Appendix B).

The Modified Compression Technique should be done once a year. In addition, women with implants are advised to do self-examination and have a physical examination by a physician. Dr. Susan Love sometimes recommends ultrasound for a very young patient at whose age the radiation could be dangerous.[10] A woman with implants should return to the same facility for all future mammograms so the procedure is always done consistently and where her records are retained.

Risks of Rheumatic Disorders

There have been a few reports of autoimmune or rheumatic disorders associated with silicone implants done prior to February 1992. The studies prior to that time did not find any data that suggested silicone breast implants contributed to rheumatic disorders.

In May 1992, the Food and Drug Administration issued a statement that "there is not conclusive evidence at present that women with breast implants have an increased risk of developing arthritic-like disease or other autoimmune diseases."[11] By 1995, the results of large-scale epidemiologic studies will be available. These will determine if there is an association of silicone breast implant and autoimmune disease. Until research can answer these questions, the FDA will not approve the silicone gel implants.

What do you do if you think you have symptoms of an immune disease? You should see a rheumatologist just as you would if you did not have an implant. The symptoms may be related to many types of physical conditions and can be effectively treated, especially if treated early.

What are the symptoms of immune disease? They are pain and swelling of the joints; tightness, redness, or swelling of the skin, hands, and feet; swollen glands or lymph nodes; fatigue and unusual hair loss. Any of these symptoms should be reported to your physician, for they can be signs of many types of health problems.

What does the FDA advisory panel recommend for a woman who already has silicone gel implants? She should see her physician or the plastic surgeon who performed the reconstruction on a regular yearly basis. She should do this even if she is not experiencing any symptoms such as muscle or joint pain.

If a silicone gel implant has ruptured, the FDA guidelines are specific: (1) The woman should immediately contact the physician. (2) The implant should be removed as soon as possible and sent back to the manufacturer for analysis. (3) The implant should be replaced.

"Silent" ruptures can occur. Therefore, it is important to have regular Modified Compression mammograms as recommended by the American Cancer Society for your age group in order to detect problems.

What should you do when a saline-filled breast implant ruptures? As we have already mentioned, saline implants are being used for breast reconstruction since the removal of silicone gel implants from the market. The saline implant deflates rapidly and the salt water is absorbed in the body within a few hours. This type of implant is covered with a silicone rubber envelope. Again, the FDA has established guidelines: (1) The physician should remove the implant. (2) The implant should be sent to the manufacturer for analysis to determine the cause of the rupture. (3) The implant should be replaced.

How do you handle any difficulty with your implant? You need to stay under the care of your physician or plastic surgeon. You can also call FDA at 1–800–638–6725 for informational material on breast implants or to report a specific problem. Have the following information ready to report: (1) The manufacturer's name of your implant and the product brand name (call your doctor for this information). (2) The date of your implant surgery. (3) The date that the problem started. (4) Nature of the problem. (5) Name and address of the surgeon. (6) Name and address of the facility where the surgery was performed. (Also see Resources in Appendix B).

What should you do if you have a silicone gel–filled implant? The FDA has stated that there is insufficient risk to justify the removal of silicone implants in women who already have them in place if there are no symptoms present. The FDA is not recommending that you have your implants removed if you have no problems. If you do experience any symptoms that you feel may be related to your implants, contact your physician or plastic surgeon as you would for any illness. It is important to know that most women do not have any problems with their implants.

How often do silicone gel–filled implants rupture? They rupture very infrequently: as low as a fraction of 1 percent and as high 6 percent of all silicone implants. There are numbers that you may call about any concerns you have. For the FDA call 1–800–638–6725, 9 A.M. to 7 P.M. EST, Monday through Friday. For the American Society of Plastic Reconstructive Surgeons, call 1–708–228–9900, twenty-four hours a day.

How do you find out what kind of implant you have? You should contact your plastic surgeon first for this information, which he or she will have on your medical record. If you are unable to contact this physician, call the medical records department of the institution where you had your surgery. You may have to write a formal request and pay a small fee. Expect to wait about three weeks before you receive the information.

What is involved in an implant removal? Breast implant removal is a simple operation. It does have the normal risks, such as infection, that are associated with any surgical procedure. You will want to discuss with the surgeon whether the scar tissue surrounding the implant will be removed. You will also want to decide on the type of implant replacement. At the present time, the only type available is the saline-filled implant. If a replacement is not made, the skin and tissue of the breasts will sag and appear flat.

The surgical fee will depend upon the extent of the needed surgery. Your insurance carrier may cover the cost of the implant removal, but you will need to check with your company in advance.

What is the position of the American Society of Plastic and Reconstructive Surgeons (ASPRS) on removal of implants? The first action you should take when you have concerns about your implant is to consult with the surgeon who originally performed the implant. However, if this surgeon is not accessible because of your relocation, his/her retirement or death, ASPRS has arranged a program called Breast Implant Patient Relations Network (BIPRN). You may call 1–708–228–9900 for information. ASPRS is the largest organization of plastic surgeons in the world. It represents 97 percent of board-certified plastic surgeons in the United States and Canada.

REACTIONS TO RECONSTRUCTIVE SURGERY

In 1990, the first national survey of women who have had breast augmentation or reconstruction was conducted to determine how they felt about the results of their breast implants. The study was sponsored by the American Society of Plastic and Reconstructive Surgeons and supported by the American Society for Aesthetic Plastic Surgery. Detailed questionnaires were completed by 592 women whose implants had been in place for an average of eight years. Sixty-five percent were for the purpose of cosmetic enlargement and 35 percent for reconstruction after cancer. Results indicated that 93 percent of the women were satisfied with the results of their surgery and 82 percent said that "without a doubt" they would choose to have the surgery again. Among women who had reconstruction after cancer, 80 percent said the implant restored their feelings of wholeness and 55 percent felt the reconstruction helped them forget the diagnosis. Ninety percent of them felt free of discomfort and the inconvenience of an external prosthesis.[12] The satisfaction with breast reconstruction reported in this study was confirmed by the women we interviewed.

Reactions of Women to Reconstruction

It had been a year and a half since Mindy Bishop had her mastectomy when, during a routine check-up, her surgeon asked her if she was dating. She replied, "No, I feel very disfigured. Even though people can't tell how I look, I know. I just can't imagine getting involved with someone because at some point he is going to find out."

"I really think you need a reconstruction," said her doctor. "It would help your self-esteem and you would have more confidence in dating."

Mindy thought about it for another six months before she began the steps of reconstruction. During the first stage of tissue expansion she felt better about how she was going to look. She bought a pretty sweater dress and hung it in the closet with a note pinned on it: "You will get to wear me after surgery."

The reconstruction process was difficult for her and she began to have feelings of regret for "putting herself through it," but when it was over, she was glad. "I don't have to deal with the external prosthesis and I feel whole again," she said. Now, several years later, Mindy is happily remarried and expecting a child.

For Eleanor Armand the external prosthesis was very uncomfortable and, being large-busted, she was bothered by the imbalance. A year later, when Eleanor decided to have reconstruction, her husband Gene was concerned about her having surgery. Her doctor recommended the TRAM procedure, using the rectus muscle from her abdomen. After it was over, her husband noticed a great improvement in Eleanor's self-esteem. She was more outgoing, looked happier, and was getting involved in outside activities. Both Eleanor and Gene are delighted with the results.

Before her reconstruction, Mary Lynn Gordon said that she did not like the way she looked. "When I took off my clothes and passed by a mirror, I looked pretty bad. I looked like I had been in a concentration camp and somebody had experimented on me," she confided. "Every rib showed; I had a big gaping hole where my breast used to be. Now it is so wonderful not to have to cart that prosthesis around and be careful about what I wear. I can put on a sweatshirt or a T-shirt or walk around in a bathing suit. I feel so good that I can do these marvelous things."

Some women reject the idea of reconstruction. They feel that they do not want to put themselves through more surgery, or they have a fear of a recurrence that would not be detectable because of the prosthesis. Some women—like Ann Jillian, who elected not to have it—are accepting of themselves without reconstruction. Jillian wrote that, "I thought I had already asked enough of my body . . . with the trauma and shock of a double mastectomy. I decided to wear my prosthesis on the outside of my body rather than going through surgeries to wear it on the inside."[13]

Reactions of Spouses to Reconstruction

Husbands also react differently toward reconstructive surgery. Some say it isn't necessary because the loss of a breast doesn't affect their feelings toward their wives, whereas others are openly in favor of it. Bill Waters said it hadn't really mattered to him, and he felt it wouldn't affect their relationship one way or the other. After his wife Phyllis had reconstruction, he confessed, "I'm glad we went this way. I like what she had done. She is satisfied with it and that is what matters."

John Reuther was definitely in favor of Cynthia's reconstruction because she needed it for her own feeling of self-worth. He thought it was amazing what the plastic surgeon had done for her and encouraged any spouse to keep an open mind about it "because it can do wonderful things for a woman."

Mel Thayer thinks his wife would have had a harder time dealing with her breast cancer without reconstruction "because she always has been very conscious of how she looks. It has been more help getting her through this than anything that has happened," he said.

Husbands respond to breast reconstruction with different degrees of acceptance. Some seem to object more from concern than from resistance. Others react with complete approval and enthusiasm about the outcome.

The purpose of breast reconstruction is to preserve breast symmetry as well as the woman's self-image, which, in turn, influences her health. The breasts have psychological importance for a woman's self-image that is deeper than mere cosmetic concern. They symbolize her femininity, fertility, and ability to nurture. This symbolism has been documented in literature dating back to the artifacts of the Neolithic Period of 10,000 B.C.

In this chapter we have given a history of reconstructive surgery, explained current procedures, and discussed the issues that must be considered in making a decision about having it. The risks have been presented and the questions concerning immune disease and problems with implants have been posed and answered. To conclude the chapter, reactions of several women who have made a decision about reconstruction as well as the reaction of some spouses have been offered.

The development of reconstructive surgery has given women a choice, and each must make her own decision about having it. We hope that the decision will be based on information and an honest examination of your own needs and convictions.

As you read on you will learn about holistic methods, or alternative treatments, that can supplement medical treatment. Most of these therapies aim at strengthening the body's immune system. They include mental and spiritual techniques such as meditation, visualization, prayer, and psychic healing. Other methods focus on nutrition, exercise, and substance used by practitioners of homeopathy. Although there is no scientific evidence that these methods can change the course of the cancer, they have enabled patients with cancer to cope and live fulfilling lives. These and other methods are examined in the next chapter.

Chapter 5

Holistic and Alternative/Complementary Treatments

Marianne Stevens and undergone her first breast biopsy at the age of 21. She had a hysterectomy and eight more lumps that proved to be benign over the next twenty years. Just before Christmas she had her tenth biopsy and this lump also tested negative, but the doctor found cancer cells in the tissue next to the lump.

She had developed a false sense of security, Marianne told us. However, her reaction to this diagnosis was not disbelief, but shock and a feeling that "her time was up." She experienced a great deal of grief because she realized it meant losing her breast. But in spite of her personal turmoil, she and her husband felt lucky that the cancer was discovered while in the earliest stage so she wouldn't be hurried into treatment but would have time to make considered decisions.

From the beginning she began active management of her disease. Her first decision was to wait until after Christmas before telling their children or anyone about the diagnosis. Her doctor assured her that a delay of a couple of months in having treatment would do not harm.

Her next step was to go shopping for doctors. The most difficult thing for her, she said, was to tell her surgeon that another doctor would be doing her mastectomy. To her relief, he was understanding and very cooperative. In a large medical center in a nearby city she had found a highly recommended surgeon who reviewed her history and did another mammogram. Dr. Thomas, known to be conservative in her treatment, recommended bilateral surgery because the type of cancer that Marianne had was almost certain to appear in her other breast. Another shock. The next few days were extremely difficult for Marianne. Now she had to accept the reality that she wasn't losing just one, but both breasts.

She requested that the surgeon send the slides of her tissue to the Mayo Clinic to make certain of the diagnosis. She wanted no mistakes. Then she and her family sought counseling. Because the young son of one of her friends had experienced a difficult reaction to his mother's mastectomy, Marianne and her husband Glen wanted to be sure their children were informed and reassured. They were especially concerned that their son, who was away at school, would have adequate support.

At the same time, Marianne began networking, talking with women who had undergone mastectomies. She particularly wanted to talk with someone who had undergone bilateral surgery; and through Cancer Share, she was able to find a woman who had. She also accepted the invaluable help of a friend who had lost a breast several years earlier and was a volunteer for Reach to Recovery.

During this time Marianne was reading "volumes" on breast cancer to learn all that she could about her disease. Concentrating on her arms, she embarked on a vigorous aerobic conditioning program. She increased her vitamin intake and abstained from any kind of medication, even aspirin, for a month before the scheduled surgery. In addition, she prepared herself mentally and emotionally so that by the time she went in for the surgery, she had dealt with "the worst part." She felt that would enable her to get on more quickly with the business of living. The two days before the surgery were "bad ones" when she and her husband grieved for the loss of her breasts.

Marianne made a quick recovery. During her first check-up her surgeon told her to do whatever she wanted. She was soon swimming and taking dance aerobics. Her arm mobility was amazingly good. The only difficulty she had in her recovery occurred when her mother visited to help her. Her mother, wanting to be protective, thought Marianne was overdoing it and resuming her activities too quickly. Unfortunately, the well-meaning parent was operating from old notions about convalescence, and she shortened her visit with the feeling that her efforts to assist her daughter were not needed.

The story of Marianne's experience illustrates how we can take an active role in our own recovery. She combined traditional medical treatment with alternative methods to increase her body's ability to heal both emotionally and physically from the loss of her breasts.

BEYOND TRADITIONAL MEDICINE: INTEGRATING HOLISTIC CONCEPTS

What accounts for the interest in nonmedical therapies, especially when their results are unproven? Our question was answered by physicians, psychologists, and therapists who have pioneered the field of holistic and complementary methods and often received considerable criticism for their beliefs. People have put great faith in drugs but are realizing that they can go beyond medication to help themselves maintain good health. Another reason for patient discontent is that health care has become more impersonal as technology and specialization have increased. Most patients want to receive encouragement and hope from their physicians and nurses despite what some may say about preferring competence to bedside manner. Machines and impersonal medical procedures can be frightening to patients who are already traumatized by the diagnosis of cancer. They need reassurance. Moreover, people have come to the realization that medical science can't fix everything.

HOLISTIC APPROACHES

Holism, a term that Jan Christian Smuts coined in 1926, is derived from the Greek word *holos*, meaning "whole."[1] It is an old philosophy that views the body as a balanced system in which spirit, mind, and body work together as a whole. When one part in this system is affected, it in turn affects the other parts, just as a faulty spark plug stalls or shuts down the engine of an automobile or lawnmower.

Those who practice holistic methods in the purist sense oppose any traditional medical intervention such as surgery and drugs. They believe that the body maintains its balanced state through proper nutrition (fruits, vegetables, nuts, grains, abstinence from meat), fasting, exercise, and meditation.

Some methods claiming holistic philosophy have cultist backgrounds. Norman Cousins, who attended a number of conferences on holism, found that they included clairvoyance, astrology, numerology, graphology, psychic surgery, and other topics. He felt that the methods were fragmented and lacking in research and evidence that related them to good health.[2] In spite of the lack of clear proof that they heal, these techniques attract some people who have perhaps been disappointed by medical treatments and are searching elsewhere for cures for their illnesses. If therapies make undocumented claims, they should be approached with caution.

Treatments that combine holistic concepts along with traditional medical practice are beginning to gain the acceptance of some medical caregivers. These professionals are aware of the therapeutic effects of a good physician-patient partnership and the need to encourage the patient to fight. The leading spokesman of this cooperative relationship between the patient and health professionals has been the late Norman Cousins. Many of you are familiar with his interesting story, but it bears retelling.

Norman Cousins' Story

Cousins was diagnosed as having a serious collagen disease of the connective tissue some years ago, and the doctor told him he had only one chance in five hundred of recovering. He refused to accept the "verdict" and believed he could beat those odds. Cousins set up his own course of positive action to "tame" his illness. As writer and editor of the *Saturday Review* for many years, Cousins was well informed about the human body and mind and was accustomed to challenges. He wondered how he could have gotten this disease and realized that he was exhausted from a stressful schedule. That, he reasoned, could have taxed his immune system and made him vulnerable to disease. With the help of one of the research assistants at *Saturday Review*, he checked out the effects of aspirin, which he was receiving in large doses for his pain, and discovered that it could be detrimental in the treatment of his illness. He also learned that there was a deficiency of Vitamin C in patients with collagen disease. After discussing his findings with his doctor, who assured him of his support, Cousins discontinued the aspirin and began taking large amounts of Vitamin C. He pondered how he could combat the pain without aspirin and began to work on maintaining positive emotions. That was when he stumbled onto the discovery that laughter had an anesthetic effect. It enabled him to sleep, so he focused on finding things that made him laugh. He recovered from the disease.

Cousins' account of that experience in his book *Anatomy of an Illness* brought him to the attention of the public as well as medical professionals and institutions. Because he spoke from knowledge and experience, he won their respect and was instrumental in bridging the gap between science and holistic concepts in medicine. However, he needed to document his hunches about healing. His opportunity came in 1978 when UCLA asked him to join its Program in Psychoneuroimmunology, a Center for Health Enhancement, Education and Research (CHEER). It was established to learn how to develop a new life-style and ways of coping with stress. Cousins' assignment was to do research in positive emotions. He accepted the offer, knowing that his ideas would be met with skepticism. In the years that he was with the program, convincing evidence was compiled to support his experience.

Cousins learned from studies done on patients with breast cancer that the natural killer (NK) cells in the immune system were less active in patients who were depressed. Also, tumors spread more rapidly in depressed patients. Additional studies indicated that the immune system becomes more active and more effective when depression is relieved.

Using relaxation exercises that he adapted from Dr. Green of the Menninger Foundation Clinic, Cousins showed patients how they could have some degree of control over their bodies. He observed that those patients who could do the exercises successfully had less depression. When they were able to free themselves of panic and helplessness, their immune systems seemed to fight illness more effectively.[3]

Cousins was convinced that the patient's will to live and belief that he or she can get well increases the healing power of surgical treatment and medication. Cousins' conviction has been supported by studies such as the one by Greer et al., who found that patients who did best had a determined attitude and generally believed they could conquer the disease.[4] Positive emotions seem to stimulate the immune system and its killer cells to attack the disease. The key to recovery, Cousins stated, is the physician's ability to give a message of hope and "invoke the patient's own bodily resources" to do the healing.[5]

Cynthia's Story

Cynthia Ruether, a young women we have followed through her battle with breast cancer, illustrates the effect of a strong will to live and the need for hope. Throughout her life Cynthia's self-esteem had been badly battered by a verbally abusive father and an alcoholic husband. She had counted on her husband being with her on the day of her mastectomy, but he neither accompanied her to the hospital nor gave her any support. Devastated, she realized that she was "on her own."

Cynthia began therapy sessions, gained the courage to divorce her husband (fortunately, she had a job), and began the struggle to overcome her sense of low self-worth. During the process she became friends with a young man with whom she worked. He admired and encouraged her; eventually their friendship led to marriage. John stood by Cynthia through reconstructive surgery and accompanied her when she underwent treatments. His support and the encouragement of a caring nurse and surgeon strengthened Cynthia's determination to overcome the disease.

She was feeling very good about herself and her life when the cancer recurred. The doctor who diagnosed it said nothing could be done. Two other doctors confirmed his prognosis. Being a fighter, Cynthia was so angry that she was determined to find someone who would give her hope. After some searching she found an oncologist who gave her the encouragement she needed and started her on chemotherapy.

We had not seen or heard from Cynthia for nearly two years when we sent her a note asking her how she was doing. This was her reply:

> John and I are doing fine and currently re-planning our life around health instead of disease. We will be moving [she included their new address]. I am well. No recurrence of the cancer. I continue with counseling, Trager Massage, jazzercize three hours a week, and visits to the oncologist. I have increased my intake of Vitamin C each day and supplement my diet with selenium, Vitamins E, A, D, and calcium. Life is good and God has blessed me greatly through this disease. Keep in touch!
>
> Love, Cynthia

MEDITATION, RELAXATION, AND IMAGERY

Techniques such as meditation (Zen, Yoga, transcendental meditation, and others) have been devised for easing the stress in everyday life. Meditation commonly denotes thinking about a problem. In the therapeutic sense it means bringing the mind under control or focusing in such a way as to close out all stressful thoughts and feelings.[6] The practice that was developed became known as Yoga in the East but takes the form of prayer in the West, where transcendental meditation (TM) is viewed as therapy.

When Herbert Benson was heading a Harvard research project to find a way to lower blood pressure, some practitioners of transcendental meditation offered to demonstrate the benefits of TM. Through this experience with TM the Harvard group discovered the "relaxation response" to be useful in conjunction with meditation. Those who practice these techniques report feelings of well-being and release of stress, thus aiding the body's internal environment. Benson points out that the "relaxation response" is useful but is not to be viewed as a cure-all for medical problems.[7] A study by Kiecolt-Glaser and associates showed that the practice of relaxation does reduce stress. Findings also indicated that relaxation may enhance one's immunity, which acute stress tends to suppress. The researchers suggest that relaxation may be a valuable aid to one's health, especially during stressful times.[8]

O. Carl Simonton, a physician who as a young man had had cancer, felt that reactions to an event that are "bottled up" can precipate a disease. Simonton and his wife Stephanie, with whom he operated the Cancer Counseling and Research Center in Fort Worth, Texas, began showing cancer patients how they could help themselves to get well. The Simontons have been criticized for making unproven claims and for instilling persons with false hope. Nonetheless, the Simontons have developed techniques that have helped cancer patients deal with stress and improve their quality of life. They have used meditation, relaxation, and visual imagery techniques, which they learned from the study of biofeedback. All these techniques require a quiet environment, a word or syllable that is repeated, a passive attitude, and a comfortable position. Those who practice them have reported less stress and a sense of well-being.

Biofeedback, from which the Simontons adapted their techniques, refers to the process of getting information about one's heart rate, muscle tension, blood pressure, or other physiological functions, and voluntarily controlling them. Sound or visual signals emitted from an electronic device enable a person to hear or see changes in her own muscle tension, for example. The person can use this information and regulate her muscle tension (or other physiological functions), which is not normally under conscious control. A part of the preparation for biofeedback is relaxation.

Relaxation Techniques

Simonton teaches relaxation techniques by asking a patient to set aside three 15-minute periods of time each day—morning, noon, and evening—to sit quietly and concentrate on relaxing. Starting with his or her head the patient gradually relaxes each set of muscles, moving from the head to the feet. When in a relaxed state, the patient pictures him- or herself in an appealing, quiet setting—by the ocean, under a tree, as long as it is peaceful and pleasant.[9]

Another advocate of meditation is Bernie Siegel, a pediatric and general surgeon whose book *Love, Medicine and Miracles* is well known. He believes that we tend to program the messages we hear about ourselves from others. If those comments are negative, we undergo conditioning about our worthiness. Because words can be self-fulfilling, Siegel believes we should reject negative ones and replace them with pictures that will enhance our lives.[10] He also suggests that if a surgeon or anesthetist does not talk to a patient in the operating room, the patient should take a tape with appropriate messages or play music while undergoing surgery. Music, words, meditation, visualization, relaxation, and prayer are among the many ways that we can communicate with our inner selves. In his book *Peace, Love and Healing*, Siegel includes meditations with instructions for using them. As preventive medicine, Siegel also recommends relaxation techniques to boost health and gain peace of mind. Just as Benson does, Siegel stresses the importance of medical treatments for cancer—radiation, chemotherapy, and surgery—along with the techniques of inner communication.

While studying the various relaxation approaches described by physicians, I have become aware that some physical fitness instructors are also using these for "cooling down" the body after exercise. At the end of an aerobic class I took, the instructor used relaxation and visualization to slow down the heart rate. Following a full body stretch, we relaxed our muscles from head to feet in the manner suggested by Simonton. Then we proceeded to imagine ourselves relaxed and weightless. Against a background of soft music, usually a melodic symphony number, the instructor provided the imagery. She suggested that we visualize ourselves floating on a cloud through the blue sky. As we imagined the sound of waves below us and the birds around us, we were slowly moved about by the wind. Gradually we drifted downward to land gently on the soft earth.

If we were all patients being taught by Carl Simonton, he would suggest, after we had relaxed in a similar manner, that we picture our cancer in whatever form we imagine it takes. Then he would ask us to visualize our treatment. He suggests that radiation therapy might consist of "millions of tiny bullets that would hit all of our cells, both normal and cancerous, in their path."[11] The normal cells would survive the attack because they are stronger but the cancerous cells, which are weaker, would die. In our last step, we would picture the white cells "swarming over the cancer cells," carrying them away and flushing them out of our systems. We would then visualize our cancer as smaller and our health as better. After the exercise, Simonton would tell us to go about whatever we wanted to do.

Jeanne Achterberg, author of *Imagery in Healing*, states: "Imagery has always played a key role in medicine" and it affects the body on "mundane and profound levels."[12] To realize its effect, imagine you are speaking before a large audience, or waiting for the arrival of someone you love dearly, or running from a burglar who is chasing you with a gun. What emotion and physical changes do you feel? Because of the effect images have, they can also affect the body's responses to illness.

Fran Humphrey's Use of Visualization

Fran was the family counselor to whom we've introduced you earlier. She was the epitome of a cheerful fighter and used all the techniques that she had learned in her study of psychology and holistic treatment. Following Simonton's suggestions, she found mental imagery very helpful. She pictured her cancer cells as "egglike things" being eaten up by Pac-men. She breathed deeply to cope with nausea, the result of her chemotherapy, and mentally transported herself to some other place and visualized being there. This and the other techniques that Fran used, along with medical treatment, may have helped her body to destroy two fast-growing tumors that appeared over a period of two years.

During our last interview with Fran we learned that she had another tumor, this time in a lung, which meant the cancer had metastasized. Her determination to keep fighting was inspiring.

PRAYER AND PSYCHIC HEALING

The healing rituals present in most American churches include prayers for the ill and bedside services. The effect of prayer upon recovery from serious illness cannot be scientifically documented, but there are many who believe in it and exemplify its power. A number of women whom we have interviewed—and, in some cases, their husbands—have attested to the importance of prayer in helping them to cope with breast cancer and to sustain their belief that they will recover. Some said the experience with breast cancer has resulted in their spiritual growth.

Kay and Daniel Sherwood were sustained by their faith and the prayers of their parishioners as well as their attitude that her breast cancer was a challenge they could handle no matter what course it took. Fran and George Humphrey also drew courage from faith and prayer, as did other couples with whom we talked.

An interest in spiritual healing and the "laying-on-of-hands," which has come to be called "therapeutic touch," has been revived in many churches. Through his or her hands, the psychic healer directs energy to the affected parts of the body. Patients reported that the experience is relaxing and conveys to them the feeling of being cared for.[13] In fact, as Dr. Susan Love has noted, some nurses use a similar approach of therapeutic touch with patients.[14] Psychic healers also use prayer, meditation, and other rituals. The trust and encouragement conveyed by the healer who touches them may do more to give patients the will to fight than any special kind of "energy" that may emanate from the healer.[15]

Tests have been done with plants, fungi, enzymes, and mice in an attempt to prove the effects of psychic healing, but findings are inconclusive. Physician Nolen, hoping to identify a person who has supernatural power, made an extensive investigation of miracle cures. Finding no such person, he concluded that in a sense all healing is miraculous and that healers help patients by relieving their symptoms and by encouraging them to think positively.

Christy's Story

When I first met them, Christy and her husband were optimistic that they had contained her breast cancer. Several months later the cancer was found to have metastasized and was in her bones. Christy had already been practicing meditation, visualization, and other alternative techniques to help herself. With this recurrence of cancer the medical treatment was much more extensive; it involved maximum chemotherapy, radiation, and long periods of hospitalization. Christy decided to go to a psychic healer. When I asked her about it, her only reply was, "I had the laying-on-of-hands. I felt nothing. It was not a good experience for me."

Christy's medical treatments and her practice of self-healing have been successful so far. When we discussed the alternative approaches she had used, she said, "It's difficult to maintain a positive attitude when you feel so badly, but I try."

NUTRITION AND EXERCISE

One of the most popular therapies is good nutrition and the use of vitamins. Although more research is needed to determine the effect of vitamins and certain foods on breast cancer, nutritionists generally agree that fat and protein intake should be reduced. Organizations such as the National Cancer Institute and American Cancer Society recommend this reduction for the general population. Fats do not appear to initiate cancer, but they may promote its growth. More studies are needed to understand this phenomenon.[16] Women who are overweight are at higher risk of breast cancer. Because both polyunsaturated and saturated fats may increase the risk of cancer, monounsaturated fats, such as olive oil, in moderate amounts is recommended.[17] For beneficial effects Dr. Brian Morgan, a leading nutritional expert at the Columbia University College of Physicians and Surgeons, recommends Vitamins C and E, and selenium (an element resembling sulphur), as well as cruciferous vegetables (e.g., broccoli and cauliflower) and foods containing beta-carotene.[18] Although abstinence from the use of caffeine is recommended, there is unclear evidence to determine its effect on breast cancer.[19] However, in the case of alcohol, several studies give some evidence that its consumption may increase the risk of breast cancer particularly if drinking occurs at an early age, before age 30.[20] What is most important is to eat a balanced diet and exercise at least three times a week.

There are many books on nutrition, some of which are listed in our bibliography. Pelletier includes a computerized Nutrition, Health, and Activity Profile for analyzing and comparing one's diet to established requirements.[21] Morgan has a special section devoted to diet and breast cancer; and Dreher has directions for designing one's own prevention diet.[22]

Although many Americans have joined the fitness craze, many do not get a sufficient amount of exercise. Stress researchers suggest that the dramatic increase in cancer is related to the unreleased stress of an affluent, sedentary life-style. Experiments have shown that physical exercise tends to stimulate the immune system. Animal studies have found that repeated stress without physical outlet results in body deterioration and that exercise decreases tumor growth.[23]

Exercise is important for the woman who has had breast surgery. It can aid in her physical and emotional recovery, help relieve tightness in the chest, reduce muscle tension and symptoms of lymphedema, and make her look better. However, exercise should be undertaken *after* she consults with her physician. Nancy Brinker, who had considerable difficulty with lymphedema after her mastectomy, undertook a regimen of exercise but was careful to be moderate and to avoid overexertion. She included instructions for some of the exercises she used in her book *The Race Is Run One Step at a Time*. These exercises have have been approved by the National Cancer Institute.[24]

For the person who is not recovering from surgery or illness, exercise programs of at least one hour in duration, three times a week are recommended for beneficial effects. Anyone who is not accustomed to regular exercise should consult with her physician, begin gradually, and follow warm-up and cool-down procedures. The type of exercise one chooses will be more effective if it is enjoyable.[25]

PEARSALL'S FORMULA FOR SUPERIMMUNITY

Dr. Paul Pearsall's approach to maintaining wellness focuses on our characteristic reactions to life events and our ability to master our emotions. As director of the Problems of Daily Living Clinic at the Sinai Hospital of

Detroit, he has counseled thousands of people and lectures widely on the relationship between illness and wellness.

Pearsall proposes that each of us can do something to strengthen our immune system by following his formula called B-A-FITER. The formula consists of *Belief* in our health, a positive *Attitude* of hope and high self-esteem, genuine *Feelings*, and the *Imagination* to visualize health where it may seem unattainable. The *T* in *FITER* stands for rational *Thinking* and the elimination of self-accusation. *Experience* represents the control we can gain over our bodies by adopting good habits of eating and providing a healthy environment for ourselves. *Remembrances* of good feelings and experiences feed positive messages to the supersystem.

He explains that our immune system, in coordination with our brain, must maintain an effective temperature. He means that if our immune system is either overactive (running hot) or underactive (running cold), it fails us when we need it most. When we are "running hot" we tend to overreact to any significant event. In contrast, if we are "running cold" we underreact. The hot-reactor feels alarmed, defensive; the cold-reactor feels victimized, defeated.[26]

Pearsall theorizes that we need to be aware of extreme emotional reactions and moderate or bring them under control. He provides tests to help us determine our predominant style as well as suggestions for cooling down or warming up our emotional responses. He also outlines a one-month immunizer program. The goal in controlling our emotions is to enhance our immunity and work toward achieving balance and growth in periods of crisis.

Rachel's Experience

Rachel Dunne had had a mastectomy a couple of years before her other breast had to be removed. She decided to have reconstructive surgery at the same time that the second breast was removed. That is when the doctor found another tumor in the area of the first mastectomy. Extensive lymph node involvement required that she also have chemotherapy again.

The most difficult task for Rachel was telling her children about her cancer. They had already experienced great trauma with her divorce from their father and the suicide of their brother. Now cancer. "My first thought," she said, "was 'how sad for them.' " She also thought that the grief she had not resolved from her son's death may have expressed itself in her cancer.

Infections complicated her recovery, but when she was healed, she felt very fortunate to have found the hidden tumor. Breast reconstruction also made her feel whole again. Rachel wasn't sure how she had gotten through the experience. What had helped was her own inner strength, the support of wonderful family and friends, and the encouragement she received from the surgeon's caring nurse.

Although she was realistic about the possibility of recurrence, Rachel believed that she could go a long way toward healing herself. When we met she had completed the surgery and chemotherapy and was taking a "pro-active" approach in her living style. She had normally eaten a healthful diet but decided a cholesterol work-up would be a good precaution. It revealed a high level of cholesterol, which she thought may have promoted her cancer. When we last talked she had been on a diet with very low fat content and high fiber, and was exercising and living more healthily. She was optimistic about finding a substantial drop in her cholesterol level with her next blood test. She was also seeking a new job on the west coast where she would be near a sister and other family members, closer to her children (away at college), and able to do things she had wanted to do. Her positive mental outlook was tempered with realism and determination.

Rachel made the move to the coast and six months later wrote us that she had actually done so without having employment. Nonetheless, she had kept a positive attitude and found a great job in her field. "I love it so far," she wrote, "and am ready for the new challenges. The fortitude it took to face the treatment (for cancer), as well as the reconstruction, has given me the courage to try these new things at this stage in my life. I know it will work out great!! I even got through the earthquake in one piece and am writing by candlelight."

Rachel probably was not familiar with Pearsall's B-A-FITER formula, but she was certainly practicing it along with the lessons of Bernie Siegel and others. She illustrates the growth that can take place in a time of crisis when one has encouragement and determination.

LAUGHTER AND POSITIVE EMOTIONS

When Norman Cousins emphasized the positive effects of humor and an upbeat attitude on health, his ideas were met with skepticism. However, researchers and the medical community are now recognizing that laughter does have a therapeutic effect on the body. Among other measurable physiological changes, it increases the heart rate, lowers blood pressure, improves oxygen consumption, relaxes muscles, reduces stress, and helps us to confront problems.[27] In *Superimmunity*, Pearsall states that it is "biochemically impossible to get sick or sicker when you are laughing."[28] Laughter, he says, demonstrates wellness. Cousins likened the blocking action of positive emotions against panic, depression, and stress to "the bullet-proof vest that protects us against the effects of emotional assaults."[29]

How do we put laughter into our lives when we are ill? We can try not to take ourselves too seriously by reading humorous books, watching funny movies, collecting jokes, and seeking out people who make us laugh. One hospital in a large midwestern city has provided a comfortable room for cancer patients and their families to sit, talk, and read joke books, listen to cassette tapes of comedians, and watch videos. A bookstore in the same city offers humorous books, tapes, and videos for people coping with illness.

Dr. Howard Bennett, who encourages physicians to laugh at themselves and keep some humility about their profession, has collected humorous stories that he has published in *The Best of Medical Humor*. Humor, he states, "reduces the emotional distance between physician and patient and, in doing so, improves communication and mutual understanding."[30]

Another physician, Dr. Benjamin Felson, who advocates humor for reducing tension and lubricating friction, states that humor makes a doctor appear "more human and humane."[31] He, too, has written a book consisting of his favorite stories, *Humor in Medicine . . . and Other Topics*. These are listed in our bibliography.

HOMEOPATHY

Derived from the Greek *homoios* (meaning "similar") and *pathos* (meaning "suffering" or "sickness"), homeopathy is based on the law that "like is cured by like." A practitioner of homeopathy studies the symptoms of illness and searches for a remedy that produces these symptoms in a well person.

The discovery of homeopathy was made by the German physician Samuel Hanneman, who was frustrated with brutal medical treatments and his inability to help one of his children who was critically ill. Turning to the translation of medical materials for his livelihood, Hanneman happened upon the key for curing sick people when translating the works of a Scottish professor of medicine. The professor claimed that the bitter, astringent qualities of quinine cured intermittent fever (malaria). Experimenting on himself, Hanneman took quinine and soon developed the symptoms of malaria. He reasoned that it was not the bitter taste that cured the fever but the fact that quinine produced the symptoms of malaria in a healthy person.[32]

Homeopathic practitioners believed that the body strives to keep itself in balance, and they regard symptoms as the body's defense against harmful forces. Therefore, the symptoms should be supported. Standard medicine, on the other hand, considers symptoms to be manifestations of a disease that need to be opposed. The goal of the homeopath is to strengthen the body to resist harmful organisms, rather than to identify and destroy them with drugs.

Homeopathic physicians, who are licensed physicians, take considerable time getting to know and diagnosing patients. Consequently they limit the number of patients they can see in a day. For example, a Dr. Panos sees only ten patients a day and spends at least an hour with each new patient. Homeopathic physicians do not treat disease; rather, they treat the whole person. Treatment is less expensive, involving fewer diagnostic tests; and prescribed homeopathic remedies do not cause adverse side effects.

Homeopathic medicine is used as an alternative treatment for cancer. One of the dangers is that some people practice it to the exclusion of conventional medicine. In doing so, patients may be limiting the resources available to them and thus lessening their chances of recovery.[33]

CONTROVERSIAL TREATMENTS

There are other treatments that we have not discussed. Among these are controversial therapies such as laetrile and immuno-augmentative therapy (IAT). Neither of these treatments is legal in the United States and both entail risk. Deaths from cyanide poisoning in laetrile have been reported. Some of the injections of blood proteins used in IAT have been known to carry AIDS and hepatitis. Before using therapies that have not been proven, one should thoroughly check them out. Each year the cost of quackery to American patients is very high.[34] Anyone wishing to try these controversial therapies can find helpful information at the local divisions of the American Cancer Society.

Holistic medicine integrates the best from mainline medicine and the body's self-healing abilities. Lawrence LeShan identifies a person's vocational, emotional, physical, and spiritual life as areas of concern in the holistic approach. He reminds us that our needs change in the different stages of our development and that what may be right at one time may not be at another time.

Holistic medicine is based on four axioms that make up a coherent whole: (1) If health is to be maintained, we must take care of the physical, psychological, and spiritual levels of our being; (2) Being unique, each of us must have individualized treatment; (3) As a patient, we should be a part of the decision-making team; and (4) We all have self-healing abilities.[35]

Norman Cousins, who was imbued in the scientific tradition, was perhaps the first influential spokesman to convey the idea that "every individual places his or her own stamp on the disease."[36] His book *Anatomy of an Illness* caught the attention of medical professionals and sparked their interest in the relationship between health and emotions. At UCLA Cousins endeavored to improve the environment of medical treatment and establish scientific support for his belief in the healing power of positive emotions combined with medical treatment. Thus, he opened the door for holistic treatment that incorporates the patient's participation and the physician's therapeutic-scientific knowledge. The physicians whose approaches we have discussed favor holistic/alternative treatment, but not to the exclusion of traditional medicine, which, although imperfect, endeavors to find scientific evidence of treatment outcomes.

In response to the insensitivity of some professionals, lack of consideration for patients' views and feelings, poor communication skills, and overemphasis on technology, more and more patients have turned to alternative or holistic methods. Dr. David Spiegel, in his book *Living beyond Limits*, points out the danger in putting too much faith in holistic practices that promise cures. Patients with cancer who believe that they will be cured by these methods may turn their disappointment into self-blame when the cancer does not disappear.[37]

The goal of most advocates of holistic methods is to help patients extend their lives and improve the quality of their days. In some cases, cancer has gone into remission, even disappears, but there is no sound evidence that the holistic practices were responsible.

Dr. Susan Love, the breast surgeon to whom we have often referred, considers the decision to use alternative therapies to be a highly personal one. Cautioning us about alternative practices that may be unsafe, she reminds us that traditional medical treatments can be supplemented with other therapies that may increase survival and improve the quality of life. She cites the example of one of her patients who has practiced holistic methods, faith healing, anything that she believes may help her. "This patient's commitment to taking control of her healing process," says Dr. Love, "has turned a terrifying experience into a triumphant challenge."[38]

We have discussed the alternative and complementary methods of coping that are practiced by many advocates of holism in conjunction with traditional medicine. What must be remembered about holistic methods of treatment is that some persons may believe it is in their power to defeat cancer by following these methods. Thus, they may believe that failure to overcome cancer reflects weakness in them. However, as scientists gradually learn the intrinsic secrets of the human body, we are discovering genes over which we have no control. The importance of practicing some of the principles of holism is to strengthen the immune system so that it can assist the treatments that scientists and researchers have developed and will continue to test. Fighting cancer with every resource available, including holism, has enabled many persons to have healthy, fulfilling lives with cancer.

Now, in the next chapters, let us consider the subject of interpersonal relationships. What happens to them when breast cancer or other life-threatening illnesses occur? How do those closest to us respond? What are our reactions? How can we work through feelings and fears together?

Chapter 6

Effects of Breast Cancer on Couple Relationships

The Taylor family (Audrey, Mark, daughters Annette and Beverly) had finished answering the questionnaires for our study and I joined them around their dining room table to ask further questions. The interview gave them an opportunity to express their feelings and disclose problems not tapped in the questionnaires.

Audrey explained that the last year and a half had been very difficult. She had had cancer of the thyroid and undergone a hysterectomy; then, acute peritonitis had nearly taken her life. She was so grateful to be alive that when the breast cancer was diagnosed it was "just another hurdle." She remarked, "It wasn't the first time I'd had to handle bad news. We just do what we have to do."

HOW ILLNESS CONTRIBUTES TO RELATIONSHIP STRAIN

Annette and Beverly agreed that the peritonitis was more frightening than the cancer. Beverly, who was a college student, said that although she was not as worried about her mother's recovery from the breast cancer, it was more "emotionally wearing" because it extended for such a long time. She thought that it had had a negative effect on her mother's self-concept and body image.

Mark intervened to explain how close Audrey had come to death and declared that the doctors had handled the cancer poorly. The doctor discussed with Mark the wisdom of telling her about another setback. Mark felt strongly that she should be told.

Mark listened carefully to Audrey and their daughters. When they finished

their explanations he released his pent-up feelings: "This is the most devastating thing that has ever happened to me. I don't think anyone realized
or showed concern for what we, the family members, were going through—
not the medical staff, our minister, or a woman we knew who had breast
cancer. No one seemed to want to talk with me. I like to think I can handle
difficult situations, but I didn't know how to deal with this. It's the first
time in my life that I didn't feel in control."

Audrey didn't say a word, but looked puzzled as he continued: "My
biggest concern was what I could do to help my wife. She's always been
very strong through her other illnesses and problems, but this time I
couldn't tell how she was handling this. When I tried to talk to her about
it, she'd say, 'Why are you so obsessed about it?' If I didn't ask her how
she was, she'd say, 'Why don't you ever talk about my having cancer? Are
you scared to death?' She was giving me mixed signals and I didn't know
which way to turn. Her behavior was so different from what I'd experienced
with her. That's why I thought she wasn't handling this well. It weighed
heavily on me that I was unable to help her."

Audrey spoke: "I thought I was handling it fine." Mark directed his next
comment to her, "You didn't realize that you put yourself in a shell. It was
almost as though anything anyone else was trying to do was never right at
the time. I thought I was going out of my mind," he confessed. "I'd been
considering going to a psychiatrist. Then I was out of town on a business
trip and visited some former neighbors. I learned that the wife had also had
breast cancer. Her husband started to talk to me about what he was going
through, and it was the same thing I had been experiencing!"

RELATIONSHIP STRAIN, DISTANCING, REJECTION

On my third visit with the Taylors, only Mark and Audrey were present.
That evening they told me they thought they had always communicated
very well, but from Mark's point of view, the breast cancer had changed
that. Audrey had not perceived the anguish that Mark was experiencing,
which he described as "total chaos." In fact, he admitted that his inability
to "get in sync" with what she was thinking or needed would have resulted
in his running from their relationship had they not finally talked about it.
Audrey had no realization of the depth of Mark's distress; she had been too
involved in working through her own feelings. Fortunately, their disclosures
to one another have made them closer and their marriage stronger.

This moving account of the Taylors' experience illustrates the impact that
an illness such as breast cancer can have on relationships. The series of illnesses had affected Audrey's normal behavior—Mark's and their daughters'
as well—so that they did not know how to interpret one another's needs.
Mark wanted to give Audrey support, but she rejected it and he couldn't
understand why. Her way of working through problems was to internalize

her feelings, she said. Perhaps she was also thinking that her silence would spare her family from worry, but from Mark's description, she seemed to be suffering from mood changes. At any rate, both were getting messages of rejection.

Women with breast cancer and their family members, especially mates, often reflect each others' reactions and ability to cope.[1] Although women vary considerably in their response to cancer, those with breast cancer tend to have difficulties in relationships.[2] Good communication, the subject of a later chapter, can help to reduce the interpersonal tension.

How the Woman's Behavior Contributes to the Strain: Rejection, Avoidance, Aversion

The stresses that the woman herself undergoes have already been discussed. A closer examination of them will help to understand how her behavior can contribute to the strain felt by the family.

The woman with breast cancer harbors many fears. She is fearful of pain, of dependency, of the effect of her illness on her family, of recurrence and death. In fact, for the rest of her life she will deal with the possibility of recurrence. She also fears disfigurement, the loss of her physical and sexual attractiveness, and actual rejection.[3]

You may recall the story about Mary Lynn Gordon, who refused to have chemotherapy because she didn't want to lose her hair. When she finally decided to have the treatment, she not only lost her hair but also gained weight, which was very upsetting to her. Not all women gain weight with chemotherapy and recuperation, but those who do say it is one of the most distressing things about treatment. Women who have always watched their weight find the added pounds difficult to accept and to lose. It's understandable that breast cancer can also affect body image and self-esteem.

The experience causes a woman to re-evaluate her life: what is important to her, what isn't, and what she really wants. It is frightening, but it can be a challenge for growth.[4] For example, we've introduced you to Joy Martin, who described the experience as similar to being on a roller coaster. After her mastectomies, she not only felt very fortunate to be feeling so well but also became more philosophical about disappointments, such as being denied the promotion she had anticipated.

Rejection is another fear of women who have breast cancer. Some sense the negative reactions of others, especially loved ones, who are afraid of getting cancer themselves.[5] A woman may also sense their aversion to mutilation and body changes. When she feels this aversion toward her illness, she may behave in negative ways. For example, she may show anger over trivial things, become uncooperative or bitter as she notices the gradual decrease in the attention she receives. As I admitted to you in the Introduction, I wasn't comfortable being around my friend Lois and consequently made less effort to see her. My behavior was not unusual.

Some people do avoid cancer patients. They may also avoid talking openly with them, just as I did with my friend. Families sometimes discourage discussion of feelings, and patients report that some professional health care workers also tend to evade intimate or negative topics.[6] It is difficult to know if the person with breast cancer wants to talk about it. Many do not, so it is helpful when a woman opens this subject herself if she wants to discuss it.

Only a few years ago the diagnosis of cancer was kept from the patient and the family maintained "a conspiracy of silence."[7] This silence "isolates" the ill person and prevents the expression of feelings. In recent years many have come to believe that knowledge of the diagnosis prolongs the patient's life and improves its quality.[8] However, as Klagsbrun pointed out in 1972, we were still talking about whether or not the patient should be told about the disease.[9] Even though we are now more open about cancer, some people still cling to the notion that silence protects the ill person.

When others try to be cheerful and optimistic, that can be upsetting to a patient, especially if she feels terrible. Nonverbal behaviors tend to convey true feelings and are more believable than spoken words, so the patient gets a mixed message from the well-intentioned person who is a poor actor. Forced cheerfulness is more disturbing than helpful. I recall seeing a friend whom I had not seen since the death of my husband. She said nothing about my loss, but talked on cheerfully as though my life were the same. Concluding that she had not heard, I asked her if she knew about my husband. Embarrassed, she admitted that she had heard but didn't know what to say to me. I was sorry to have embarrassed her and wished she had just given me a hug or said only two words, "I'm sorry."

Another unfortunate reaction is that others, often family members, blame the ill woman who is fearful and depressed for not trying to get well. This releases their frustration, and perhaps relieves them of feeling guilty about being unable to help. It also results in conflicting emotions that are painful for both the ill woman and family members.[10] Another reason for avoiding patients who discuss their problems is that we think they are not coping well, that they should not upset their families by discussing their fears and complaints.[11]

An example of avoidance in a spouse occurred when Claire Vosburg was told she had breast cancer. Her husband, who was with her when the doctor gave the diagnosis, made no comment until they were outside his office. Then Claire's husband said, "Well, I could have done without that news." He was unable to say anything about how she must feel, never mentioned her breast cancer again, and had not seen her scar when I talked with her some time after her mastectomy. She assured me several times that her husband was a man of few words and that his silence didn't bother her.

An instance of aversion is Mindy's husband, who told her very bluntly that her scar repulsed him. Mindy was devastated, and while she was still recovering they were separated and eventually divorced. We have heard of other cases of spouses who found their wives' mastectomies repugnant, but fortunately most men are compassionate and supportive.

Although a number of researchers, such as Grandstaff, discuss the problem of rejection, withdrawal, and avoidance, there is little systematic investigation of how often it occurs.[12] Lichtman et al. found that 40 to 42 percent of the seventy-eight women with breast cancer that they studied had experienced rejection or isolation from at least one person. Of that number one-third of the husbands had conveyed an attitude of rejection.[13]

Wortman and Dunkel-Schetter reviewed the studies that have examined the nonverbal avoidance/rejection behaviors of the able-bodied toward patients with cancer.[14] In the 1960s and 1970s researchers were stressing the importance of nonverbal behavior in medical settings where health care professionals have the opportunity to help patients and family members. Current training seminars on communication and cancer, such as those offered by Hospice in Cincinnati, may be continuing this practice.

Grandstaff suggests that a couple experiencing this problem must work toward resolving it themselves. However, some may need the assistance of a professional. Some physicians, nurses, and social workers are especially attuned to the problems of families and offer intervention. For example, Dr. Rosenbaum, author of *Living with Cancer*, invites couples and families for interviews in which he gives personal as well as medical support. He realizes, of course, that issues can be sensitive and that the patient and her family must have the wisdom and courage to accept help.[15]

Strains on the Partner/Spouse

The problems that husbands experience are similar to those of their wives. The effect of breast cancer on the spouse has been studied by a number of researchers.[16] Fifty-six percent of the husbands in Baider and De-Nour's study reported increased tension and almost the same number of problems as their wives were having. Maguire studied fifty-two men whose wives had had simple mastectomies. Three months after the surgery, some of the husbands had problems that included moderate to severe anxiety and a few suffered depression. Although a moderate to marked deterioration in their sexual relationship was reported by 21 percent of the men, the majority felt their marriages were not impaired. However, a year later 10 percent reported a deterioration in their marriages and over half of them (56%) thought the mastectomy had had an adverse effect on their lives. Many of them (76%) thought having someone with whom they could talk would have helped them.

Grandstaff interviewed and counseled families with breast cancer at Stanford University School of Medicine and observed that spouses and family members tend to feel anger, frustration, denial, fear, depression, and grief.[17] Their fear that the patient may die also brings about anticipatory grief and sets off the processes of denial, recoil, and depression identified by Kübler-Ross.[18] These reactions correspond to the emotional kinds of coping responses found in women diagnosed with breast cancer, which we discussed earlier.

CRITICAL EVENTS FOR THE COUPLE

What are the most traumatic experiences for the couple? Many husbands in Grandstaff's study said that when they were told that the breast had to be removed, they went into emotional shock.[19] Spouses in other studies have reported that the time in the waiting room, when they fear their wives may die, is the most difficult for them. The time during hospitalization is also particularly stressful.[20]

Viewing the Scar

Two other events that can have a major impact on the woman's sexual identity and her self-concept may also adversely affect the marital relationship.[21] Following the shock of diagnosis, a significant threat comes when the scar is viewed for the first time.[22] It is a moment that both spouses dread. Often the patient sees the scar first. Some women do not want their husbands to be there. However, a woman's concealment from her husband may make it difficult for her to accept the change in her body. The spouse must condition himself to see his wife's disfigurement and accept it.[23]

Daniel Sherwood's account of his experience illustrates a perceptive husband who knew he must prepare himself to view his wife's incision. Daniel wanted to be present when the doctor removed the bandages, but he had great anxiety about it. When he had heard Kay's diagnosis, he immediately feared she was dying; but when the lymph nodes were found to be clear, his fear of death was replaced by the anxiety of seeing the scar. Being a compassionate man who obviously adores his wife and openly expresses his feelings, Daniel knew how critical his reaction would be for Kay. He also knew Kay would be watching his face and his expression could be devastating for her. He prepared for the worst and prayed he could control his response.

It was a tense moment. Kay was indeed watching Daniel intently. When the doctor lifted the bandages, Daniel's face broke into a smile. It was a pleasant surprise. The scar was neat and looked much better than he had imagined. For them the anticipation had been far worse than the reality, and Daniel's positive reaction did a great deal to help his wife through another traumatic moment.

Ann Jillian had not wanted her husband, Andy Murcia, to be present when her bandages were removed, but he insisted. He, too, had expected the scars to be much worse than they were. In fact, he said they gradually almost disappeared. Murcia and his friend Bob Stewart, who wrote about their wives' breast cancer experiences in their book *Man to Man*, said that they were not concerned with "scars" and "mutilation" but with their wives' survival. Bob called his wife's scars "beauty marks."[24]

The two men admitted that their gratitude in having their wives alive does not diminish the sense of loss that they feel. Rod Emerson, one of the husbands we interviewed, said, "I'll confess I loved Paula's breasts and I miss them, but I admire her strength and I could not get along without her."

Glen Stevens felt the loss keenly and urged Marianne to have her breasts reconstructed, but Marianne didn't want to undergo more cutting. Her bilateral mastectomy (both breasts were removed at the same time) was her ninth surgery, and that was enough. When we met, Marianne and Glen told us about their disagreement over the issue of reconstructive surgery, and we were concerned about its effect on their relationship. Recently, I asked her if she had reconsidered her decision. "No," she responded; "Glen and I have worked through it and find it's okay for me to be flat-chested."

Breast reconstruction has improved the self-esteem of many women, but some, like Ann Jillian, have chosen not to subject their bodies to additional surgery. Their spouses, if caring and wise, find other compensations. Andy Murcia says nothing is "more pleasurable than seeing your wife happy, content, alive, and secure in your love." What makes Ann sexy, he says, is "what's in her mind."[25]

Breast loss can be especially traumatic for single women who want to date and marry. Because the breast is such an erotic symbol in our culture, women fear that it may be a turn-off for some men. For example, Betty Trautenberg told me she had worried about how men she dated would react when she told them about her mastectomy. To her surprise, it was never an issue. Nor was it a problem for Judy White, who did not tell the man she dated about her breast loss until their relationship became serious. Then she decided she had to tell him and discovered that he had known about it through mutual friends even before he began to date her.

Effect on Self-Esteem

The level of a woman's self-esteem often hinges on her husband's or partner's assurance that losing a breast doesn't affect his love for her. Her healthy recovery depends on his ability to reassure her of her femininity and desirability. Although patients with cancer may report a decreased desire for sexual intercourse, they have an increased need for touching and other physical contact.[26] Studies document the fact that women who have unsympathetic partners have particular difficulty adjusting to the scar. Along with the phantom breast sensations they may feel, the husbands' lack of compassion is a constant reminder of the loss of their breasts.[27]

In some cases, insecure women who "devalue" themselves will thwart their spouses' efforts to give them reassurance. Researcher Gates presented the stories of four women in which each had made her husband a victim by attacking him in ways to which she knew he was sensitive. To protect himself each husband withdrew from the closeness that both he and his wife needed. Gates interpreted the wives' behavior as a call for help and suggested that husbands refuse to allow their mates to "give in" to their negative feelings.[28]

During an interview with Joanne Moser, she confessed that she had become overly emotional and had developed a "poor me" attitude about her breast cancer. Her husband John told her there were far worse things that could happen and ordered her to quit feeling sorry for herself. His "tough love" approach worked. She now has an accepting, cheerful attitude and is honest about having indulged in self-pity.

Sexual Adjustment

Sexual adjustment is probably the most critical time for spouses following breast removal. It may also be the most difficult adjustment for the couple.[29] Much of their adjustment will depend on how the woman feels about her femininity after a mastectomy, and on the quality of their relationship prior to the illness. It also depends on their ability to communicate about feelings, such as his concern that he might hurt her and her fear of his rejection. These issues are sometimes "very difficult for people to verbalize."[30]

Joan and Robert Parker have candidly shared their experiences and feelings in a book they wrote together entitled *Three Weeks in Spring*. In it Joan discusses her anxiety about getting a prosthesis and viewing the scar. These had been two big hurdles for her. The third was how she and Robert would resume their sexual life. Robert was worried, too, but hesitant to make the first move. Joan decided that she would have to take the initiative. Fortunately, because she and Robert were able to talk, they made the adjustment more easily than they had anticipated. Their story can be helpful for couples who feel fearful and awkward about this part of their relationship.[31]

Fobair and Mages investigated three modes of treatment for patients who experienced adverse effects of breast cancer on their sexuality: crisis intervention, group support, and team care in the hospital or home.[32] The role of the therapist or facilitator in each of these methods is to encourage the couple to talk about their fears and feelings and to anticipate changes. Several researchers have reported some success with these approaches.

Witkin, who did psychosocial counseling, found that most of the forty-one women with whom she worked welcomed and benefited from the counseling. Furthermore, most of the women's partners were eager to help. Witkin stated that "sex therapy in the usual sense is as effective for the mastectomy couple as for any couple, that is, as effective as the couple will allow."[33]

Because of the sensitivity of this subject, we addressed the sexual and marital issues in our questionnaires, but sometimes the women brought them up in the interviews. For example, Marion Prince rather hesitantly confessed the effect of her mastectomy on her sexual adjustment. She explained that her flat side made her self-conscious and inhibited her enjoyment of sex. She asked her husband Charles if he had been aware of this. He denied that he was, but he was very understanding of her feelings (his first wife had died of breast cancer). It did not appear that Charles and Marion had talked earlier about this subject, and we hope that Marion's disclosure has enabled them to express their feelings more openly.

In another instance, Kathryn Lathrop, whose husband did not participate in our study, volunteered information about her inability to have intercourse. Her difficulty was not the result of her mastectomies but of an earlier unrelated physical problem. Kathryn had had a radical mastectomy, with considerable disfigurement, fifteen years prior to the second mastectomy. Although she had not had reconstructive surgery after her first surgery, Kathryn had the second breast reconstructed to bolster her self-image. She did it without her husband's approval.

EFFECTS ON THE MARITAL RELATIONSHIP: WITHDRAWAL, COUNTER-WITHDRAWAL, DISPLACEMENT

How do these critical events affect the marital relationship? If a woman thinks of herself as mutilated and therefore less sexually attractive, she may withdraw from sexual intimacy for fear of rejection. Her mate's desire may also be decreased by fatigue, worry, and fear of hurting her. He may respond to her withdrawal with counter-withdrawal, and each may perceive this as rejection.[34]

Another reason for a woman's withdrawal may be a treatment regimen that causes her great discomfort and fatigue. Not all women suffer complications with chemotherapy and radiation, but many do. Nausea may result and can cause hormonal imbalance. Although it can be a psychological response, nausea more likely results from the combination of drugs and individual reactions to them.

These and other factors may affect the sexual relationship that had been satisfactory prior to the mastectomy.[35] The woman's desire and ability to function sexually may be impaired by her lowered self-image and her anger at being dependent. Her attitude may cause him to lose interest. In addition, the importance she places on her marital-sexual relationship and the quality of that relationship seem to have a bearing on her sexual adjustment.[36] Moreover, women who are more satisfied and feel that their husbands understand their needs are better able to confide in their husbands.

A husband may withdraw when he feels displaced by his wife's cancer or when he feels his role in her recovery is overlooked. Two spouses raised this issue with us. Warren and Kit Bradley had two children at home and one at college. Kit's bilateral surgery came at a time when Warren's administrative job was very demanding. Between his job, housekeeping, meeting his children's needs, and caregiving, Warren was exhausted and stressed. He said that all the attention was focused on his wife's welfare and that no one seemed to be concerned about him. Mark Taylor expressed a similar feeling of unimportance in his wife's recovery. He needed someone to understand what he was going through emotionally and found no one who would talk with him about it.

In another instance, cancer displaced the spouse. Brian Campbell was trying very hard to be helpful when Nancy was experiencing side effects with each chemotherapy treatment. He was, in fact, trying to be a "superhusband." They discussed with us some of the conflicts they were having over his compulsion to complete household tasks. He said that Nancy was very particular about the house, so he was spending a good deal of time on cleaning chores in an effort to relieve her of worry about it. She said she needed for him to be more sympathetic with her. Nancy explained that Brian could not talk about his feelings, could not stand to have her cry, and tended to get angry. She complained that he also said hurtful things to her.

Brian and Nancy hadn't been married very long, and breast cancer complicated the normal adjustments that newlyweds must make. Brian seemed a little resentful but wanted to be helpful. Both of them admitted that her moods changed frequently, and he said that he could not seem to please her. As he walked with us to our car, Brian confided why he felt that Nancy's complaints were difficult for him to manage. He said her behavior with breast cancer "was like having [his] mother go through menopause." Some of Brian's responses to Nancy's illness were being replayed from earlier family experiences that had been unpleasant for him. His inability to talk about his feelings and her mood swings resulted in tension between them.

THE MARITAL ADJUSTMENT

Lichtman concluded from her research that husbands' reactions to breast cancer are related to how well their wives cope.[37] Husbands in a well-adjusted marriage will have a better reaction to their wives' illness than those in an unstable marriage. Furthermore, good or strong marriages are likely to remain good after breast cancer.

Family counselors Stinnett and DeFrain have identified the characteristics of a good or strong marriage. These are empathy, commitment to and promotion of one another's welfare, good communication, and mutual satisfaction with their relationships and life-styles. A strong family has a sense of purpose and has developed positive strategies for handling life stresses.[38]

We asked thirty couples to rate their satisfaction with their emotional and sexual relationships before and after the breast cancer. Eighty-four percent of the women reported their emotional satisfaction prior to breast cancer to be "high." After the breast cancer, 68 percent said it had become even more satisfactory. Likewise, before the appearance of breast cancer, 85 percent of the men reported "high" emotional satisfaction and 47 percent said it had improved after the illness.

Of the women Janet and I have interviewed, only three divorces appeared to be the direct result of the breast cancer, although the disease may only have been the breaking point in an already troubled marriage. In another case separation had occurred prior to the breast cancer, and the illness did not bring about reconciliation. In a fifth instance the wife was unaware of the instability of her marriage until after the breast cancer was found. Separation resulted. With another couple, we do not know what impact the breast cancer had, but divorce came during the wife's recovery from the disease. When Lichtman et al. asked women with breast cancer why their spouses reacted as they did, responses were: "because of his qualities," "because of mixed reasons," or "because of the situation itself."[39]

Several explanations may account for a spouse who reacts badly. His typical method of coping with any adversity may be anger, avoidance, or denial. Expressing feelings may not have been acceptable in his upbringing. He may have learned to displace his feelings and blame others. Or he may have grown up in an environment void of compassionate behavior. Had he been able to witness compassion, he would have learned "that reality, including problems and human limitations, is accepted and even cherished rather than abhorred, diluted and denied."[40]

Communication and sexuality can be a problem for couples experiencing breast cancer. Some husbands have expressed a need to talk with someone about their worries but do not find the opportunity or anyone who is willing to listen. Furthermore, a couple's misperceptions of what one another is thinking and feeling and their failure to verbalize their thoughts can lead to unnecessary tensions. Because experiences and interpretations are private and often below the level of consciousness, what one imagines the other to be thinking and feeling can be very inaccurate.

Heinrich and associates suggest that teaching methods for reducing stress and improving communication to couples could help them with sexual adjustment.[41] Schover proposes a brief counseling session with a couple to facilitate their sexual adjustment and other problems related to the breast cancer.[42] A number of other psychologists, such as Simonton and LeShan, help patients and family members work through the problems that cancer presents.

Researchers have found that "marital quality appears to be important in psychologic well-being."[43] A supportive relationship provides a buffer for stressful events by reducing its adverse effects on the body's immune system.[44] Couples who have enjoyed a stable and satisfying marriage prior to the breast cancer and who are able to keep open the lines of communication are apt to find that the breast cancer experience bonds them more closely. As families have told us, the experience has caused them to re-evaluate their lives and appreciate one another.

We have explored how the stress that a woman's breast cancer creates for both her and her spouse or partner can contribute to relational strain. Reasons for avoidance, rejection, aversion, and other kinds of distancing have been examined. Specific critical events, such as viewing the scar and making the sexual adjustment after breast cancer, can affect a woman's self-esteem and the relationship.

How does breast cancer affect the other family members? From the perspective of family systems theory we continue with an examination of the effect that breast cancer, or any serious illness, can have on children and other family members. The ages, developmental stages, and individual characteristics determine the reactions and coping efforts of each group. The young child, the preteenager, teenage daughters and sons will often react quite differently. Little study has been done on the effects of breast cancer on a woman's mother or sister. Being aware of behavior that is often typical of each age group may enable you to help them cope.

Chapter 7

Effects of Breast Cancer on Children and Other Family Members

In the previous chapter we related the story of Mark Taylor's turmoil when his wife Audrey had breast cancer. Neither Audrey or his daughters were aware of his feelings but his disclosure prompted Beverly, who was studying nursing, to talk about the dilemma she was also having.

"I didn't know what to say to Mother either," Beverly confessed. "I should have known—we learn this in our courses—but when it's your own mother, it's different, so I just kept our conversation light. I think mother was pretty emotional and it affected her more than she realized or admitted. I talked about it with a teacher at school. I had to talk with someone."

Beverly explained that her inability to do or say anything therapeutic had led to conflicts with her mother. Hurt, frustrated, and frightened, Beverly became angry with herself because she didn't know how to make it better for her mother. She felt that she was a failure and couldn't talk to her mother without crying. That, of course, upset her mother.

In contrast, Beverly's younger sister Annette was also worried, but she confided in her boyfriend and went on with her life. She believes she handles crises well without getting depressed or withdrawn. Because she was unaware of the medical implications, she thinks she worried less than her sister and father.

During an illness, when family members need one another most, they may find it difficult to be open with one another and to maintain closeness. Some members may be unable to face cancer or talk about it, so they withdraw or "run."[1] They also may be afraid of "catching" cancer, or of facing the pain of seeing the changes in the ill person or of losing her. Depending on their ages, children may be frightened or unaware of the dangers and more preoccupied with their own interests and needs.

THE FAMILY SYSTEM

To explain interpersonal strains that arise in a family, it is helpful to look at the transformation that occurs in the family structure as a result of a traumatic event. If we view our family as a unit made up of smaller parts and subsystems, we get an idea of the complexity of its composition. The subsystems are the various relationships, or alliances, existing between the family members. There is a unique relationship between the parents, the father and each child, the mother and each child, each child with one another, and special relationships with various extended family members. When one member is ill, each of these relationships is affected.[2]

The diagnosis of breast cancer has an immediate impact on the family system and its ability to function in its normal manner. In fact, as Parkes noted, "cancer invades the family in much the same way that it invades the human body."[3] While the mother is undergoing treatment she cannot carry out her usual tasks as the head of the house. The father will probably have to assume her household and childcare duties, in addition to making hospital visits and carrying out his job responsibilities. Depending on the length and difficulty of his wife's recuperation, he may also be part-time nurse after she is home.

Less attention has been paid to the effect of breast cancer on the children and young adults than on the spouse. However, in the last decade or so a few studies have given us insight into the reactions of children. The illness creates a number of fears, inconveniences, and conflicts for children. Their needs cannot be met as easily as when their mother was juggling schedules, providing transportation, and reminding them of duties and deadlines. Each offspring is experiencing fears and anxieties about the mother's illness, and at the same time has his or her own agenda of goals, activities, and needs, which the illness has temporarily upset.

In families where parents have divorced and remarried and there are stepchildren, the situation is even more complex. If members are highly dependent upon one another, they may have more difficulty than if they are independent. The disruption caused by illness compounds the normal stresses of family living and can result in interpersonal tension.

The ability of the family to maintain its stability depends on the characteristics of the individuals in it, the extent to which they customarily work together, and their patterns of coping. Their support from outside sources also has a bearing on their ability to function well.

According to their ages and developmental stages, each child will be affected differently and each will have his or her own set of problems.[4] In her interviews with families, Grandstaff observed that a child's first concern is fear of the mother dying.[5] She advocates giving a child a realistic explanation and reassurance to allay the fear. When the emotional upheaval that the parents are obviously undergoing is not explained, the child is left to his or her own imaginings, which may be far worse than the reality.[6]

An example of feeling "left out" occurred not with a young child but with a teenage son, who, of course, knew that his mother was having a breast removed. However, he had no idea how her body would look after the surgery. When she came home from the hospital, the mother took her daughter, younger than her brother, into the bedroom to show her the scar. The son, who visualized his mother with a big hole in her chest, was never shown the result of his mother's surgery. He disclosed to us and his family that he felt like an outsider and expressed his anxiety and hurt.

The Young Child

Parents naturally want to protect children from traumatic events, but secrecy may arouse more misgivings than the child already has. He or she needs some explanation but should be spared details.[7] The young child needs a great deal of reassurance that he or she did not cause the illness. Children usually feel that they are somehow at fault when a traumatic event occurs. LeShan points out that a child whose parents divorce or whose parent dies will often say, "If I'd been a better boy, Mommy would love me enough so that she would never leave me."[8]

Children of different ages have different conceptions of death and, consequently, react differently to the possibility that a parent's illness may mean she will die. The universality of a child's belief that a parent's death is his fault cannot be overestimated, LeShan states. He advises that this should be dealt with as early as possible by a parent, relative, minister, school nurse or counselor, or physician. A young child may also have a negative image of doctors and needs to be reassured that the doctors are trying to help his or her mother.[9]

The age and maturity of the child will, of course, determine how much he or she should be told. For example, Mindy Bishop could not hug or pick up her toddler after her mastectomy and had to explain why she could not. She gave him enough information to help him understand why it hurt her and showed him the bandages. Later, as he began to ask questions, she explained more. She was cautious about telling him anything that would increase his apprehension. He was already upset about the losses that were occurring in his family (his parents' divorce and the death of his favorite uncle) and had become very protective of his mother. As he grows older, he still cautions her to drive carefully when she leaves for work so nothing will happen to her.

The School-Age Child (Age 7–13)

In a study of members of families who were interviewed over an eighteen-month period, thirty children under age 12 openly discussed their feelings at being told of their mother's breast cancer.[10] They described their feelings of sadness, of being sorry for their mother, and of not understanding what would happen or what to expect. Thirteen of them were worried, scared, afraid to see their mother, fearful that she might be different. One was angry that her mother had gotten cancer. Four children said they were "confident that everything would be all right" or they related a feeling of being unconcerned. As the interviews progressed, the children revealed a variety of both positive and negative changes in their families' lives.

In our study of families, Janet and I did not include any children under the age of 9, and several mothers chose not to have older children participate. Of the nine who were ages 10 through 13, we found only two who sometimes feared that their mother, or grandmother in one case, would die. Four "worried a lot," one was "afraid," three were sometimes "angry," two were sometimes "depressed," one "thought about it a lot," and four "prayed a lot." One 13-year-old girl could remember very little about her feelings when her mother's cancer was diagnosed because it occurred about the time of her parents' separation. However, her mother's recurrence had made a deep impression. Her younger brother reacted to their mother's illness by having stomachaches and other maladies that kept him home from school.

We found that with the exception of one 12-year-old boy, children of this age were reticent to talk. Two boys seemed the most concerned about the cancer recurring. In all cases, the mothers appeared to have been open and considerate of their children's feelings.

Children who are having difficulty with any stressful event may exhibit behavioral disorders. They may have nightmares, become aggressive, have problems in school, undergo changes in appetite, and display other antisocial behaviors. The well parent or another perceptive family member should be watchful for indications of these symptoms of stress and seek to help the children.[11]

The Adolescent

Medical psychologist Wellisch found that the psychological stresses of a parent's cancer can be unusually intense for the adolescent. He or she may be expected to take more responsibility for household and child care duties and feel forced into a parenting role. This reversal of the developmental process may lead to conflict. The adolescent may "act out" distress by using drugs, arguing frequently with parents, becoming promiscuous, or even running away.[12]

Relationships with preteen and early teenage children can remain intact, even improve, if the parents talk openly and honestly about the breast cancer. Giving responsibilities while taking into consideration the child's obligations and commitments in school also helps to sustain relationships. Even when it is difficult to arrange transportation for children's activities, it is important that their needs not be ignored. It should be remembered that these children are at an age when they are beginning a gradual emotional withdrawal from the family.

The Teenaged and Older Daughter

The relationship between a woman who has breast cancer and her daughter becomes vulnerable, especially if the girl is an adolescent. Because some breast cancers appear in families, the daughter may fear that she will also develop it.[13] In addition to that fear, Lichtman and her fellow researchers suggest that the mother's demands on a daughter for support can lead to a difficult relationship.[14]

There were six teenaged daughters and one granddaughter (ages 14–18) who participated in our study. One granddaughter, Sarah, reported that she handled her grandmother's illness by ignoring it and becoming more social. Sarah also stated that since her grandmother's breast cancer, family conflict had increased and her parents were less attentive and less supportive of the children. Sarah seemed distant from the family and we later learned from her mother that Sarah was lacking in self-confidence and was becoming difficult. In another instance, Sally Waters, also age 16, whose parents were divorced, was very close with her mother. Sally commented that she was often fearful, worried, and had a tendency to cry since her mother's mastectomy. She had withdrawn from others but had one "best friend" with whom she could talk about her feelings.

One 18-year-old daughter was always fearful for her mother and of passing breast cancer on to the children she would have some day. Her emotions ran the gamut of fear, anger, and depression; she had not yet reached the stage of acceptance.

An initial reaction of most of the daughters we interviewed was anger. Some of them had experienced conflict with their mothers, but that seemed to have been resolved. In one instance, Betty Sawyer expressed her anger that she hadn't known what "malignant" meant at the time of her mother's diagnosis and had taken the surgery too lightly. When she heard a rumor at school that her mother was dying, she felt very remorseful.

How well the parents "break" the news and explain the situation appears to determine how their children will handle it. Judith Viorst reminds us in her book *Necessary Losses* that adolescents are in "the letting-go stage of life" and that they are experiencing their own kind of grief as they renounce childhood and move toward adulthood. They have feelings of isolation, loneliness and confusion.[15] Recalling this period in our own lives may help us to understand, in part, the reactions of adolescents.

Thirteen older daughters (20–39 years of age) also took part in our study. Christine, the daughter of Margaret Muncy, said that her mother's breast cancer was traumatic for her because her paternal grandmother had died of it. Christine grew up with a terrible fear of breast cancer and found it very difficult to practice breast self-examinations. She was afraid of finding a lump.

Christine explained that her grandmother had had a poor self-image and a low sense of worth. Christine was proud of her mother for having struggled to find employment, which had enabled her to become happy with herself. "If I have learned anything from these experiences," Christine wrote on her questionnaire, "it's that you must be in charge of your own life. If you are not satisfied, you must bring about proper changes as soon as possible—not merely wait for someone else to make them for you. I also feel that a positive outlook is much healthier than a negative one, that physical exercise on a regular basis alleviates a lot of life's tensions/stress, and that proper nutrition is a big key to our health."

Millie Davis's daughter Ann experienced great fear not only for her mother but also for herself. She told us of her dream in which she had been diagnosed with breast cancer and was lying in the hospital. "It really frightened me," she confessed, "especially because I know I'm not as emotionally strong as my mother."

Cindy Moser was away at college when her mother's cancer was diagnosed. Like Christine, Cindy always feared breast cancer because it had taken her maternal grandmother's life, and Cindy is convinced she will have it. She had put off going to get a check-up because she didn't want to know if she had cancer. Her attitude has been "I'm going to die anyway, so just let me." Fortunately, her mother has helped her change her perspective and accept the importance of early detection.

Cindy admitted that she has a strong sense of guilt because she didn't quit college and come home to be with her mother Joanne when she was recovering from surgery. Joanne had hoped Cindy would volunteer to come home, but she didn't want to ask her. Cindy feels that her failure to be with her mother then put a barrier between them that has taken them some time to overcome.

The most touching disclosure of a daughter's reaction was Mary's story. Kit and Warren Bradley's only daughter, Mary, was at college when her mother had bilateral surgery. The shock almost caused Mary's world to fall apart. She was angry, depressed, and sad about her mother's illness and suddenly became very insecure about her own future. The trauma shook her faith in her church, which she felt had failed to give her "practical" support. She resented the fact that many people, even close friends, were too fearful to reach out and help them.

The year following the diagnosis was extremely stressful for Mary, a time when she never felt in control of what she was doing and everything seemed disorganized. She now worried that her parents would die before she could accept their deaths. Furthermore, she had been forced to re-evaluate every-thing she had believed. In her struggle with overwhelming questions, she had experienced strength as well as weakness many times and was grateful to have people who cared enough to let her handle it in her own way.

Out of this emotional turmoil Mary and her family have come to appre-ciate one another more, to share responsibilities, and to adopt an attitude that enables them to enjoy each day. They have learned to relax, be open with one another, value their time together, like one another, and have fun together. In other words, they have used the traumatic experience as an opportunity for growth.

Teenaged and Older Sons

The effect of a parent's breast cancer on sons has also been neglected. Grandstaff noted that the adjustment for sons around 15–16 years of age appears to be unusually difficult.[16] She cited a case in which a teenaged son refused to visit his mother in the hospital or talk to her about her illness. In another family of five sons and a daughter, all the children made a good adjustment except for the 16-year-old. He did not want anyone to be told about his mother's mastectomy and began to develop various illnesses fol-lowing her surgery. Grandstaff observed similar patterns among other teen-aged sons.

Four sons between the ages of 14 and 19 participated in our study. Esther Seifert's 15-year-old son Walter seemed very concerned about his mother when we first met with them. He indicated that her breast cancer sometimes made him depressed, bitter, and often fearful and worried. Sometimes he also had the fear of the cancer recurring and his mother dying. He com-mented that there were some positive family outcomes since her illness; family members had become more considerate, closer, and more caring. Furthermore, his religious faith was stronger.

The Bradleys' oldest son, John, a 17-year-old, was going through a teen-age crisis prior to his mother's illness. He had used alcohol to deal with the anger he felt over his mother's surgery, but he seemed to have emerged from this period when we met him. He attributed his rebellion to poor peer relationships and lack of recognition of his athletic abilities. He indicated that his self-esteem had improved, that the family had grown closer, and that he had begun helping other people since his mother's illness. His sister Mary verified John's improved relationships with his family.

These cases support Grandstaff's observation that teenaged sons may have a difficult time with their mothers' breast cancer. When the family is able to remain intact and work together and discuss their feelings, it may help them in their adjustment.

Mothers and Sisters

We have found no information about how mothers and sisters react when a daughter or sibling has breast cancer. However, we can relate several stories told to us by the women we interviewed.

Marianne Stevens, whose bilateral surgery we discussed earlier, took a very rational and thorough approach to the loss of both breasts. She prepared her children, concentrated on her physical and mental health, and talked with women who had undergone mastectomies. As a last step, she mourned with her husband Glen for the loss of her breasts. Marianne made a remarkable recovery and soon returned to her normal activities. However, her mother, who had come some distance to help her, thought Marianne was resuming her activities too soon. This caused conflict and the mother shortened her visit.

In another instance, Ann Schneider's mother reacted in a way that was very disturbing to Ann. In fact, Ann said that she had coped with a mastectomy, two recurrences, the nausea of chemotherapy, and the skin irritation of radiation far more easily than with her mother's reactions. Ann's mother was very critical, often making hurtful remarks to Ann. When Ann most needed encouragement, her mother's gloomy outlook was an additional stressor, making it difficult for Ann to maintain hope. Because her mother lives alone, Ann worries about her reactions and dreads telling her about her problems. Fortunately, Ann's husband is very understanding and supportive about the mother-daughter relationship. They realize that they cannot change her mother's behavior.

Whereas Ann's mother was overly responsive in a negative way, Mindy's mother seemed unconcerned. She told friends how worried she was about Mindy but did not express her concern to her daughter. Fortunately, Mindy was able to turn to friends for the encouragement she needed.

Breast cancer can change the relationship with a sister. Some sisters become closer and more supportive; others distance themselves, refusing to acknowledge that the disease has occurred. Their denial may be their way of dealing with the fear that breast cancer could happen to them. The siblings of both Ruth Thayer and Peggy Thompson seemed unconcerned and unsupportive, which, of course, strained their relationships. At first Ruth and Peggy were hurt by these reactions, but then they realized that their sisters simply could not face the possibility of having breast cancer themselves.

Close relationships can be fragile, easily hurt by misperceptions, fears, misunderstandings, and stresses. Family support is vital to each member's well-being, especially that of the person who is ill. It is helpful to understand why and how relationships become strained and damaging in a time of crisis such as breast cancer.

Using family systems theory to explain the complexity of relationships, we have discussed how the illness of one member can affect the other members. The impact on each person will differ according to age, developmental stage, and perceptions of the illness. If parents are aware of childrens' typical behavioral responses to a serious illness, they can be better prepared to maintain the family stability. How children and other members cope with the illness may depend to a great extent on what they are told and how well their needs are met.

In the next chapter we will examine relationships with health care professionals who will be the primary caregivers during the woman's treatment and initial recovery. We explain what patients and families expect of physicians and nurses and reasons for unsatisfactory relationships between them. The importance of clear and empathic communication on the part of professional caregivers as well as the family's responsibility to the relationships is discussed.

Chapter 8

Relationships with Health Care Professionals

Although many of the women and their families have shared their satisfaction with doctors and nurses, a number of them have been frustrated by what seemed to be insensitivity to their feelings. Because a woman becomes acutely distressed when the need for a biopsy is mentioned, the attitudes of health personnel can greatly affect how she will adjust to the diagnosis of breast cancer.[1]

The physicians who treated Fran Humphreys exemplify the effect that attitude can have on the patient. Fran, who underwent multiple surgeries, chemotherapy, and bone marrow transplant before her eventual death, appreciated the warmth and humor of two of her physicians. "I had young doctors who were very quick to let me have input into the decision making," she said. "They gave me more freedom than many doctors do and I think that made a difference. I used humor to get me through the experience and they picked up on my clowning and clowned with me. I'm sure not all doctors do that, but mine did and it was very helpful to me."

Fran went on to explain the emotional support she had: "I felt very close to my plastic surgeon with whom I could discuss everything, especially how to get through this. When I left his office for what might be the last time, I felt sad and alone. I never felt that way toward a doctor before."

On the other hand, some women we interviewed did not have such good experiences. Carol McNeil said, "One thing that bothered me right after the diagnosis was the distance some of the hospital staff kept when I was a patient. My surgeon, who was a wonderful surgeon, never used the word 'cancer,' nor did any of the nurses. No one ever said to me, 'This must be pretty frightening for you.' I never felt that I could get support from the professionals in those early stages. The only support I had was what I initiated with certain other people. I think this lack of sensitivity to my feelings had a lot to do with my loneliness. No one ever asked me how I felt about this cancer. Not even the nurse in my surgeon's office ever said, 'How are you doing? How are you feeling? How are you coping?' I finally met one nurse who treated me in a way that helped. She spent time with me, even getting tears in her eyes when we talked. From my experience she is unique, not the norm."

When Nancy Campbell first found a lump, she felt the doctors were callous in their remarks. In fact, she changed from both the surgeon and oncologist to physicians who were more understanding. Nancy also found the treatment at hospitals to be humiliating, particularly the lack of privacy. She felt she was being treated without any consideration for her feelings. For example, curtains were not closed when she was put in a dressing room with other patients, including a male.

PATIENTS' EXPECTATIONS OF PHYSICIANS

A woman with breast cancer is under the care of several specialists. This could include her family doctor, gynecologist, surgeon, anesthetist, oncologist, or oncology radiologist, in addition to nurses, possibly a social worker, and sometimes a psychotherapist. Of course, a patient expects all these professionals to be competent, but for some women competence alone does not help with the emotional effects of the disease.

Because of the trauma of being told that she has breast cancer, a woman needs some empathic acknowledgment of her feelings. The physician who has determined that a lump is likely cancerous and should be examined by a surgeon needs to be especially aware of the shock a woman will experience at hearing a confirmation of one of her greatest fears—cancer. Once she hears "cancer" or "malignant," she will not likely comprehend another word.[2] At that point, the physician should do whatever he or she can to reduce the emotional distress that the woman is experiencing.

Some physicians give the diagnosis and treatment information in a blunt or insensitive manner. Their tone of voice, facial expression, and body language may not convey concern or caring. They may keep a wide distance between themselves and the patient and divert their eyes from her. Because she puts her confidence in her physician, this initial encounter is crucial. If this meeting is unsatisfactory, the devastation she feels may make her adjustment difficult. The findings of a study by Dr. Peter Houts suggest that when emotional help is provided early, just after diagnosis, there is a greater possibility that the patient will cope better if the disease progresses.

Dottie Corcoran, who was still undergoing chemotherapy when we first saw her, said, "I don't want the doctor to be a friend, but I do want some expression of caring, certainly a more personal relationship than I have had. My primary care physician answers my questions and I feel I get accurate information, but he doesn't relate to me as a person. Even though other health care staff have treated me in a more personal way, there is still a distance. They seem to be in such a rush all the time. As a result of this depersonalized treatment, I feel angry, impatient, and dissatisfied."

Another patient, Sue Norton, said of the surgeon who performed her mastectomy, "to call him 'cold' is an understatement." She became concerned when no one told her the results of her bone scan. When she inquired, the nurse told her everything was all right but later she learned that the scan showed spots on her sternum. Her oncologist was also aloof and abrupt. When she asked questions, he replied, "Oh, you don't need to know; don't ask." She said, "I felt that he just hung me out to dry. I was so angry I had a discussion with him and told him that I resented how I was being treated. After that, he seemed more concerned. Thank goodness, my plastic surgeon was very caring and different from the others."

A poor approach to a patient who was to undergo chemotherapy is illustrated by the experience of a woman who was recovering from a mastectomy and reconstruction. Without identifying himself, an oncologist whom she had never seen appeared in her hospital room and told her that she was scheduled for several tests and that her chemotherapy would begin the following week. Then he departed as abruptly as he had appeared. His aloofness and curt manner upset the patient, but she was too intimidated to make a complaint. Upon learning of the scheduled tests, her plastic surgeon, who thought it was too soon for her to have tests and chemotherapy, cancelled the tests. The patient didn't want to see the oncologist again but wasn't assertive enough to break her appointment. A relative who was a nurse intervened, cancelled the appointment, and made one with another oncologist whom she recommended.

In addition to treating patients with consideration, doctors and nurses should be honest and trustworthy. Shari Lovell maintains that her physician was not being truthful when he told her he had given her the estrogen-receptor test. This made Shari somewhat bitter toward physicians, because five years earlier she had had a radical mastectomy and had received no information about reconstructive surgery on that mastectomy site. She warns other women to get a second opinion before consenting to surgery.

Woman and their families also expect that physicians will listen to what they say and that they will explain the treatment options that are available. Some women would like a physician to suggest what he would do if he were recommending treatment for his wife.

Professional caregivers should also acknowledge the worry and emotional turmoil that husbands and close family members are experiencing. Although Fran Humphrey was very pleased with her physicians, her husband George did not receive the same consideration. After Fran's first operation, George said, "The surgeon should have talked to me about what I might expect to go through and what I might need. Actually, the only time he talked with me was after the surgery to tell me what he had done and how it turned out."

In summary, patients and families not only want physicians to be competent but many of them also expect some compassion and recognition of the emotional impact of breast cancer. Patients would like to be treated as persons, not as medical cases. They want doctors to listen to them, explain their treatment options, and be honest, truthful, and trustworthy.

PATIENTS' AND FAMILY MEMBERS' EXPECTATIONS OF NURSES

Nurses are a primary resource for the breast cancer patient. To make decisions the woman needs information, explanations, and support, which nurses can provide. In an article on making decisions about breast reconstruction, Zanca quoted Jane Hunter, an oncology nurse who works with women with breast cancer. Hunter stated that "nurses can help the patient clarify and process information. Nurses should encourage the patient and family to ask as many questions as they wish and as often as they wish." Hunter emphasized that "clarification and reinforcement should be given as often as needed, even if the patient has already been given the same information in previous contacts." Moreover, a nurse should give the woman and her family permission to express what they feel at this time.[3]

What Kinds of Information Does the Nurse Give the Woman Who Is Having Breast Treatment?

In addition to answering questions about procedures, medications, and the many other things that trouble a patient, the nurse should inform her of support groups. Even before a woman is hospitalized the office nurse can supply phone numbers and information about the American Cancer Society, hospital breast centers, and other support groups. If a woman is informed prior to having to make decisions about treatment, she can share her concerns and worst fears with others who have the same apprehensions. Hunter also urges all women to attend a support group, even those who say, "I don't need a support group. I've handled other crises and I'm strong. My husband and family are enough support." These women will benefit from being in a group where they don't have "to keep up a front for everyone else."[4]

By showing concern and caring, nurses can make a great difference in how well a patient responds to treatment. When her physician told Ruth Thayer about the option of having reconstructive surgery, she experienced many emotions. After several nurses sat and talked with her, explaining everything about the procedure and assuring her that her feelings were normal, she felt less anxious.

Having a nurse whom a woman can call when troubled about anything related to her breast cancer can give her a sense of security. For example, Sue Norton explained what it meant to her to be able to call her plastic surgeon's nurse. She said, "When you are in the doctor's office you hear what they say but you don't absorb it. After you leave and you are miles away, all of a sudden these silly fears crop up and you think, 'Oh no, I don't know what to do!' When I call the doctor's office, his nurse Francine has always made me feel that she is delighted that I call her about my concerns. She is willing to answer any of my questions. In that office, they genuinely care and make me feel as though I am the most important person who ever lived. I'm not a number or just another patient, but part of a family or team."

Another woman in our study, Peggy Thompson, found nurses in the hospital where she was waiting for her breast surgery to be exceptionally thoughtful. "Two nights before I was scheduled for surgery two nurses entered my room at 10 o'clock and asked if I had any street clothes," Peggy told us. "When I told them I had indeed brought clothes they said, 'You need to get dressed; you are breaking out. We're taking you out for some real food. We'll be leaving at 11 o'clock on a four-hour pass.' " Along with seven other nurses, they went to a restaurant, ate good food, talked, and didn't return until 2 A.M. These nurses made Peggy feel so special that she shared her fears and felt less apprehensive about what was ahead for her.

How Can Nurses Help the Family?

First, nurses need to be aware of families' past experiences with cancer. They also need to be aware of the families' traditions and rules, especially for ethnic groups other than their own. Nurses can gather this information in casual conversation and by asking probing questions. They should then incorporate this knowledge in the patient's care.

Dyck and Wright, both R.N.s, conducted a study to determine what families expect nurses to do throughout an adult's cancer experience.[5] The answers included explaining tests and procedures, giving honest information, keeping the family updated as to the status of the patient, and contacting the physician for the family. Although the nurse is not considered to be the primary caregiver, family members rely on her (or him) to clarify and expand on information that they need. Families can expect and should be able to feel comfortable with the nurse in this role.

Family members value a nurse who is genuine, honest, friendly, cheerful, compassionate, and competent. If he or she can plan ways to make it easier for families to talk about what they want to know, and if the nurse is friendly and approachable, the family members receive the emotional support and sense of caring that helps them cope.

Klein has outlined the following steps for health care professionals to help the patient and her family through a crisis: (1) Help the patient to express her feelings. (2) Do not give false assurances. (3) Help the patient to anticipate the future. (4) Involve the family. (5) Help the patient to consider how and what to tell the most significant persons in her life.[6]

REASONS FOR UNSATISFACTORY RELATIONSHIPS BETWEEN PATIENT, FAMILY, AND HEALTH CARE PROFESSIONALS

Earlier we discussed some of the difficulties that members may be having within the family. Each is preoccupied with his or her own needs and may be making wrong assumptions about how other members act and feel. Family rules, habitual ways of talking, fears of losing control, and difficulty in expressing feelings may inhibit their communication. In addition, the stress of illness may cause unresolved family issues to resurface.

Professional caregivers, particularly surgeons, experience different kinds of pressure. Forgetting that the surgeon is only human, the patient and family often perceive the surgeon as "godlike" and put great faith in his or her ability.[7] The responsibility of curing or arresting the disease and giving the patient hope rests with the surgeon.

Dr. Richard Hillier has described the common anxieties that doctors may experience. They may have feelings of discomfort with dying patients and pessimistic attitudes toward curability of a disease. Because each person reacts differently to drugs, physicians have concerns that narcotic painkillers may either cause too much sedation or fail to relieve pain adequately. They may also have apprehension about overlooking a curable condition or the belief that death is a failure on their part.[8]

In addition to the differences in perceptions and pressures, there are other reasons for difficulties in the caregiver-patient relationship. Misunderstanding can occur when a professional caregiver's verbal and nonverbal messages seem contradictory. For example, the patient may interpret the physician's nonverbal message (which may be communicating fatigue and worry) as being contradictory to the reassuring words he is speaking. If a doctor does not listen or pay enough attention to the patient's complaints or does not explore the effectiveness of pain medications he has prescribed, a breakdown in confidence can occur. Moreover, some physicians think that the less a patient knows, the less she will worry. This attitude can be upsetting to the patient.

Breaches can occur in the relationship in other situations. The health professional may become defensive rather then dealing with a patient's complaint. A physician may believe he or she is being honest by giving a woman the plain truth about her diagnosis and/or prognosis, but the manner of telling her may be insensitive. A caregiver may fail to convey hope, give the woman too little information for making decisions about treatment, or make an inaccurate estimate of her life expectancy with the disease. These failures can result in an unsatisfactory relationship.

THE STATUS OF COMMUNICATION

A group of researchers studied communication patterns in a medical setting and found that considerable conflict arises at all levels of health care among the health professionals themselves.[9] Because the relationship between doctor and nurse is a serious one based on openness, truth, and trust, conflict may occur when any of these elements is violated. Conflict also arises from their desire to protect their territory.

In relation to patients, physicians and nurses often see themselves as the sole agent responsible for the patient's recovery, whereas she may wish to exercise autonomy in her own progress. Moreover, when family members try to impose their wishes, conflict may result. According to researchers, some physicians tend to view verbal discourse as having the potential for conflict, so they avoid it as much as possible. Avoidance is also a means of keeping emotionally uninvolved. Overworked surgeons, whose schedules give them little time for more than a fleeting relationship with a patient, may view communication as a waste of time.

Despite our awareness of the importance of good communication in the health care setting, the quality and quantity of communication and interaction have not been improving.[10] In an effort to bring about positive changes, an organization called the Cornerstone Group offers seminars and consultation to the medical community on topics relevant to improving health care. Included in the available seminars is "Communication and Cancer: Knowing What to Say When You Don't Know What to Say."[11]

COMMUNICATION BETWEEN PHYSICIAN AND FAMILY

If it is possible for the spouse to accompany his wife in her consultations with the physicians prior to her surgery, he should do so. If not, some other family member or close friend should be with her and either take notes or tape-record the instructions. That person can ask questions and clarify what the physician says.

Then, after the surgery, the surgeon should talk with the spouse and other family members who have been waiting. He or she should explain the patient's condition, the outcome of the surgery, and what complications might be expected and suggest the kind of support and care she will need from them. The physician should also convey an understanding of the stress the family is experiencing. He could suggest that they call his office nurse if they have further questions.

Patients who are satisfied with the excellent care that their health care professionals have given them are quick to express their appreciation. Paula

Emerson, who had a double mastectomy and reconstruction, shared her feelings about the care she received. She said, "There are going to be set-backs. The doctors are human beings and unbelievable demands are made on them. If you listen and have patience, you will find them to be right. After all, they are the best in the world."

One plastic surgeon who realized the importance of the woman's emotional reactions to breast cancer and reconstruction preferred to entrust this responsibility to his nurse. A compassionate, competent person, she handled patients' questions and emotional concerns. The sensitivity with which she did this earned her a large following of grateful women.

Lynn Robbins has much praise for the surgeon who performed her reconstructive surgery. "He was marvelous," she said. "I wasn't just a patient; I was a definite person. We joked and laughed together and I cried a lot. He would say, 'Here comes Lynn, get out the Kleenex.' He and his nurses were great."

FACILITATING COMMUNICATION WITH HEALTH CARE PROVIDERS

As the patient and family, you have a responsibility in building a good relationship with health care providers. They cannot know your needs or dissatisfaction unless you make them known. It is far better to talk over concerns with the nurse or doctor than to remain unhappy. If the problem cannot be resolved, you are free to change doctors.

When you talk with your health care providers, you'll find them more open if you are aware of how you are making your requests or voicing complaints. Rather than making demands, ask many questions so that you understand why a procedure or test is being done. Ask for written information about your alternatives for treatment of the cancer. At the time of the diagnosis, request the names and phone numbers of support groups that are accessible in your area. For a list of specific questions to ask at the time of diagnosis, see Appendix C.

Physicians, nurses, and other health care professionals have emotionally and physically demanding jobs and work under extreme pressure. They witness a great deal of suffering and grief and often experience "burn-out." When they treat you well, they need to know that their efforts are appreciated. Tell them how grateful you are. The person following you will enjoy the same attention and concern, making their recuperation easier. By encouraging and helping someone else, you also benefit.

Dr. Rosenbaum wrote in his book, *Living with Cancer*, "Listening and talking, an atmosphere of openness and candor, are the means by which an enduring, supportive relationship is developed. . . . But to make such a relationship a reality, a patient must have the wisdom to know his needs and the courage to articulate them to his physician."[12]

In this chapter we have explained the effect of relationships with professional caregivers upon the woman's adjustment to breast cancer. The patient's expectations of physicians and nurses and reasons for breakdowns in communication and confidence are identified. Caregivers as well as the patient and her family have a responsibility in facilitating satisfactory communication. As patients increase their demand for more decision making and participation in their health care, effective communication becomes a necessity.

As we move on, we emphasize the importance of openness regarding the feelings and issues that arise with breast cancer and other stressful events. We explore how beliefs, patterns of interaction, and misperceptions may inhibit empathic communication. Methods are suggested for improving communication through self-disclosure, empathy, expressing feelings, effective listening, and nonverbal messages. Finally, what is communicated to children must be carefully considered.

Chapter 9

Communicating about Breast Cancer

Lawrence LeShan, a psychotherapist with more than thirty-five years of research experience involving several thousand cancer patients, has observed
that most patients and their families cope far better if they can communicate
openly and honestly. He believes that honesty conveys respect for the patient's strength and ability to cope with the truth and increases the family's
ability to manage a crisis.[1] It also establishes trust. Physician Cournos tells
a heartrending story of one family's efforts to shield their 80-year-old father,
who had cancer, from upsetting news.[2]

The father had been having a great deal of pain, and when he attempted
to take his life, it was assumed he could not endure the suffering. Under
questioning, he disclosed that the family's secrecy about another matter had
caused his despair. He could not bear being excluded from his family. His
sister had died the week before, and the family decided it would upset him
too much to be told. He learned of the death from a distant acquaintance
who called to express sympathy for his loss. Feeling that his family was
treating him as though he were already dead, he had no reason to live. The
family explained that they had meant well and assured him that they still
needed him. Their reassurance gave him another four months of life. As the
story illustrates, it can be less devastating to know what is happening than
to feel excluded.

DISCUSSING CANCER WITH OTHERS

Why do some women and their families keep their breast cancer a secret?
Joanne Moser explained her reasons for secrecy: "Cancer is not something
that people want to talk about. We who have it don't want others to know

it because they are afraid of catching it. They think it's a disease like measles or chicken pox. I didn't tell anyone when I had my mastectomy." Joanne has now become more open about her cancer and has been helping others as a volunteer in Reach to Recovery.

Another reason for secretiveness is the fear of death that the word "cancer" engenders. The Adamses have been very private about Jane's cancer. In fact, no one in Larry's family knows about it and only Jane's siblings and parents have been told. It has not been shared with friends. Jane and Larry told their children that their mother was having surgery but did not mention cancer. Because Larry's father had died of cancer, they thought their children would be frightened to know their mother had it. The Adamses believe that they are open with one another and discuss issues in family meetings, but they are obviously closed with extended family members and friends. The ability to communicate with one another has enabled them to cope without the support of others.

Mel and Ruth Thayer, on the other hand, were able to talk about Ruth's breast cancer and also share with others. They maintained the open communication they already had and, unlike the Adamses, learned that close friends and other who had experienced cancer were important to their coping. Mel was very concerned about Ruth, who worried about recurrence and would awaken in the night, panic-stricken that she had another lump. She was tearful when she talked about it and somewhat resentful that after all the other illnesses she had been through, she had gotten cancer. Mel did not believe in psychotherapy, but he did want her to find a support group or someone with whom she could talk. She had not done so, but fortunately the oncologist and her surgeon's nurse had been helpful.

Mel himself found that others enabled him to deal with Ruth's fears and discouragement as well as his own. He said, "Talking with others makes you realize that you are not alone, that many other people go through this fear of recurrence. Some mask it better than others; but if you talk with them, you know that the fear is normal and that somewhere down the road it tapers off." Mel went on to tell us about a good friend who had cancer in his lymph nodes years ago. "This friend went through hell for a long time—on the day of his check-ups he would break into a cold sweat. Gradually his apprehension went away. I definitely think it is helpful to talk with others who have had the same experience." As Mel hoped they would, Ruth's fears have finally subsided and she says she seldom thinks of the cancer now.

Couples who have established good communication are better able to help one another when severe stress occurs.[3] If they normally talk openly about their feelings, they have less difficulty addressing sensitive issues.[4] However, the nature of some situations, such as a life-threatening illness, can inhibit them from being open and candid. Such was the case with the Taylors and Princes, whose stories we have related to you. Both couples

were very satisfied with their marriages and claimed to have good communication. But after Audrey's breast cancer, the Taylors suddenly found themselves unable to talk. The Princes also had difficulty discussing a sexual issue
that was troubling her after her mastectomy.

WHAT HAPPENS TO COUPLE COMMUNICATION

In his book *The Fragile Bond,* family therapist Napier discusses the expectations and patterns of interaction that develop between a couple and
challenge a marriage. He explains that we tend to behave and communicate
in ways that we learned from our parents. A couple can fall into repetitive
patterns of interaction without being aware of it. Unfortunately, in many
marriages communication diminishes as couples get used to one another
and become involved with the tasks of everyday living and raising families.
Budgets, schedules, and practical matters demand their attention and they
begin to lose touch with one another.[5]

Dr. Nolen, author of *The Making of a Surgeon,* wrote in his later book
Crisis Time! that he and his wife had not sat down for years to discuss how
they felt or whether they were satisfied with their marriage. Like many couples, they had been taking one another for granted and behaving as if they
could read one another's minds. It took a mid-life crisis to make them realize
what had happened to their relationship. Nolen believes that what became
a major problem for them might have been minor if he and his wife had
been really communicating. He has observed that "once two people are
married, they immediately run out of things to say to one another." From
then on, he says, the "bulk" of their conversations consist of "monosylla-
bles."[6]

One explanation of the interpersonal distance that occurs with couples is
found in the theory of R. D. Laing, a British psychiatrist.[7] He explains that
our experience with another person is based on our perception of that person's behavior and what we imagine he or she may be feeling, perceiving,
or thinking. Because we cannot really know what goes on inside the other's
mind, we make guesses. At the same time, the other person is doing the
same about us. Both of us may be making inaccurate inferences. Married
couples often assume they understand the other so well that they do not
need to clarify their perceptions with one another verbally. If we do not
check our interpretations of the other person's feelings and thoughts and
exchange honest responses, we may not only misunderstand the other but
we may also feel misunderstood. Laing's theory gives us some insight into
how distancing can occur between couples.

There are other ways in which misunderstandings occur in a relationship.
First, we often send one another more than one message by saying one
thing verbally and another nonverbally. Because 90 percent of our messages

are nonverbal and the other 10 percent verbal, the meaning that the partner gets can be confusing and inaccurate. It is a mixed message. Second, misunderstandings can occur because of the setting or context in which the communication takes place. Third, the response of one partner to the other's comment may be unrelated to what was said.

Finally, when the emotional responses to one another do not match, or bond, misunderstanding can take place. If one displays warm concern and the other responds with cool rejection, their dissimilar behaviors may be misinterpreted. One husband told Scoresby, author of *The Marriage Dialogue*, the only time he and his wife shared the same emotion was when they were "mad."[8]

DISCUSSING FEELINGS AND PROBLEMS

It is clear from studies and the families we have interviewed that some members, particularly men, avoid talking about sensitive issues such as cancer. In fact, a number of spouses who declined to participate in our study stated that they had no need to discuss the topic with others. One spouse's opinion was that talking about cancer makes you dwell on it. He thought you should put it behind you and move on with your life. He had a good point; cancer *can* become an obsession that dominates thoughts and conversation, but the fear of recurrence and the need for vigilance makes it difficult for a woman to forget. Keeping the communication open can help a couple and their family to work through their fears in a supportive manner.

Patients who have been able to discuss problems with families and friends have said it provides them "reassurance, support, empathy, and information."[9] Therapist Simonton, who counsels families, believes that in order to deal with cancer, members must talk about it, get to know others who have it, express their fears, and reach out for support.[10] If family members are not able to communicate, especially on crucial issues, Dr. LeShan suggests that close friends or professionals help them.[11] Physician Rosenbaum realizes that it is not easy for some people to talk about "their deepest concerns," so he meets with family members together, usually in late afternoon or evening. He encourages them to bring up problems and ask questions.[12]

Not all families are agreeable to discussing feelings and problems. Family rules and cultural traditions may prohibit them from talking about personal issues. In this case, the physician must respect their privacy. All he or she can do is offer them an opportunity to meet if they have questions or want more information.

As patients become more involved in the decisions about their medical care, communication becomes more important. Moreover, with attention now being given to psychosocial effects of disease, the importance of being supportive requires verbal interaction.

HOW WE COMMUNICATE

As we are aware, we communicate by sending and receiving messages through words and body movements. Even when we have not spoken a word we have transmitted a message through our actions, facial expressions, and attitude. Eye contact, closeness or distance from the receiver (proximity), gestures, posture, and touching are important elements of the nonverbal message. Our communication is effective if the recipient of our message interprets its meaning as we intended it. What stronger messages can we give than a warm hug or hand clasp, and receive the same in return?

The tone, quality, pitch, and volume of the voice carry an additional message. These vocal components also convey meaning, adding to or distorting our message, sometimes contradicting it. As an example, if a person says, "I feel fine" in a tone that reveals weariness, and with body posture that indicates fatigue, we believe the strongest message. We believe that he isn't feeling "fine" but doesn't want to admit it or is trying to mask his true feelings.

As Rosenbaum has observed, each member of a family experiencing cancer "is searching for the most tactful way to deal with the other."[13] They can handle the stress better and strengthen their relationships if they can convey feelings and concerns clearly in verbal and nonverbal ways. How can they do so more effectively?

A couple can change their communication by making a conscious effort to do so. Unless they can be aware by talking about their "talk" and attempt to improve what they say and how they say it, they will continue to have misunderstandings and may drift apart.

Improving Communication

Self-Disclosure. By disclosing information about ourselves we encourage communication. We also help the other person to know and understand what we are thinking and feeling. Disclosing personal information is a part of developing trust, intimacy, and understanding. It should be done gradually, with consideration for the other person's reaction to what we tell him or her. For our relationship to continue, the other person should reciprocate by disclosing to us.

Using a hypothetical example, let us suppose that Harry has never told his wife Ann of the unhappiness he felt as a child because of his mother's mood swings. His mother was never diagnosed or treated, but her changeable moods caused great anxiety and pain for his family. After Harry's wife has surgery for breast cancer, her unpredictable moods remind him of his mother's. His reactions to his wife are similar to those he had toward his mother. He always had the feeling that his mother's moods were a way of manipulating him and his father; he begins to feel the same way about his wife. Ann is now the target of the anger and resentment that well up in him. He often gets into conflicts with her, especially when she is having difficulty with the side effects of treatments.

Being a sensitive person, Harry reflects on his reactions to his wife's illness. Images of his childhood help him to realize that he is responding to her as he did to his mother. He decides to take the risk of telling her about his feelings. After listening attentively, Ann tells Harry about a childhood experience that left her with a great deal of insecurity. By sharing their experiences Harry and Ann move into a deeper level of understanding. Had Ann not shown empathy for Harry and reciprocated his disclosure, their relationship probably would have remained strained and difficult.

Empathizing with Others. Communication experts agree that the basis of effective interpersonal communication is empathy.[14] Empathy is the ability to put ourselves in the other person's place so that we understand and share what he or she is feeling. A vivid description of empathy appears in a touching scene in Harper Lee's book *To Kill a Mockingbird*. Atticus, a small-town lawyer in Alabama, has the formidable task of bringing up his daughter Scout and her brother Jem without their mother, who had died. On her first day in school, Scout has been made to stand in the corner and has had such a miserable time that she begs her father to let her stay home and take her lessons from him. After hearing her account of her day, Atticus explains why she must attend school and learn to be tolerant of others.

"First of all," he says, "if you can learn a simple trick, Scout, you'll get along a lot better with all kinds of folks . . . .You never really understand a person until you consider things from his point of view—until you climb into his skin and walk around in it."[15] If Scout didn't understand what that meant then, she eventually learned the meaning and the importance of empathy from a father who practiced it.

Empathy requires that we care about the other person's feelings and that we be perceptive. We empathize by listening carefully, maintaining eye contact, lessening the space between us and the speaker, observing nonverbal messages, and withholding judgments. The last point is very important because of our natural tendency to become judgmental. To empathize, we listen carefully and go through a process of imagining how that person is feeling. Then we respond in a way that conveys our understanding and support.[16]

Most of the couples with whom we talked demonstrated the ability to empathize, but there were several spouses who did not. As you recall, Claire Vosburg's husband Hugh said to her after the doctor told her she had breast cancer, "I could have done without that news." Mindy's husband reacted with, "You are repulsive to me." Their statements carried no understanding of how their wives were feeling. Their statements were, in fact, very hurtful. These spouses were probably focusing on their own feelings about their wives' loss of attractiveness and desirability to them. If Hugh had said, "This is terrifying for you. I want you to know that I will love you just as much without your breast," he would have been empathetic and supportive. Had Mindy's husband remarked, "You must feel devastated," he would have at least shown some consideration for her feelings, although he would be offering no support or willingness to help her.

In contrast, many of the men we interviewed were understanding of what their partners were experiencing. For example, John Seifert wept when he heard the doctor's diagnosis. Although John could not talk about it, his emotional response at that time told his wife that he cared. Jack Young knew what the disfigurement would do to his wife's self-esteem and assured her that he understood and loved her. Mel Thayer felt as torn up as Ruth was and made it clear that he, too, was devastated. Their husbands' expressions of empathy and support were important to the women's recovery.

Some people possess a high degree of empathy. Others are not easily attuned to the feelings of another person. They can increase their sensitivity by listening carefully, observing, and by putting themselves into the other person's situation. Empathy is an important quality in all our relationships. Napier emphasizes the need for developing it if we want to maintain or improve them.[17]

When Empathy Is Especially Important. An important time for showing empathy is when an ill person talks about dying. Death is not a comfortable topic and we often say something like this: "Oh, you're not going to die," or "You shouldn't talk like that." Such comments encourage denial.[18] An appropriate empathic comment to someone who says she is dying is to reply, "You must be feeling as though the treatments will never end and you'll never get well. Would it help you to talk about it?" Or, "You have endured the treatments and the pain for so long. It must be very discouraging. How can I help you?" Your response acknowledges her feeling and indicates that you understand, you care, and you want to help.

Fear of death is a real and frightening concern for the ill person as well as for family members. It is important that they be allowed to talk about their fears and other negative emotions. Once they have expressed their feelings, you can move the conversation on to more positive, comforting topics.[19]

Another time for showing empathy occurs when the woman (or family member) needs to talk about the loss of the breast, her diminished self-image, or other losses resulting from cancer. The grief that the woman feels over her losses is similar to what we experience with the death of a loved one, or with a divorce and other interpersonal losses.[20] We need to mourn for them. For some, grieving is a very private experience that they do not wish to share. Others reach out and talk more openly with empathic listeners.[21]

What do we say to a woman like Lynn Robbins, who felt such anger after losing both breasts that she lashed out at others more fortunate than she?

We don't say, "Be grateful that you found the cancer early." Rather, an appropriate response could be something like this: "Of course you are angry, and you have a right to be. You have lost an important part of yourself. You've been very courageous about this." Touch her or hold her hand if she allows it. Then offer to help her in some specific way. Suggest that you take her children after school, drive her to treatments, or do some shopping. Communication is not a panacea for dealing with grief, but talking with empathic others can help the grieving person work through emotional turmoil.

Expressing Feelings. Baider and De-Nour studied the adjustment of couples to breast cancer and found that those who were less able to adjust had difficulty expressing their feelings.[22] When persons do not give us verbal clues as to what they are thinking or feeling, we don't know how to treat them. As we've noted earlier, we must guess; and because our only frame of reference is our perception of their behavior and our own experience, our guesses may be inaccurate. To deny and repress feelings can force them "underground" only to emerge in other ways.[23] Furthermore, one of the outcomes of repressed feelings can be depression.

Researchers have discovered that persons with cancer often suffer from repressed feelings.[24] Klopfer, in an early psychological study of cancer, measured the amount of denial of patients. Some had a strong need to deny their emotional pain in order to look good or show that they were coping well.[25] Simonton found that when feelings—particularly the anger and fear prevalent with cancer—are experienced fully and expressed, they tend to lessen or "dissipate."[26] Moreover, being able to own and describe our feelings, rather than withholding or expressing them in negative ways, causes less defensiveness in others.

What is the difference between expressing and describing our feelings? We express feelings when we yell, cry, remain silent, curse, pound the table, and demonstrate them in other ways. We describe them when we explain what and how we are feeling and reveal the source of the emotion. First, in describing feelings, it is important to acknowledge that the emotion is ours by saying "I am feeling sad" (or whatever the emotion is we are experiencing). Then tell why. For example, a family member might express his fear that the patient will die by being cantankerous with other members. If he could say, "I'm worried that she may die," he would have explained the feeling (worry) and the reason for it. In doing so he would probably have verbalized the emotions that other members are experiencing and would be opening the way for them to discuss their concerns.

On one of my visits with Kathryn Lathrop we could hear her husband in another room talking with someone over the telephone. Kathryn commented, "One of the difficulties I have had in the forty-two years of being married to him is that he does not share his feelings with me. He keeps them inside, but he can express them to a total stranger. It used to be very hard for me when I heard him pour out his feelings to someone he didn't know and would probably never see. I have always had to guess what is going on inside him." Kathryn spoke with resignation and some sadness.

It is not always easy to identify our feelings, nor can we expect to change the other person—only ourselves. Our intention when we express our feelings is to clarify our position so that other people can understand and know how to treat us.

Like Dr. Rosenbaum, therapist Simonton believes that communicating feelings within the family is crucial to their overall health. It creates "a healing attitude" and helps the patient to gain the "psychological strength" she needs for recovery.[27]

The Value of Open-Ended Questions. One of the best ways to open the lines of communication is to ask questions that will encourage the other person to talk. The questions should be open-ended; in other words, they should not evoke a "yes" or "no;" answer, and they should not be evaluative or judgmental. For example, when Audrey Taylor asked Mark why he was obsessed with her cancer, he reported that she said, "What's the matter, are you scared to death?" Mark, who is a tall, strong man, a former officer in the army, and accustomed to handling difficult problems, was not in the habit of admitting that he was "scared to death." Instead of challenging him as she did, suppose that Audrey had said, "Mark, you're bringing up my cancer so often that it makes me feel you are very concerned about it. Is there something about it that is troubling you?" The question is worded so that she does not threaten Mark's masculinity or ability to handle crises.

Suppose that Mark's frustration had not reached a point at which he was willing to admit his feelings and he replied "no." Then Audrey could have said, "Oh, I just thought you might be worrying. If you are, please let's talk about it." She has given him an opening, shown sensitivity to his feelings and respect for his wishes to remain silent. She has also created a climate in which he can feel less hesitant to reveal his concern. When Mark is ready to talk he can say, "Audrey, you asked the other day if something is troubling me. As a matter of fact, there is. It's hard to express, but I'll try."

We realize that both Audrey and Mark were emotionally upset and not in the frame of mind to think about how they were communicating. However, if a couple can get into the habit of wording questions so they do not threaten the other's ego, the reward will be more open communication and "a healthier, more intimate family."[28]

Effective Listening

Effective listening is important in receiving and absorbing information and establishing trust. You may recall Ellen Barkley's difficulty in comprehending and remembering what the physician said to her after he told her she had breast cancer. Effective listening requires concentration; but when a person is emotionally upset, she only concentrates on the message that has the greatest impact. After that, she may hear what is said but be unable to focus on or absorb its meaning. In fact, when a message evokes negative emotions in a person, he or she may close out further messages.[29]

As we discussed in relation to empathy, good listening is essential in developing sensitivity to others and in conveying a caring attitude. Combs and Avila, who have examined the therapeutic methods used in the helping professions, say that listening carefully to a person pays him or her "the highest form of compliment."[30] Listening conveys caring. Often what an ill person or family member needs most is someone who shows, just by listening, that they care.

Communicating Affection Nonverbally

The need for affection increases when we are ill and plays a significant part in our healing process. For a person who has difficulty expressing affection verbally, touching and holding demonstrates love and caring. The fear of contagion makes some people hesitant about having physical contact with cancer patients. The fear of hurting a patient who has had surgery may keep loved ones from hugging or holding her.[31] Thus, a person with cancer may not receive the affection she needs.

Some patients withdraw from being touched because of low self-esteem, depression, or other psychological reasons. They want and need affection but may feel they haven't earned it. Simonton suggests an appropriate response to the person who withdraws: "I think I understand that you don't want to be held right now." Then go on to assure her that you care for her and want her to know that you do.[32]

TALKING ABOUT YOUR SEXUAL RELATIONSHIP

Those who have experienced or treated chronic illness advocate open communication when there is anxiety about sexuality. If a couple ignores the issue and fails to resolve it, they tend to become distant from one another. When Joan Parker had breast cancer she and her husband shared in their book, *Three Weeks in Spring*, their concern about resuming their lovemaking.[33] Because the Parkers were able to talk, they made the sexual adjustment more easily than they had anticipated. However, not all couples can talk comfortably about their sexual relationship even "under the best of circumstances."[34] For example, Kim, a young woman with one child, told me that her husband was very supportive and caring when she had her lumpectomy, but that they were never able to talk about the effect of the cancer on their relationship. In fact, her husband never utters the word "cancer." He refers to her breast cancer as "the thing you have." She realizes that their sexual adjustment was easier than if she had had a mastectomy, but she could never discuss it with her husband. When the doctor became concerned about swelling in her lymph nodes some time after her lumpectomy, she told her husband that she was going through some tests for some suspicious spots. He retorted, "You're all right" and became belligerent toward her. Finally Kim said to him, "I know you're upset. So am I, but I need your support, not your belligerence." Her comment made him aware of his reaction; he was concealing his anxiety by being antagonistic toward her, which can be a normal reaction. He changed his behavior toward her and became more empathic. Suppose he had not?

How to Approach Sensitive Issues

When sensitive issues and difficult problems need to be resolved, several approaches have been suggested by experts. Miller and associates, who developed a workshop for enriching relationships, advocate that you set up a time and place for this serious discussion.[35] Explain to your partner that you want to set a time when you will not be disturbed so that you can talk about something that is bothering you. Tell him the nature of your concern and choose a time when you will not have external pressures. If you are initiating the discussion, consider factors that affect your spouse's receptiveness—certainly do not choose a time when he is tired, hungry, or has had a bad day at work. Also consider a comfortable setting conducive to an intimate talk. For example, one of my friends found that she and her husband usually got into an argument when they talked in their family room, which was carpeted in red. This would not be an appropriate place, particularly if you were aware of its effect on you. (My friend changed the carpet.)

Before the appointed time you can mentally prepare yourself to stay with the issue that is troubling you. Be determined to avoid bringing up other problems or complaints. Above all, resolve to show that you value and respect your partner's feelings. In the meantime, if your concern relates to your breast cancer, get some information from the library or the American Cancer Society.

A woman who realized the importance of obtaining and sharing information about sexual adjustment to illness is Beverly Kievman. She explained in her book *For Better or For Worse* that she read all she could find about sexuality and chronic illness when her husband developed severe diabetes, which required amputation of both legs.[36] She suggests that you and your spouse read the information together. It helps both of you to feel that you are not alone with this problem and gives you some points to discuss. Kievman also suggests that you disclose your discomfort about bringing up the subject and your reason for doing so. Explain that it is important to your relationship. You should also express your feelings openly and honestly.

In the event that your partner refuses to talk about your sexual life, respect his refusal. It doesn't mean he doesn't care; it probably means he feels very uncomfortable talking about it. You have opened the way and he may decide later to bring up the subject himself. If he doesn't, you have several other alternatives. Talk with your doctor; he may be willing to counsel you or make recommendations for a therapist. One of the oncologists with whom we talked advises her patients about sexual adjustment. If your oncologist does this, arrange to have your husband go with you when you have an appointment. You could also call Reach to Recovery or one of the other support groups, as Carol McNeil did, to find a volunteer who would be willing to talk with you.

TALKING WITH CHILDREN

There should be no question about telling children that their mother has breast cancer; they will be aware that something is happening. As we have emphasized, not telling children can be more detrimental than telling them. Simonton observed that an older child "may sleuth out the truth" but a younger child who is not told may become "extremely anxious and threatened."[37] Serious repercussions can occur if children are protected too much. A young mother in Texas told me that the greatest mistake she and her husband had made in handling her mastectomy was not telling their children that it was cancer. When they were visiting a relative, a young cousin told their daughter her mother had cancer. The daughter became so upset that she had nightmares for months and lost trust in what her parents told her. It is taking them a long time to rebuild that trust and allay her fears.

How children should be told is determined by their ages and levels of maturity. They can be spared the frightening details, but giving them information about the illness helps dispel their anxiety.[38] Simonton suggests that you begin with a statement that you have learned you have cancer. Then answer their questions honestly. Explaining to them does not require that they be given "a college course in cancer," nor should a parent "dump" her anxiety on her children.[39] Because they tend to assume the blame when upsetting things happen in the family, assure young children that they are not responsible for the illness.

As we have discussed earlier, older children, especially teenaged daughters who will relate the disease to themselves, need more information. In our limited contact with teenaged sons, we have learned that they also may have great anxiety. Therefore, they may need to be included in discussion of the cancer as much as daughter.

What children's peers say to them will have a tremendous impact. You may recall the case of Betty Sawyer, who was told by friends at school that they heard her mother was dying of breast cancer, which was not true. Betty felt very guilty that she had not realized the seriousness of her mother's condition and experienced unnecessary guilt and emotional turmoil.

It is important that children be helped to express their fears and other feelings. Kievman suggests that parents watch for warning signals of depression, such as eating and sleeping problems, low self-esteem, negative behavior changes, dropping school grades, and problems with peers. Other symptoms of their anxieties may be drinking, using drugs, driving too fast, and other forms of hell-raising. Being included in the family discussions may avert behavior problems, although there is no assurance that this will work with teenagers who are undergoing their own traumas. A child's emotional "acting out" of distress complicates the recovery of the ill parent who feels responsible, a situation that happened in the Kievman family.

A very helpful pamphlet written for children, entitled "When Someone in Your Family Has Cancer," is available through the National Cancer Institute (see Resources, Appendix B). Also, librarians can often suggest reading for children.

In summary, clinicians and therapists stress the importance of communicating openly when cancer occurs. What family members communicate to the patient and to one another affects her recovery as well as the family members' ability to cope with the illness. Words and actions should reassure the breast cancer patient of love, concern, and support without diminishing her feeling of competency and without emphasizing her dependence on them. Most important is that the family communicate unified support and hope to the woman and to one another. Methods are suggested for communicating more effectively to convey support and to resolve sensitive issues. The needs of children should not be overlooked. They should be informed and helped to express their feelings.

In the next chapter we address the concept of coping and the resources that are available to families. The individual can draw from his or her physical, psychological, and competency resources as well as material, community, and professional resources. We review coping strategies of families who have low amounts of stress and Lerner's theory for managing anxiety. The charactcristics of good copers and coping strategies reported by woman and spouses in our study are also discussed.

Chapter 10

Coping with the Breast Cancer Experience

Donna Sargeant felt her life was falling apart when her husband told her he was leaving her. Finding breast cancer was another major blow that put her at risk of losing her life and her job. Her husband's insistence on proceeding with a divorce further demoralized her. She had hoped he would consider reconciliation after her breast cancer was diagnosed. Their children were her greatest concern, particularly her 11-year-old son, who was having stomach pains and problems with school attendance. Her daughter, age 13, appeared to be blocking out her feelings. Donna herself was experiencing brief periods of panic and depression. Discouraged about her health, she worried about her self-image, her sexuality, and how she would support her children.

How was she handling this stress? First, being a nurse, she sought information about the disease and the help of a counselor. She took charge of her life and, fortunately, had several friends with whom she could talk frequently, as well as a very supportive family. She began attending a support group. However, she indicated that she was using alcohol to help her cope.

Another woman, Laura Mills, owner of her own business, called her staff together, explained her diagnosis and radiation treatment, and told them she did not want them to treat her any differently than before the illness. She expected them to carry on in their normal manner as she would do. Laura had accepted the fact that she had breast cancer, but she still experienced disbelief that it had happened to her.

In another instance, Lynn Robbins, to whom we introduced you in the discussion of anger, let out her feelings and cried "buckets of tears." Then, as time passed, her outlook changed and she drew on her sense of humor to get through some of the most difficult periods.

Having had large breasts and being very comfortable with her body image prior to the surgery, Lynn had difficulty accepting her loss. In fact, she was not able to look at her body in a mirror after her double mastectomy.

Although she didn't have reconstructive surgery immediately, Lynn never considered not having it. Then, after she had the tissue expansion, the next procedure was to reopen her breasts to insert the implants. The day she was scheduled for this operation she was particularly apprehensive and decided to lighten things up in a dramatic way. After the nurse showed her into the operating room, she pulled from a bag an inflated bosom which, with the nurse's help, she attached over her chest. The IVs were inserted and Lynn, covered with a sheet, was lying on the operating table when an attending physician, whom she had never seen, entered. He observed the large mounds but maintained a straight face and noncommittal manner. Then the plastic surgeon entered, looked at her, and said, "Okay, lady, sit up." As Lynn did so the sheet fell to her waist, exposing her enormous plastic falsies. A camera clicked (the nurse had slipped out to get it), and the attending physician's face relaxed in relief that the job was much smaller than it had looked. Both men broke up in laughter. Lynn knew that her surgeon, who has a good sense of humor, would appreciate her prank, and indeed he did!

As we know, the woman with breast cancer must cope with many problems associated with the disease. Making decisions about treatment can be very upsetting when physicians whom she is consulting have differing opinions about the best procedure for her. She must cope with acceptance of the illness, uncertainties about her future and mortality. She must contend with the grief of physical changes and losses. She may also be worried about finances and, perhaps, employment if she has to give up her job.[1] Because the family is affected, coping also becomes a "collection of individual responses" and certain strategies will require input from most or all of its members.[2]

THE CONCEPT OF COPING

In an earlier chapter we defined coping as the efforts people make to tolerate physical, emotional, and psychological stress. Coping is what one does to avoid being harmed by life-strains. Weisman and Sobel describe it as "an active problem-solving process" in contrast to defending oneself by avoiding a problem.[3] It is viewed by some researchers as a process because a person's efforts change as the stresses of the situation increase or diminish. Marked alterations in a person's behavior can indicate that the stress is overtaxing his or her normal mode of coping.

As we have discussed, illness often becomes a crisis because it disrupts established routines and life-styles. Stressful events that happen quickly allow no time to plan how we will cope, whereas it is possible to prepare for other events in advance. An immediate response of denial when crisis occurs gives us time before we consider more rational strategies. Moreover, how we meet a problem the first time may not be the same on later encounters.

In a crisis our habitual ways of solving problems are often inadequate for restoring our sense of balance, and we experience fear, guilt, and other unpleasant emotions. The tasks imposed by the cancer involve managing the symptoms of the disease, the stresses of treatment and hospital procedures, and negotiating relationships with health care providers, family, and friends. In addition, we must handle the disturbing feelings associated with the illness and adjust to an uncertain outcome and the threat of losses. These tasks require coping skills that relate to both emotions and problem solving.[4]

Coping behavior can be protective in several ways.[5] It can eliminate or change the conditions causing the problems. It can alter the meaning of the experience, and it can control or manage the emotional consequences of problems. For example, fatigue is a problem for a woman with breast cancer. The fatigue cannot be eliminated without sufficient time for recuperation, but family members can cooperate in assuming the patient's duties until she is able to regain her strength. What the breast cancer means to the woman and her family can be changed by looking at it as a challenge rather than a tragedy. Many families have used the experience as an opportunity to grow closer and appreciate one another. Family members can cope with emotional consequences by sharing feelings, working together to maintain a positive outlook, attending a support group, or seeking professional help.

A woman's first coping efforts, as we have noted, are self-protective; this enables her to deal with the shock. As you recall, denial is the most common of these defense mechanisms, which include stoicism-fatalism, projection, displacement, faith, and prayer. Problem-solving efforts, such as obtaining information and seeking other opinions, are rational actions that help in making decisions about managing the event. As we saw in the case of Ann Schneider, the two kinds of coping can facilitate or hinder one another.

Coping also encompasses the resources that are available to persons and the strategies they use that make up their normal coping traits. Families are constantly facing stresses and strains to which they must adjust in the normal course of life. Many families manage these challenges amazingly well. However, difficulties arise when their resources and coping strategies are inadequate for the situation.

From the stories of Donna, Laura, and Lynn, we see that for the most part they have used problem-solving strategies that helped them to tolerate, minimize, and accept the stress. Emotional strategies, such as releasing feelings by crying or talking about them, are essential; but then a person should move on to confront problems directly. The person needs to redefine the problems so she can return to a "new" normalcy in life. Coping with emotions by using alcohol, as Donna did, could interfere with rational thinking, develop into a dependency, and lead to harmful interactions with prescribed medications.

RESEARCH ON COPING

For many years researchers have studied the coping problems of families who have undergone the stress of war, the Great Depression, unemployment, chronic illnesses, and other such events. They are now studying the families who cope successfully to determine what strengths and resources increase their ability to do so. For example, family researchers Olson and McCubbin have examined the stresses that occur in each of the life-cycle stages. They have classified the stages as (1) young couples without children, (2) families with very young and school-age children, (3) those with adolescents and children being launched into independent lives, (4) empty nest couples, and (5) retired couples. Families, especially those with more than one child, are going through several or all of these stages at the same time.[6] The changes that occur in the family life cycle occur to most families, can be expected, and are usually short-term. Stresses occur with each transition.

Olson and McCubbin asked husbands and wives to identify the stresses they had experienced during the year prior to their participation in the study. Financial and business stressors were found to underlie many of the strains that persisted throughout all stages of the family cycle. Medical and dental expenses, job and career changes, loss of employment, retirement, family illnesses, and death were other common stressors that they identified. A rather persistent strain experienced in many families resulted from the father's absence. As would be expected, pregnancy can be a major stressor during the childbearing years. Having children leave and return home is a strain in the launching stage.

When normal stresses are unresolved and an unpredictable crisis event—such as a life-threatening illness—occurs, the family must contend with a "pile-up" of difficulties.[7] Many of us have experienced these periods in our lives, and they have been trying times. A crisis threatens our family relationships, roles, communication patterns, individual and family goals, as well as our feelings about the changes that the crisis entails.[8] What resources do family members draw upon in order to cope?

Physical, Psychological, and Competency Resources

As family researchers point out, the number of resources is impossible to catalogue but major categories have been identified. First are the physical, psychological, and competency properties of a person: health and energy, positive beliefs, and problem-solving and social skills. Health and energy are particularly important when the stressful problems, such as chronic illnesses, endure over time or when the situation is extremely demanding. Coping is certainly easier when one feels well, but the ill person has less energy for coping than other healthy family members. However, a number of researchers have observed that people who are weak and ill have a surprising capability for coping "when the stakes are high enough."[9]

An important psychological resource is to have a positive regard for one's self. A sense of confidence and mastery of skills is formulated on the beliefs that we have constructed from authority figures, experience, and efforts to find meaning in life. Feeling good about ourself increases our confidence that we have some control over an event, and it affects the way we view that event.[10] If we have a sense of control, we may be more likely to approach the crisis with hopefulness than with helplessness.[11] This will reduce its impact.

For example, some women react to the diagnosis of breast cancer with an attitude that it is their fate. Others react optimistically, with conviction that they have some control over their bodies and confidence in their medical team. They have a hopeful outlook as well as a strong sense of survival.

Competencies, the third set of resources identified by Lazarus and Folkman, are the rational, problem-solving skills that we use. We get information about problems, then weigh it before making decisions and taking a course of action. To illustrate, Beth Evans, who was diagnosed with breast cancer several years ago, obtained as much information as she could before deciding on treatment. She learned that a mastectomy was not the only treatment option available to her and chose to have a lumpectomy. To make sure she did not awaken to find her breast had been removed, she signed papers requesting the doctors' compliance with her wishes. Beth also did not want chemotherapy and learned that she could have iridium implants. By employing the skills she had developed through her experience, knowledge, and ability to think critically, Beth had taken control of her disease.

Social skills make up another form of competency. These include one's ability to communicate with others and behave toward them in an effective, appropriate manner. In the case of illness, as more medical information is being made available to the general public, patients are insisting on being involved in their own health care. Professional caregivers are becoming more open to this change. This makes competence in social skills very important.

Material Resources

In addition to the resources that are properties of the person, material resources are a part of coping. With the high cost of medical care, people with money are better able to afford the professional goods and services they need. In most situations, having an adequate income and insurance coverage increases the ability to cope. Knowing that we have comprehensive insurance and sufficient funds to take care of expenses not covered by insurance can alleviate worry and increase options for treatment.

Cancer care is expensive. One woman said she could never have afforded her medication had she not been working and had her own insurance. Some women have changed their insurance to a carrier that would pay for reconstructive surgery. Because they consider reconstruction to be cosmetic surgery, some companies do not cover it. When the cancer recurs and expensive treatment extends over a long period of time, a family's financial resources can be depleted. Several families we have interviewed have been forced into bankruptcy by the high cost of treatment and loss of employment.

If you have problems with insurance, read *Cancervive* by Susan Nessim and Judith Ellis. These authors have compiled information and resources about medical insurance that should be helpful. See Appendix A for more information about the book.

Community and Professional Resources

A number of agencies and professional programs and services are available for women and their families, some specifically for families with limited income. These agencies provide information, counseling, and support for individuals and family members.

An example of a family-centered program was the weekend retreat held for cancer patients and their families by the Cancer Services of North Memorial Medical Center in Minnesota in the 1970s. Families attending the weekend retreat participated in various social, informational, and physical activities to increase morale and develop friendships. The aim of the program was to improve family problem-solving techniques, strengthen self-esteem, and increase interaction skills.[12] Whether that program was continued is not known, but many support programs have been developed for women with breast cancer. Attention is also being paid to the needs of children and spouses. With the increased awareness of the psychosocial effects of cancer, more family-oriented programs may be appearing.

Social Support

The support received from family, friends, and community is considered to be one of the most important resources for coping with illness. For this reason supportiveness is the subject of the next chapter.

PERSONAL AND ENVIRONMENTAL CONSTRAINTS

Sometimes resources are available but pride or certain other constraints in a person's belief system and cultural values may inhibit him or her from seeking assistance.[13] An example is the cultural norm and the stigma that causes women to be secretive about cancer. A friend told us of her mother who had not revealed to her family that there was something wrong with her breast. When the other breast developed symptoms, she finally sought medical help. By then the breast cancer had become very advanced. In this case, the lack of pain enabled the woman to endure and hide the disease. As we become more enlightened about breast cancer, we hope women will no longer feel secretive or stigmatized by breast cancer and realize the importance of early treatment.

Other constraints against disclosing breast cancer may be that a woman lacks insurance, is too intimidated to seek help, or does not know how to go about getting it. Some women may not know how to find help. Assistance is available if women will seek help through local family or social services such as Cancer Care, Inc. (See Resources, Appendix B).

FAMILY COPING STRATEGIES

In the same manner that they identified stressors, Olson and McCubbin investigated important coping resources of families who experienced stress, but only in low amounts. Although coping resources varied somewhat in each life stage of these "low-stress" families, some resources occurred frequently. Among them were family accord, satisfaction with financial management, and communication. These families also expressed satisfaction with their health practices, child rearing, and the support they received from family. In addition, "low-stress" families tended to have a supportive social network as well as leisure activities they shared. Couples had resolved personality issues and were satisfied with their marital and sexual relationship. Finally, families with "low stress" had a positive view of the quality of their lives.[14]

Although each individual uses specific strategies to protect or manage his or her stress, the nature of the family unit requires that their efforts be cooperative. Consider the following illustration. To cope with their mother's illness a teenaged son may increase his physical activities, a daughter may withdraw from friends and spend more time at home, and the spouse may cut back on his overtime hours at work. Each is coping individually. Collectively they agree that they will work together on cleaning the house, preparing the meals, and spending specific times together to discuss their needs and share their feelings.

A THEORY FOR COPING WITH ANXIETY AND LOWERING STRESS

In her book *The Dance of Intimacy*, Dr. Harriet Lerner, a staff psychologist at the Menninger Clinic, applies the systems theory to explain the complexities of family relationships and the management of anxiety. The family system, which we discussed briefly in the chapter on relationships, is in a continuous process of maintaining its unity and of developing independence and individuality. Families vary greatly in the degrees of connectedness and separateness they allow and achieve.

Even as the family, with its individual systems and subsystems, or alliances, is working to stay connected, each member is also striving to develop individuality and self-identity. Guided by traditions, values, and beliefs, members impose limits on one another through spoken and unspoken rules. Between members there is a normal tension resulting from their desire to be both independent and connected with one another.

Conflict can arise when individual and family needs and goals are thwarted or come into conflict. Some members seem to need more space, whereas others want closeness.[15] Some strive to fulfill family goals; others do not. As an example, in a family that emphasized education and professional achievements, the father was asked about his adult children. He proudly enumerated their careers except for one, his oldest. Of him, the father said, "Like the one chick who never cracks open the shell, my oldest son has never left home."

Events, such as life-threatening illnesses, that change the family's normal pattern of functioning increase the tension. Previously unresolved issues can intensify the anxiety that results from the cancer or other stressors. Members may be unaware of the impact of these previous issues, which may be the key to their reactions and coping behaviors. If they repeatedly react in the same unproductive manner, Dr. Lerner calls the predicament a "stuck" position.[16]

Lerner identifies six "stuck" patterns of coping: overfunctioning, underfunctioning, fighting, pursuing, distancing, and other-focusing. For example, the overfunctioner takes charge without regard for his or her other responsibilities or needs. In contrast, the underfunctioner takes a "laid back" approach and lets the others take responsibility.

To illustrate, let's suppose the mother of three daughters has bilateral surgery that entails a longer-than-usual recuperation. The two daughters who are in high school are quite capable of handling the housekeeping chores and are willing to take turns before and after school to meet the family's needs. Their father can arrange for a visiting nurse or a friend who has offered to help during school hours. However, Mary, who is away at college, insists that she drop out of school for the rest of the quarter and come home to take care of things. Although her father insists that it is neither necessary nor advisable, she quits school, comes home, and takes over. Mary is an overfunctioner.

Her sisters now do very little to help Mary and become more involved in activities outside the home. In this situation, they become underfunctioners. Two younger sons in the family cope by fighting and, thus, add to the tension.

The other reactive patterns—distancing, pursuing, and other-focusing—can be demonstrated by another family experiencing breast cancer. In this instance, the mother chooses to have immediate reconstructive surgery, to which her husband is opposed. As she pursues or tries harder to convince him, he begins to withdraw from her. The more she insists, the more distant he becomes. She accuses him of not caring about her feelings. He begins to turn his attention to their teenaged son, who is having behavior problems at school. In this situation the mother is reacting by pursuing, and her husband retreats from her and focuses on a son who is "acting out" his anxiety by making trouble.

Understanding and Changing Our Reactions

To break these unproductive patterns of dealing with anxiety, Lerner suggests that the only person one can change is the self. She advocates looking at one's own strengths and vulnerabilities rather than dwelling on the behaviors and faults of the other person. In the case of the couple who disagree on reconstructive surgery, they should remain emotionally connected and examine other stresses that may be coloring their reactions. They should clarify their positions with one another. If she is not too emotionally upset to think rationally, the wife may become aware that she fears that the loss of her breast will shatter her self-esteem, which has never been strong. Her spouse may also examine his vulnerabilities and gain insight into his reactions. Because his former wife had died after a recurrence of breast cancer, he may fear that reconstruction will increase the likelihood of recurrence or make recurrent cancer difficult to detect.

How can this couple regain the closeness that both of them need? By empathizing and showing concern for one another and disclosing their fears, the couple can begin to understand one another's positions.

Why We React as We Do

Because reactions are often triggered by past experiences or parental views and coping patterns learned early in life, examination of our reactions can help us to understand them.[17] In the example of the family just described, the husband may withdraw because, as a child, he learned his behavior from a father who gave his wife the silent treatment when he couldn't impose his will on her. Then his father focused his attention on one of the children.

Other forces that intensify our reactions are current stresses that we are ignoring or have failed to resolve. We may be dissatisfied with a job or a relationship. We may not have worked through our grief after the death of someone close to us. We may hold resentment toward a parent who has never shown us warmth or love. Children may feel that they are not accepted by their peers, or that siblings are favored by their parents. The point is that each family member reacts differently because each has different experiences that shape his or her perceptions of a situation.

Dr. Lerner's Suggestions

Lerner suggests that we can work toward changing our reactions by examining our beliefs, values, and goals. The daughter who insisted on dropping out of college to run things at home may have done so because she really wasn't doing well in school and wasn't sure about what she wanted to do with her life. In other words, if her goals for herself had been clear, she may have realized that it was best for her to let the family manage without her and prepare herself to be financially independent.

Lerner's next step in changing is to take a position of responsibility and have a plan of action. For instance, the spouse who opposes his wife's reconstructive surgery should verbalize his fears and say something like this: "I understand how important your appearance is to your self-esteem. I want you to know that the loss of a breast will not affect my feelings for you and I will support you in whatever decision you make. I do have one condition: that you get another physician's opinion and consider this very carefully. This is a very tough decision for you, but I know you will make the right one."

Putting into practice Dr. Lerner's suggestions for changing our ways of coping with anxiety may seem impossible when we are emotionally upset. It will be particularly difficult for the patient whose illness puts her at the low end of the marital seesaw. A sensitive, empathic spouse can take the lead and help both of them through this process.

CHARACTERISTICS OF GOOD COPERS

Because of the varied circumstances, the wide range of coping behaviors, and the time at which they are observed, as well as other factors, there is much on the subject of coping that remains to be explored. The theories and findings we offer here represent the work of respected researchers whose observations are helpful in understanding the challenges of life-strains.

Before we summarize the resources and strategies that are characteristic of good copers, it should be noted that coping strategies are judged to have value if they work.[18] In other words, they work when they help members to manage the stress and enable a family to function satisfactorily. Olson and McCubbin suggest that stressful events occurring in the earlier stages of life can be managed best by acknowledging responsibilities and taking charge. In later stages of life, it is more helpful to accept circumstances and be less reactive.[19]

Other methods of coping are suggested by researchers. Pearlin and Schooler found self-reliance to be "more effective in reducing stress than seeking of help and advice," especially in family relationships.[20] McCubbin and associates studied coping patterns of wives during long wartime separations. The researchers found that women who coped most successfully directed their actions toward strengthening their individual resources.[21] Others who have studied stress have found that informal support networks of family, friends, and co-workers are valuable resources for coping with it.[22] Lazarus and Folkman consider a person's appraisal of a situation to be a crucial factor. Persons who see the event as a challenge will put forth great effort to maintain a positive outlook and substantial effort.[23] This supports Lipowski's observation that viewing an illness as a challenge "inspires generally adaptive coping strategies."[24] There is considerable agreement among researchers that good copers are flexible and can adapt to change. Good copers also draw from a wide range of resources and strategies.

THERAPISTS' SUGGESTIONS FOR COPING

What do therapists who have helped patients cope with critical and prolonged illnesses suggest for survival? For individual coping, Simonton et al. advocate regular physical exertion and some form of mental concentration. That can be meditation, relaxation, self-hypnosis, or imagery, in which one visualizes a positive expectation. They claim that these combined activities will decrease fear, change attitudes, and strengthen the "will to live" and the immune system. They will also decrease stress. For coping with the fear of recurrence and death, therapists suggest that we confront the fear and examine our feelings and attitudes about it. They recommend a six-week program of exercise, reading, relaxation, and mental imagery during which one examines the cancer's stresses and benefits.[25]

In *The Healing Family*, Simonton and Shook suggest that family members, including young children, work as a team to develop a family game plan. They should set goals and focus their energy in a positive direction. The patient, unless too ill, should be the team captain. Members can maintain a file of information they gather on medical treatment, psychological and community resources, nutrition, exercise, and other pertinent data. They should share an attitude of hope, which can be reinforced by finding a physician whose belief system matches theirs and whose competence gives them confidence. Therapists also stress the importance of each member taking care of themselves, increasing physical touch, and respecting each person's autonomy. A very practical suggestion is that some family member always accompany the patient to the doctor with a tape recorder or notepad for taking notes.[26]

In a study of families with breast cancer, Thorne found that those who coped effectively had a general family philosophy in regard to the cancer experience. Although they used a variety of coping methods, these families have strived to maintain family dignity and normalcy. The confidence they have had in their medical care providers helped them maintain a "positive attitude" of acceptance and hope.[27]

Beverly Kievman, whose husband died of diabetes after a long period of debilitation, also advocated making a plan and working to keep one's own balance. She kept a private notebook in which she wrote her feelings and shared with her husband the anger she felt toward the illness, not toward him. Her honesty, she believes, gave him the dignity of being treated as an equal in their relationship. In a second notebook Kievman listed questions about the illness and tasks that needed to be done. She called it her action plan.

Hardest of all for her, Kievman admitted, was coping with the "foreverness" of the long and difficult illness that had completely altered their lives.[28] Dick and Beth Thornton, who fought breast cancer for over ten years, also described their most difficult coping effort as the "foreverness" of it.

In their book *Compassion and Self-Hate: An Alternative to Despair*, the Rubins tell us that knowing and accepting the fact that life is tough makes living easier. They also remind us that human beings are strong and resourceful. They believe that fighting for the right to fail increases our flexibility and enables us to bend under adversity without breaking.[29]

EXAMPLES OF COPING

Throughout these chapters we have referred to a number of coping behaviors. We close this discussion by sharing more of the resources used by the women we have interviewed. Kathy Mayer, whose cancer was diagnosed just after the birth of her baby, was helped by the positive attitude of her husband and the comment of a friend. The friend said, "It doesn't matter how long it would be, two or two hundred years; if I were going to worry every day about cancer, I wouldn't be *living* my life. To the best of my ability I would have to assume things were going to be fine, then live my life as I would want to live it." The friend's words made a strong impression on Kathy, who took a new perspective about what she wants to do with her life. She has reorganized her priorities and decided that she will pursue her career with less intensity. When I last saw her, she looked radiant and happy.

Joy Martin, a naturally exuberant person, said that her father had instilled in her "the work ethic and need to keep busy. When you come from stock like that, you develop a get-up-and-go, fighting spirit." Joy coped with the loss of both breasts by searching for the positive things in her experience and helping others with breast cancer. She, too, has re-evaluated her goals and takes career disappointments more philosophically than she did previously.

Gertrude Strader tried to keep her mind occupied and went on with her life. Seeing others who were worse off than she made her realize that she was fortunate. In Cynthia Ruether's case, her survival instinct and the need to take control of her life helped her to cope. "You never know what you can do until you go through it," she said.

Rachel Dunne, who demonstrated great inner strength through her divorce and son's suicide, was determined not to let things "totally throw her." She has taken a pro-active approach to her health and, as the Simontons have advocated, directed her energy toward new challenges and personal growth.

When we first met Margaret Muncy she and her husband were still adjusting to the shock of her breast cancer and the feeling that this was one of the worst things that could have happened to them. Margaret was doing well when she had a terrible fall down her basement steps and narrowly missed striking her head on a sharp object, which could have cost her her life. As it was, she was almost immobilized with a broken arm and other serious injuries. Recuperation was far more difficult than her breast surgery had been. She was tempted to give up the struggle, she said, when someone reminded her that "no one dies from a broken arm." That gave her the determination to pull together all of her forces and get through it. She drew strength from relaxation and visualization techniques as well as her religious faith. On our last visit she recounted the mishaps that had brought her to the realization that there could be things worse than breast cancer.

How did spouses cope? Jack Young said that he and Shelley did a great deal of reading about breast cancer, the options and the procedures. He believed that gaining knowledge and realizing that they had to accept the illness had helped him. Mark Taylor, in his effort to reach out to his wife, almost reached the point of despair until they were finally able to talk openly with one another. In the case of the Mayers, Alan took an optimistic view and firmly believed that Kathy would be fine. Some men refused to dwell on it and went on with life, whereas others helped their wives by making plans for the future.

Coping is a complex concept that is related to personal factors such as age, beliefs, and self-regard. According to researcher Bandura, good coping results from mastering challenging tasks, which in turn develops one's competence and the expectation of a good outcome.[30] Effective coping also consists of using practical, realistic ways of solving problems and of being resourceful in getting information and support. In addition, we cope more effectively if we draw from material, community, and professional resources that are available to us. We can change unproductive strategies of coping by applying the suggestions of therapists and those who exemplify good coping.

The life-strains experienced by many of the women whose stories we relate have tested their resources and coping skills. Common to most of them has been their inner strength and the support they have received from family and friends.

In the next chapter we explain what it means to be supportive and receive support. Of course, the woman who has breast cancer needs the most support while undergoing treatment. However, she also has a responsibility in making known her needs and in giving support to her family members. By maintaining as much independence as she can, she will aid in her recuperation. The voluntary support of friends and extended family as well as support groups and community resources can relieve stress for an overworked spouse and children. Suggestions are given for friends who will listen and do the thoughtful little things that say "I care."

Chapter 11

Supportiveness of Family, Friends, and Community

From his years of experience in treating many patients with breast cancer, Dr. Clinton Ervin observed that every woman experiences some emotional trauma. He found that the long-term damage a woman suffers depends on the support of family and friends as well as her inner resources and a caring, supportive physician.[1] Because considerable research verifies the positive effects of supportiveness, this important resource has been studied extensively.

Most studies have found that people who have close personal relationships during illness are more likely to cope effectively than those who do not have such relationships.[2] The social support she receives helps a woman having a mastectomy to make a better adjustment.[3]

Ronnie Kaye, a psychotherapist, learned the importance of support when she had a mastectomy and then a recurrence. The experience was so traumatic for her that her emotional recovery was long and difficult. In her fight to recover she reached out to people who would understand and treat her "gently." She discovered that many people feel uncomfortable and are "completely unaware of how to be supportive or helpful."[4]

What does it mean to be supportive? We are supportive when we give a person the feeling that he or she is accepted, loved, and needed. Support conveys that a person is valued and is a part of a network with which he or she has mutual obligation and understanding.[5] Keeping in mind the feeling we want to instill, let's examine ways in which family members and friends can give support to a loved one who is fighting an illness that could take her life.

Because of the potential erosion of a woman's self-esteem and sexual identity, we know that her husband's or partner's support is crucial. Being keenly aware of the spouse's role, Dr. Ervin developed an approach for helping women manage the complex problems of mastectomy. In each step he involved the woman's husband or partner. Several days after the surgery he asked the husband to come to his office, where he explained the effect of the mastectomy on his wife's femininity, her fear of his rejection, her depression, and her need for reassurance of his love. Ervin stressed the importance of the husband taking her hand, telling her that he loves her, and assuring her that "a change in contour is not going to matter." Ervin realized this is not easy for many husbands and also knew that when a husband does not make this move, "the road ahead is rough!"[6]

The spouse's support and physical contact becomes even more important during treatment if his wife's condition is critical. Critically ill patients have a greater desire and need for the comfort of touch and closeness even though the desire for sexual intercourse may decrease.[7]

Dr. Ervin provided spouses with comforting words. But what of those men who find it too difficult to express their feelings verbally, even with Dr. Ervin's comforting words? A nonverbal message, such as a hug, can convey their feelings. In 1971, when Marvella Bayh, whose husband Birch was then senator from Indiana, was told that she had breast cancer, he took her in his arms and wept. After the mastectomy, when her greatest fear was that he would be repulsed by her disfigurement, he assured her that nothing had changed. "Do you think I married you for your breasts?" he asked her. "I married you for who you are."[8]

THE WOMAN'S RESPONSIBILITY

Women, especially those who are trying to be brave and strong, may not be making their needs known. When psychotherapist Kaye had breast cancer, she realized that she needed to take the responsibility of expressing her needs and of asking for help. When she was recovering from her mastectomy, she felt she had no privacy and too many visitors who meant well but saw her at her worst. She felt resentful about that experience, and when she had her recurrence she decided she could do something about it. She called family members and friends and told them that she would be going through a difficult time. She explained that she was feeling "very alone" and "terribly frightened" and would need their help. She asked them to call her at least once a week and tell her that her being alive "mattered" to them. They responded to her request. Each day during her recovery she received phone calls that reminded her she was loved. The calls were a great source of comfort. By making her needs known, a woman with breast cancer can help those who want to reach out to her but don't know how.[9]

WHAT THE SPOUSE AND FAMILY MEMBERS CAN DO

First, it is important to establish "honest, open communication" and then to accept the patient's mood swings.[10] As Nancy Brinker noted, "This is a disease that makes a person feel completely out of control."[11] Lynn Robbins described the loss of her breasts as such an emotionally draining process that the emotions sometimes outweighed the physical trauma.

Anger, fear, and helplessness can overwhelm the woman with breast cancer. She needs to be allowed and encouraged to express her feelings even though they are painful for loved ones to hear. At the same time the family can express their anxieties and help the patient to sort out what is real. Sometimes all the ill person needs is for someone to listen without judging or telling her that she should not have the feelings she has. As the Simontons have observed with their patients, "the willingness to go through this experience with their loved one" is the most important kind of support a family can give.[12]

If a woman is "emotionally distraught," the Simontons suggest that you ask if there is anything you can do. Should she reply "you can take this damned cancer" or "leave me alone," or other words to that effect, you will probably feel angry and upset. Your natural inclination may be to make an angry retort or walk away. Try to empathize with what she is feeling and explain that you understand her frustration but that you are hurt by her reply. If she does make requests that are unreasonable, explain why you cannot fill them, and then continue to provide lots of closeness.[13]

Often a woman with breast cancer will endure the crisis without crying; and psychotherapist Kaye says that it's "perfectly okay" not to cry. However, weeks or months later, she may experience anxiety attacks, cry easily, and feel very lonely. That, too, is normal. As Kaye explains, "cancer is a lonely disease." The woman should be helped to realize that the grief she feels may not be entirely for the loss of her breast. It can result, in part, from unresolved grief, such as a death or some other loss or change in her life— as was the case with Rachel Dunne, who realized she was still grieving for her son. Grief becomes more bearable when we understand it and let ourselves express it.[14]

Husbands and partners do not always understand why a woman, once recovered from treatment, continues to worry about her health. Sandy Palmer told me that her husband rather impatiently asked her why she could not put the disease behind her and go on with life as he was doing. Her reply was, "Every six months I have to go in for a check-up, and each time there is the possibility of finding more cancer cells. That thought terrifies me and will be with me for the rest of my life." However, as time passes, Sandy finds that she worries less.

Instead of giving support, some men react to their spouses' anxiety in a destructive way, as did the son-in-law of Betty Williams. When her daughter Constance got upset over her mother's breast cancer, her husband became angry. Not only does Constance have to conceal her feelings, but she finds it difficult to talk with her husband. Fortunately, she has a sister with whom she can talk and brother-in-law who is supportive of all of them.

Family members tend to adjust better themselves if they assist the patient in her tasks, such as exercises prescribed for arm mobility. However, it is important for the patient to become as self-sufficient as possible, so family members should avoid rescuing her, thus making her dependent and helpless. Nor should they interfere with her right to make her own decisions and with her methods of coping.[15] The patient will make a better recovery if she uses her own resources, if her family rewards her with encouragement, and if she feels that she is providing support as well as receiving it.

Another important supportive endeavor is to help the patient anticipate the future and involve her in activities outside of her illness. For example, when Beth's breast cancer was diagnosed, the Thorntons were told that it had metastasized so much that the outcome for her was bleak. She and her husband decided that while she was able, they would do the things they had planned. Their first trip was a tour of Europe. After that, they traveled by car so they could stop when she needed rest, and visited many places in the United States. As the cancer progressed, they made weekend trips within 100 miles of their home. As she became more confined, they traveled vicariously by reading books together. They also kept in close touch with family members, who willingly carried out the plans Beth made for family gatherings. Setting goals and making plans helped the Thorntons prolong and enjoy her life far beyond the expectation of her physician when her breast cancer was first diagnosed.

Ann Jillian's husband, Andy Murcia, and his friend Bob Stewart have also made suggestions for ways that the husband can be supportive. He can strengthen his religious faith, be ready to make changes, see that she gets exercise and good nutrition, and fight his own stress and depression. He can also help her take care of her appearance.[16]

Another means of being supportive is to share experiences and lighten the serious with humor, as Daniel Sherwood, the minister in our study, did. When Kay Sherwood had breast cancer, she and Daniel decided that he should tell their congregation (which they regarded as their huge family) what was happening. During the Sunday service he explained their week's events, from Kay's mammogram and diagnosis through the medical consultations and her mastectomy. He concluded by saying, "Some of you have already asked what you can do to help us. I have made a list of suggestions for you. There will be washing and ironing and the housecleaning, window washing, and so forth. We'll be grateful for your help." His tongue-in-cheek humor drew chuckles from the congregation and broke the somber mood.

Later the Sherwoods learned that as a result of sharing their experience with candidness and humor, a large number of women went for mammograms over the next few months. When Kay recovered, she became active with Reach to Recovery so that she could help women who were diagnosed with breast cancer. In this way she has fulfilled her own need to provide support.

Family members can maintain their supportiveness if they take care of their own needs so that they do not become burned out and resentful of the sacrifices they make. Because information gives them understanding and confidence, they may find support groups that provide this resource. It is also important to seek close friends outside the family with whom they can talk.

Good relationships outside the family can help relieve the stress for families. In fact, in a study of school children, Rutter found that good relationships with peers and other adults can lessen effects of stress.[17] It is wise to turn to more than one friend for comfort, as it may be too stressful for one person and may cause him or her to withdraw support.

BEING A SUPPORTIVE FRIEND

Recently a colleague and good friend, with whom I had worked over the years and who had given us assistance on our study, died of cancer. His cancer first occurred a number of years ago. Therefore, he had great interest in our work. After we completed our study, I learned that his cancer had recurred and I called him immediately. Not quite sure of what to say or do, I expressed my dismay at hearing he was ill. He immediately put me at ease by telling me about the seriousness of his condition and his hope that the cancer could be arrested long enough for him to complete a project he had undertaken. He told me how much he appreciated the concern and support of family and friends. Because of his selflessness and generosity with anyone who sought his expertise, Roger was rich in friendships. There were some who avoided him because they didn't know what to do or say, but he understood and was deeply appreciative of those who reached out to him. They, in fact, received far more from him than they had given.

Joan Parker, co-author of *Three Weeks in Spring*, described the occasion when two friends visited her in the hospital. Not knowing what to expect of Joan's appearance or attitude, they walked into her room hesitantly, then "burst into tears." Joan said they had conveyed the powerful message that they cared.[18]

Amy Harwell, who had cervical cancer, found friends so important that she has written a book, *When Your Friend Gets Cancer*, to help friends know what to do and say. Harwell's first advice is to examine how you feel about cancer and your friendship. Friends who look upon cancer as a death sentence or as a contagious disease may not be helpful to the patient, who needs hope and acceptance. Harwell suggests that a friend needs to know how much time and energy she really wants to give to the friendship and how much it means to her. Friends with a negative attitude can say unkind or thoughtless things and act in a hurtful way.[19] Marie Wernke told us about a friend who recounted the stories of women who had died of breast cancer.

The thoughtless friend added to the fears that Marie was already experiencing.

During her husband's long illness, Beverly Kievman categorized friends according to the depth of their support. Among her husband's close friends were some who didn't come around or stay in touch. His closest friend was the most disappointing. He disappeared, making only "stilted," infrequent telephone calls. During one of those calls Kievman told him of the hurt they felt over his avoidance. They both began to cry, and the friend confessed that he was ashamed. He felt deeply about her husband but was unable to deal with his illness. Kievman's confrontation helped him to express his feelings, and he became a great support to her and her husband before his death.[20] Unfortunately, some friends do drop us when life becomes rough for us.

Harwell's most emphatic advice for friends is to reach out immediately and boldly.[21] The person with breast cancer has a need for support that is as great or greater than for any other illness. The stigma of cancer makes her feel alienated. She can cope with this feeling of alienation if family, friends, and health care providers make an effort to let her know she is important.[22]

A number of women have commented on the rejection of others. Marianne Stevens said that at first, her friends treated her as though she had the bubonic plague. Her doctor, who had prostrate cancer, told her that he had a similar reaction from his friends. When Marianne sensed that a friend was uncomfortable, she handled the situation by breaking the tension and bringing up the subject of her cancer herself.

Friends can help a woman cope with the "loss of control" she feels and her fears of death.[23] They can reach out with phone calls, prayers, cards, visits, flowers, and offers to help her as well as her family. One woman who was recuperating from her mastectomy was especially touched by the thoughtfulness of a friend who left a small package for her at the end of her visit. In it was a prosthesis (a bra filled with a breast form) for her to wear when she went home from the hospital. June Nelson, another woman who had undergone a mastectomy, also had a considerate friend who herself had recovered from the loss of a breast. When June returned home from the hospital, her friend came to see her and brought a soft prosthesis, balls attached to a string to exercise her arm, and literature about caring for her incision. Having an active person who had experienced breast cancer come to see her gave June the encouragement that she needed that day. As Mindy Bishop said, "Just knowing friends are there is a tremendous help."

When we ask a friend with breast cancer what we can do to help, the ill friend is more apt to accept a specific and immediate offer than "What can I do?" For example, the offer can be made in a way such as this: "I'm stopping at the drugstore on my way to visit you. Can I bring you anything from there?" Or, "I can arrange any morning of the week to take you for your treatments when you are home. I'd like to do that for you."

The patient also feels supported when friends offer to help with the family's needs. Taking a meal, driving a child someplace, or doing an errand can be a great lift for the stressed caregiver and will reduce the patient's worry about the tasks she is unable to do. As Daniel Preston jestingly told his congregation, there are many things in a household that friends can do.

After she has left the hospital and when she is regaining her strength, the woman recuperating from breast cancer should not be forgotten by friends. She still has the need for support—perhaps an even greater need. She is on her own when she is home, where she faces the reality of the change breast cancer has made in her life. A thoughtful friend can find other resources such as support groups and encourage her to keep busy. She can invite her to lunch or a movie.

Friends can make a difference to those who are unmarried, newly married, or widowed. If she is single, an overnight or weekend visit is especially appreciated. Women in less established marriages need more support than those who have been married for some time. For example, a friend of Mindy Bishop, whose marriage began to crumble after her mastectomy, invited her to spend a couple of weeks visiting her in Florida while Mindy was recovering from her chemotherapy treatments. Also, older women, especially widows, are often very lonely and friends may be their only source of support. For more ways to reach out to them, Harwell's book is full of ideas. Many take very little time, energy, or money and can mean a great deal to someone who needs to know "she matters."

Husbands also need the support of someone who will talk with them. Mark Taylor said he was so upset about his wife that he could not think, was totally unproductive on his job, and "felt as though he was in quicksand." Those from whom he attempted to get help did not respond until he found a former neighbor whose wife had just had a mastectomy. In contrast, Dennis McNeil had a friend who sat with him through the surgery, prayed with him, and let him talk.

SUPPORT GROUPS

Many support groups exist, although some are not easily accessible to women who live in suburban and rural areas. Some women find support groups very helpful, particularly for discovering that many of their feelings and concerns are common to others with breast cancer. Some women, like Evie Simon, think the support groups are "terrific" because you share with those who have also gone through the breast cancer experience. As Sandy Palmer said, "There is a special bond between women who have had breast cancer." However, other women, such as Paula Emerson, prefer to share on a one-to-one basis. Each woman will react differently to support groups and may find that a few meetings are helpful, but beyond that they keep her from moving on. In those cases, the family support system may be sufficiently strong to help her through the rough times.

OTHER COMMUNITY SUPPORT RESOURCES

With the increase in breast cancer, new programs are being formed in communities. Many of these support groups are sponsored by hospitals. You can obtain information by calling your local hospitals.

Organizations such as Cancer Care and I Can Cope offer information and services for breast cancer patients and their families. Local units of the American Cancer Society, which are located in many cities, can give you information on support groups and other resources in your area. If there is no local unit near you, the national headquarters in New York City can be contacted. Also the Office of Cancer Communication of the National Cancer Institute, or the U.S. Department of Health and Human Services, both in Bethesda, Maryland, can provide information. See Appendix B, Resources, for additional programs and services.

A new community resource available in several cities in Ohio is a Family Success Consortium (FSC) formed by a group of psychologists. The Consortium sponsors a program entitled Facing a Cancer Trauma: Psychological Support for Women (FACT). This program for women who are dealing with cancer addresses issues such as coping, psychological distress, self-esteem and femininity, marital and sexual problems, and death and dying. If, in a free initial consultation, the program is not found to be appropriate for those seeking help, referrals to other community organizations are made.

Just as the support of her family and friends is an important resource for the woman's recovery and adjustment, so is it for spouses and family members. It is not uncommon for them to go through periods of depression. As Allan Mayer said, "We have had overwhelming support and that has made a critical difference in our attitudes and ability to cope."

We have defined supportiveness and examined the needs for support that a woman with breast cancer has, as well as her responsibility to make known her needs. We have explored how family members can help her deal with emotions and make other adjustments. By accepting the help of others, keeping a sense of humor, and maintaining some close friendships, family members can give her support without sacrificing their own needs. We conclude with suggestions for being a supportive friend. What follows?

Looking and feeling attractive, the subject of our next chapter, may seem too much effort when a woman is coping with the effects of treatment; but those who have had breast cancer say it is important. Wigs help women to go on with their lives; paying attention to their wardrobes, makeup, diet, and exercise can make them feel better and bolster the morale of their families. In fact, preserving a good image may increase treatment success. We describe a nationwide program, "Look Good, Feel Better," sponsored by the American Cancer Society and two other associations, that helps women look attractive and feel better about themselves. See Appendix B for more information about this program.

Chapter 12

Coping by Looking and Feeling Attractive

When chemotherapy makes you feel nauseous and weak, you hardly have the incentive or energy to worry about your appearance. Looking in the mirror, you see the reflection of someone who has undergone changes that may be distressing to you.

Some chemotherapy drugs cause the loss of hair, which for some women is more devastating than losing a breast. Before undergoing chemotherapy, your oncologist can advise you about certain drugs that do cause hair loss. If you should lose yours, realize that it does grow back. Until it does, you must deal with your feelings about being seen by your family, especially your spouse, and friends.

Fortunately, a variety of wigs are available. You should purchase a wig that matches your hair before beginning your chemotherapy treatments. Many wigs look so natural that others are unaware you don't have your own hair. Some women who find wigs uncomfortable, especially in hot weather, devise becoming ways of tying a scarf around the head. Both solutions to the loss of hair enable you to go on with your life.[1]

Another side effect of chemotherapy that some women experience is weight gain. For example, Sophia, who has had both breasts removed and takes a drug by mouth daily, gained a good deal of weight during her treatment despite her efforts to control it. Mary Lynn Gordon, an athletic person and avid swimmer, could not tolerate the weight she gained. By limiting her caloric intake, eating a balanced diet, and exercising she finally began to return to her normal size. Weight gain may be caused by factors other than drugs used in chemotherapy. Researchers who did a study of the weight gain in women on adjuvant chemotherapy concluded that the gain in half of them could be attributed to fatigue, weakness, and decreased activity rather than the chemotherapy drugs.[2] Not all women gain weight; but those who do find it to be one of the most upsetting effects of breast cancer treatment.

BENEFITS OF MAKING THE EFFORT TO LOOK ATTRACTIVE

Nancy Brinker and others advise women with breast cancer that making themselves look as attractive as possible while undergoing treatment is well worth the effort. Wearing makeup, paying attention to your wardrobe, watching your diet, and doing exercises have their reward. You simply feel better. Brinker noticed that the women who have been most successful in their treatment have made the most effort to preserve a good self-image. If you look as attractive as possible, you will also give a boost to your family and friends. They'll ask fewer anxious questions about how you feel. They'll know you're better because you look it.[3]

"LOOK GOOD, FEEL BETTER" SEMINARS

The American Cancer Society; the Cosmetic, Toiletry, and Fragrance Association; and the National Cosmetology Association Foundation are sponsoring a nationwide program of free seminars, which they call "Look Good, Feel Better," for female patients with cancer.[4] The purpose is to "help women renew self-esteem by enhancing your 'outside' appearance." Certified hairdressers and makeup artists volunteer for training to discuss hygienic guidelines and teach women with cancer the effective use of makeup, wigs, and turbans to look attractive. The volunteers are also trained to promote sensitivity and understanding about what a person with cancer goes through during treatment. Women who take the seminar share information and problems, laugh together, and establish a camaraderie. Each woman goes home with a free bag of cosmetics, supplied by cosmetic companies, and a free wig unless she is happy with her own. Program materials such as information pamphlets and videos are provided without cost to the participants.

Designed to give information and bolster morale, the program has been attended by thousands of patients nationwide. In 1988, pilot programs for this endeavor were tried at the Memorial Sloan-Kettering Cancer Center in New York and at the Vincent T. Lombardi Cancer Research Center in Georgetown University Hospital in Washington, DC. In a short time the program had been developed in forty states, and it continues to expand. In 1990 alone, 20,000 women had the benefit of the program, which is being expanded to include men and children.[5]

An article in a local newspaper featured a "Look Good, Feel Better" seminar at the American Cancer Society with photographs of one woman who was being treated for breast cancer. The before-and-after shots show a dramatic improvement in her appearance. Makeup and a new wig turned her from drab and skeptical into a very pretty and much happier looking woman.[6]

Information about these seminars is included in Appendix B on Resources. If such seminars are not available in your area, a visit to a small shop with a skilled cosmetician who understands the effects of cancer could be worthwhile. A little makeup can conceal spots that appear with chemotherapy, bring out your best features, and generally enhance your appearance. Family members and friends who want to do something for a woman during her recovery can make a gift of cosmetics, cologne, nail polish, a pretty scarf, or some article that will aid her in looking and feeling pretty.

AN EXEMPLARY WOMAN

When Shirley Temple Black was Chief of Protocol under President Ford, I had an interview with her in regard to her public speaking. She had been treated for breast cancer and was one of the first women to go public when she invited the press to her hospital room to tell them about her mastectomy. Her public gesture contributed to the openness about breast cancer that exists today. She also set an example by keeping up her self-image and going on with her life in a constructive manner.

The day we met she greeted me at the door of her office in the State Department building. Dressed in a royal blue suit and standing very tall, she radiated the warmth and vitality that had made her so appealing as a child star. In fact, she was absolutely adorable and I told her so. She beamed and responded to my spontaneous comment by telling me that I was honoring her. Gracious, eager to assist me, she had prepared information that she thought would be useful and shared her plans for the future when her assignment with President Ford would be over.

Anyone who did not know would never have suspected that this vital, attractive woman was the survivor of breast cancer. She had made the effort to preserve her attractiveness and exuded the enthusiasm that comes with feeling good.

We have pointed out the benefits if a woman who is undergoing treatment makes an effort to look her best. Not only will she feel better, but her looking attractive will also be a boost for family and friends. Seminars that aid women in improving their appearance and exchanging experiences with one another are available in some cities.

In the next chapter we consider the problem of medical insurance, filling out forms, understanding and paying bills. Several approaches that may be taken when you are faced with high medical costs are suggested. The professional help of medical social workers and financial advisors who specialize in health care finances is often advisable.

Chapter 13

Coping with Medical Forms and Insurance

Several women have stated that the worst part of their experience with breast cancer was the paperwork, getting bills and insurance straightened out. For example, just prior to learning that she had breast cancer, Betty Williams experienced the death of both parents and her husband. She also suffered complications during her surgery and was forced to resign from her job because of her treatment regimen. For Betty to state emphatically that the medical bills and insurance "mess" were a very difficult part of her breast cancer, the situation had to be serious.

COPING WITH STATEMENTS AND BILLS

How do you make sense of the statements that read, "This is not a bill," and the numerous other pieces of correspondence that you receive from the hospital and physicians? One woman, Phyllis Clarke, who had taken care of the financial matters of family members as well as her own for many years, could not resolve the payment of one bill that was being persistently sent to her. In desperation, she called the bookkeeper where she had been hospitalized for an appointment to get help. The bookkeeper complimented her on the meticulous file she had kept. Statements and receipts from each doctor and institution were matched by number, stapled together, and kept in individual files. By keeping a record of dates, invoices, and payment numbers, Phyllis had found other discrepancies, but this one bill confounded her. Because she had done such a good job of organizing her statements and receipts, the bookkeeper was able to discover the problem rather quickly. The bill should not have been sent to Phyllis at all, but to another patient. Even persons who are accustomed to numbers and complicated forms are frustrated by medical bills and insurance forms.

The cost of cancer care steadily increases. As Mary Lynn Gordon said, "My most agonizing moments were dealing with my insurance company. One time I completely broke down and cried on the telephone," she elaborated, "much to the embarrassment of my secretary. Had I not had a good job, I couldn't have afforded to pay what the treatments cost me after my insurance had taken care of their part."

INSURANCE COVERAGE FOR BREAST CANCER

Not only is it tedious and exasperating to try to understand bills and keep straight invoices, statements, and payments, but you may also find that your policy does not cover your illness. Furthermore, premiums have become so high that insurance is unaffordable for many.

Getting coverage for reconstructive surgery is especially difficult. Audrey Taylor cancelled her insurance when her company declared reconstruction of her breast to be "cosmetic." Fortunately, she found a company that would cover reconstructive surgery. A number of women who have encountered the same restriction in their policies have protested to their carriers. It is a good idea to check your policy before contemplating reconstruction.

Once you are considered to be "high risk," your ability to buy insurance protection is greatly diminished. Susan Nessim was threatened with the loss of her medical benefits when her position was eliminated in a company where she had worked for eight years. Having already been treated for breast cancer, Susan knew she would have difficulty getting another insurance carrier. In order to keep her benefits she was able to stay with her place of employment by stepping down from management to a sales position. This meant that she was underemployed, but retaining her insurance was more important to her.[1]

Risk Pools and Organizations

A solution that some states have adopted is the creation of risk pools. In these states legislation mandates that all insurance companies and health maintenance organizations pool resources to give "high risk" individuals comprehensive coverage. Another alternative is the insurance offered by fraternal, professional, and other organizations to their members. For information about agencies and associations that offer group insurance, see Appendix B on Resources.

HIGH COST OF CARE

The current costs of medical care can rapidly deplete a family's savings. Patients who have been wiped out by astronomical bills have had to turn to Medicaid or declare bankruptcy. Two women in our study have gone through bankruptcy because it was their only solution to the debts they had incurred with treatment of their breast cancers.

Preparing for the Worst

There are several measures that a family should take when they are first faced with breast cancer or any catastrophic illness. First, they should know what is covered by their health insurance. Second, they should seek professional advice about the options they have and other sources of money for paying their health bills. Medical social workers and financial advisors who specialize in health care finances can provide help. Third, they can share problems with immediate and extended family members who may be able to help, if only in small ways. It is important to prepare for the worst possible scenario by making sure that you have taken care of financial and legal issues.

The high cost of medical treatment and the confusing state of billing and insurance procedures lead to additional stress for a patient who needs to keep a positive outlook for her recovery. It can also put a tremendous strain on the marital relationship and the family as a whole.

In his book *When a Loved One Is Ill*, L. Felder devotes an informative chapter to the financial challenges of illness.[2] We have already mentioned the helpful information about these matters in the books of Beverly Kievman (*For Better or For Worse*) and Susan Nessim and Judith Ellis (*Cancervive*).

In summary, we have addressed the problems of filling out forms and dealing with medical bills and insurance, which for some women can be as stressful as the disease itself. The discussion covers understanding statements and bills, having insurance coverage, and coping with high costs. Several approaches that may be taken when you are faced with medical expenses are suggested. In many cases, probably the safest approach is to seek the professional help of social workers and financial advisors who specialize in health care finances.

The next chapter addresses the problems of making the transition from illness to wellness. The woman who is dismissed from treatment finds that she cannot slip back into her former normal life. It has changed and she must adjust to a new state of "normalcy." In her frustration with the problems she encounters she may experience post-traumatic stress disorder (PTSD). Women who have successfully met this challenge offer suggestions for other survivors who must find their own way.

Chapter 14

Coping with Recovery

The second time I saw Dottie Corcoran she had completed her chemotherapy and no longer had to see her physician on a regular basis. Her hair was growing back and she appeared to be much more energetic than she had been six months earlier. She told me it was a relief to have finished the treatments; at the same time, she was apprehensive. As long as she had been having chemotherapy she felt that the cancer was under control; she had a sense of security. However, without the treatments she felt vulnerable and anxious.

Dottie was describing the symptoms of post-traumatic stress disorder (PTSD). A survivor of cancer, Dottie was no longer a patient; and although she had continued with her job while getting chemotherapy, she was now trying to fit back into a normal life. The problem was that her former normal life had changed and she was adjusting to a new state of "normalcy." Her family, friends, and work associates expected her to act like a "well" person and resume doing what she had done before her illness, even though she did not feel up to par. It was difficult to fit into her previous roles, which had been partially filled by others during her illness. Moreover, she had lost an important support group, the hospital staff members who had made decisions and cared for her. Slipping back into one's former routine can be as much of a challenge as dealing with the diagnosis and treatment of cancer.

Susan Nessim found this transition from illness to wellness so disturbing and frustrating that she began to talk with other survivors about it. She discovered that many women experienced the same anxiety, demoralization, and rejection that led her to seek psychotherapy. Then she met Lisa, also a survivor, who was having experiences similar to hers. After sharing their experiences, they decided there was a need for a support group and organized Cancervive for others who were finding the return to wellness difficult.[1]

In the opinion of her employer, cancer made Susan ineligible for a promotion. It also affected her relationship with her husband, which eventually led to the breakup of their marriage. She was turned down for medical insurance and soon learned that being a recovered cancer patient was making her life very difficult. She found Jill Ireland's experience to be true. After surviving her first breast cancer, Ireland wrote in her book, *Life Wish*, "I was changed. I had cancer. Everyone reacted to me differently."[2]

Susan Nessim talked with many other survivors whose accounts she has shared in her book, *Cancervive: The Challenge of Life after Cancer*. Being a cancer survivor stigmatized Susan and presented unexpected obstacles. No one had prepared her for the emotional, psychological, and physical problems she would encounter when she recovered.

MAINTAINING SELF-ESTEEM

Cancer often results in changes in how a woman feels about herself and how others feel toward her. It also leaves some long-term effects with which she must learn to live. Her self-esteem, which plays a critical part in her recovery, has probably suffered with the loss of a breast and other physical changes that treatment has caused. She may have many negative feelings about her body image, her sexual life, her sense of worth, her ability to have and nurture children. The effect of her disfigurement on others, as well as the financial burden of her illness and her difficulty in coping, may cause her to feel negatively about herself.[3]

A survivor needs strong support to help her maintain her self-esteem. Essential to self-feelings is the sense of belonging, usefulness, and value she receives from family, friends, and health personnel. They need to share information with her and encourage her to express her feelings. To do otherwise reinforces her feelings of inadequacy.[4] On the other hand, to treat her as a responsible person, letting her share in decisions and tasks, helps her to maintain her dignity and self-esteem.

A woman's positive adaptation to the breast cancer is also related to her ego strength, her overall capacity for adaptation, mastery, and coping. Those with high ego strength tend to cope by seeking information, by using humor and laughter. They redefine problems. They are less apt to have a fatalistic attitude and do not tend to blame others.[5] In addition, a woman whose partner reassures her that the loss of her breast makes no difference in their relationship will make a more positive adjustment.

MAINTAINING RELATIONSHIPS

Unfortunately, relationships are sometimes impaired during the course of the treatment, or rifts that may have already existed become widened. In a study of 447 homebound married cancer patients, of whom 29.2 percent had breast cancer, researchers found that 20.8 percent had mood disturbances in the family, 17.4 percent suffered impairment of family relationships, and 11.4 percent reported role difficulties.[6] Some women may find it difficult to deal with the attitudes of family and friends.[7] Furthermore, once the woman has recovered, the support of family and friends lasts only a short time. They may be weary or resentful of the inconvenience and disruption the illness has brought to their lives and are impatient to return to normal. The recovered woman is expected to return to business as usual, and the family may soon overlook the effects of the illness and treatment on her energy and emotions.

How a woman reacts to being a survivor, especially when she manifests negative moods and depression, may affect how her family and friends respond to her.[8] Children may not understand, may even fear changes in her emotional behavior, or may not know how to handle them. A spouse's caution about hurting her with sexual advances may be interpreted as rejection. She may be very self-conscious—particularly if there is noticeable disfigurement—and withdraw from social contacts, as Betty Williams did after her mastectomy. Her daughters confided that they were very concerned about their mother's refusal to see anyone other than family members.

Stress and anger can result from role changes that have been made to accommodate the mother's treatment and recovery. Having been dependent on her family during her illness, the well patient may find it difficult to fit back into her role. Children may have become more independent, making their parent feel less needed. Or the fear of losing their mother may make them overly protective and indulgent, and they may continue to treat her as an ill person.

Marital Relationships

A couple's relationship may need repair, as we have seen in several cases. In the instance of Mindy Bishop, her marriage fell apart during the most difficult period of her chemotherapy treatment. In marriages that were already troubled, separations and divorces have occurred several years after the wife's recovery. The cancer may have been the breaking point for a separation that was destined to happen. Women have discussed the impatience of their spouses who do not comprehend the difficulty of living with long-term effects and the fear of recurrence.

What can be done to rebuild a marriage? Psychologist Lerner suggests that we can best achieve more closeness by working on ourselves. We need to clarify our own values, beliefs, and life goals. We need to face and deal with emotional issues when they arise. She explains that when we focus on the other person's behavior in an attempt to fix or change him or her, the relationship becomes "too intense" or "too distant." Lerner notes that over time, a gap widens in a married couple's relationship. When this happens many men tend to distance themselves or leave the marriage rather than work toward a change. One way to enhance closeness with our partner, she says, is to work on our self. We need to keep our own behavior congruent with our beliefs and priorities and take a position on issues important to us.[9]

Relationships with Friends

Having friends let us down when we need them most can be very upsetting. Several women reported that when they were diagnosed with cancer, some of their friends dropped them. For Margaret Muncy the loss of a close friend was very hurtful. Two other survivors have been disappointed in the loss of their sisters' closeness. In both instances the cancer survivors feel certain the reason is their sisters' fear of having breast cancer themselves. Nonetheless, it leaves the survivor with a deep sadness.

If a friendship is important enough to try to salvage, the survivor probably must take the initiative with the realization that she may be rebuffed. Friends who abandon the recovered cancer patient are probably afraid and embarrassed. Becoming informed and reading books such as Amy Harwell's *When Your Friend Gets Cancer* would help the friends who take flight when they encounter cancer.

It is important for a cancer survivor to continue to make new friends. Opportunities can be found in support groups and workshops such as those being offered by the American Cancer Society. See Appendix B for support groups that are available.

Relationships with Physicians

Ending the relationship with a doctor in whom you have put your trust and care can also be an emotionally difficult separation. When a doctor releases you as a patient, he may seem to become brusque and distant as he turns his attention to other patients. This may leave a survivor with a sense of being left adrift. Nessim points out that women sometimes "project romantic feelings onto doctors as a sort of coping mechanism."[10] A fantasized relationship makes the separation more difficult.

Nessim suggests having a debriefing session with your physician in which you obtain information about your diagnosis and treatment. You can ask questions and learn who in the health care team will be available to address concerns you may have in the future. Be well informed and tape-record your discussion during this debriefing session.[11] Thereafter, it is important to follow your physician's directions, have check-ups, and maintain good health habits.[12]

One physician, whose patients have been a part of this study, has a nurse who is always available to his patients when they have questions. The fact that this nurse has had breast cancer herself and possesses a compassionate manner gives patients a great deal of confidence and a sense of security.

STIGMA

Just as Susan Nessim felt the pain of being refused a promotion because of her cancer, others have experienced the stigma of cancer in the workplace. Peggy Thompson was working for a physician when her breast cancer was diagnosed. She not only lost her job because of it but was ostracized by her associates. Fortunately, she found another job in a physician's office where the attitude toward cancer was informed and open-minded.

In another account, related by Susan Nessim, a survivor named Veronica found that in her absence other office personnel were spraying disinfectant on and around her desk. She discussed the situation with her employer, who suggested that he call an informal meeting of the office staff at which he would ask Veronica to talk about her recent illness. She handed out pamphlets, explaining that there might be questions that she would be glad to answer. Her candidness squelched the fears and prejudices of those who were clinging to the myths about cancer. Nessim believes that myths will gradually be dispelled by the influence of a growing number of cancer survivors.[13] Although women with whom we have talked have not often reported a problem with stigma and prejudice, several have been emphatic about its existence. As we become more open about cancer we hope that the stigma, along with the myths, will be eliminated.

ANGER AND RESENTMENT

Anger often surfaces as a result of the long-term effects of cancer. Some women's struggle with weight gain, or the panic they feel with any ache or pain, can arouse anger. Anger can also result from the constant vigilance one must keep without appearing to be a hypochondriac. Moreover, the frustration of finding clothes that fit and other problems with appearance can make a woman angry. When we interviewed Marie Wernke, she confessed the anger she felt toward her husband because she was putting on a brave face in an effort not to worry him even though she was having constant pain. It is normal to strike out at the ones closest to us; and they must understand that the anger is directed toward the cancer, not them.

Family members may also feel anger, which may be mixed with resentment that their lives have been disrupted. Because our culture discourages expression of "sadness, grief, anger, and hostility," we often deny or suppress these emotions.[14] This suppression can cut family members off from one another or erupt in family conflicts. Communication can be beneficial in resolving these issues, providing the family is willing to discuss them, disclose their feelings, and work through problems.[15]

PHYSICAL AFTER-EFFECTS

Body Balance

Unless the weight of the natural breast has been replaced after a mastectomy, there will be an imbalance that causes one shoulder to droop downward and inward while the other shoulder remains up. This can cause tension and discomfort in the shoulder, neck, and back. A breast form that has been designed for a woman's life-style will correct the imbalance and help to keep the bra in place.[16] Information about companies that supply breast prostheses can be obtained from hospitals, nurses, doctors, and the American Cancer Society.

With a prosthesis some women have difficulty finding clothes that fit. Many shops that sell prostheses also handle a variety of bras that may help to solve the problem. Also, it is quite acceptable nowadays to wear casual and oversized garments. The colors should be complementary and the garment becoming.

Many women have chosen reconstructive surgery, and those with whom we have talked say it has helped their self-concept as well as their body balance. A woman who considers reconstruction should discuss this with the surgeon who will do her mastectomy and a plastic surgeon prior to her mastectomy. She may want to have the entire procedure done in one operation. When she discusses this with her doctors, she should question them about the procedure, risks, and other pertinent details so that she can make informed decisions. She could also be prepared for possible complications that might occur.

Lymphedema

Swelling and collection of fluid in the arm on the side of the mastectomy can be a serious problem for women who have undergone the removal of a breast and adjacent lymph nodes. When a tumor and the adjacent lymph nodes and vessels are surgically removed, the natural flowing of lymph fluid through the system can be blocked. Lymphedema can occur immediately after surgery or several years later and can be difficult to treat. There are a number of preventive measures, including a low salt diet and regular exercise of the arm. These important precautions are listed in Appendix E.

The warning that you should avoid injury to the arm should be taken very seriously. Lymphedema usually starts with swelling in an extremity, such as the hands and feet. Injuries such as cuts and bruises can easily become infected, causing the arm to swell like a balloon. If this happens, you should seek immediate medical attention. If untreated, infection and irreversible complications can result.

Nancy Brinker relates her experience with lymphedema. Nancy had waited almost two years after her initial surgery to have reconstruction. Everything had gone well until a year later, when she accidentally burned her arm on the stove. It became infected and the arm inflated to three times the size of her other arm. In her words, it was "grotesque." Because lymphedema is often an irreversible condition, her physician was doubtful that she would recover. His pessimism challenged her to make a complete recovery. She wore an elastic sleeve, took antibiotics, and saw a physical therapist every day. Over a year later, her arm had finally returned to normal.[17]

Even for the most cautious person, an accident to the arm on the side of her mastectomy can result in a painful infection. Should this happen, it is well to remember that determination, such as Nancy Brinker has, can help bring about recovery.

Fear of Recurrence

Sophia Wellins told me, "I feel that the possibility of recurrence is always riding on my shoulder. It is always with me." Kathryn Lathrop said, "You learn you're never out of the woods. It's always there." Mary Lynn Gordon described it as "an obsession."

Even though she tries to forget that she has had cancer, any survivor must always be aware of changes in her body and regularly follow the American Cancer Society's procedures for breast self-examinations, clinical exams, and mammograms. (See Appendix D for procedures.) It is no wonder that these women have a fear of recurrence. Depending on the extensiveness of their cancer, when it was diagnosed and treated, some women are able to repress this fear much of the time—except when they go for a check-up. Then the anxiety becomes intense. Phantom breast sensations (usually pain), which were experienced by 53.7 percent of the mastectomy patients in the Jamison study, can have emotional repercussions and be a reminder of possible recurrence.[18] Wabrek and Wabrek observed from their research that "every ache and pain triggers a fear of recurrence."[19]

How does one cope with recovery and the after-effects of breast cancer? The ways of coping vary with each woman. If there is one common theme, it is their desire to help other women who are having the breast cancer experience. As Nancy Brinker expressed it in the title of one of her book chapters, they join "the race for the cure."[20] Some of them work with organizations such as Reach to Recovery; others give workshops; still others become counselors and therapists. Many savor the time with families and limit their activity to things that are most fulfilling to them. After her mastectomy Ellen Barkley kept busy with service in her church, her family, golf, and other activities. Since a recurrence and other demands being made on her time and energy, she has decided to resign from her church duties and do more of the things she enjoys. She does not dissipate her energy in worry about the cancer or the future, but has learned to enjoy each day.

Energetic survivors like Nancy Brinker and the late Jill Ireland increase their pace of living and take risks they might not have taken before the cancer. Although they work to keep healthy, they follow an active life-style in order to live as fully as they can. Nancy Brinker takes seriously the advice of the late Rose Kushner, who advised her to "always keep a full calendar. Don't give yourself a chance to worry, and don't ever plan for a time when you might not be around to fulfill all the obligations you have made."[21]

We have discussed the problems of post-traumatic stress disorder (PTSD) when a woman is dismissed from treatment and returns to what she expects to be her normal life. However, now she must adjust to a new set of problems: employment, insurance, self-esteem, altered relationships, stigma, anger, and physical after-effects. Each woman must find her own way with the guidance of those who have been successful and now offer to help other women undergoing the same experience.

In the next chapter we explore the subject of growth, a change in perspective and life-style that enables a woman with breast cancer and her family to improve the quality of their lives. We discuss how therapists and physicians help patients with cancer who wish to make positive changes and find new meaning in life. Included are examples of women who have been motivated by the cancer experience to enrich their lives.

Chapter 15

Opportunity for Growth

Beth and Dick Thornton had a special bond of respect, love, and commitment that was put to test by years of battling the cancer that started in her breast. Watching her suffer was very difficult for Dick, and he began to rely on alcohol to ease his pain. When Beth needed him most he was letting her down. She pleaded with him to restrict his drinking. Denying that it was a problem that he couldn't control, Dick curbed his use of alcohol but didn't give it up. Beth realized how difficult her illness was for him and became more understanding, but still worried. She was especially worried about how he would handle her death.

To the end Dick expressed his love in many thoughtful ways and, with the help of Hospice, kept Beth in their home until she died. As you recall, when they first learned of Beth's cancer, they lived as fully as her illness permitted; and when her condition worsened, they faced her death openly and bravely. Dick arranged for a memorial service that enabled Beth's mother to accept the idea of cremation and resolved Beth's deep concern for her mother's feelings. In every way Dick assured Beth of his love and helped her to die in peace.

Except for his reliance on alcohol, both Dick and Beth coped in positive ways. They bore the years of suffering by becoming closer and more appreciative of what they had. The tributes paid to Beth by those who knew her were evidence of the meaning that, with Dick's help, she had put into her life.

How did Dick handle Beth's death? Those who knew of his problem feared that he would drown his sorrow by drinking. Instead, Dick decided to make some positive changes. With the sedentary life that the illness had imposed on him, he had gained weight. Now he was determined to lose unwanted pounds and he gave up alcohol. "I don't need that stuff," he said, and committed himself to control it. He was taking a step toward growth.

DEFINING GROWTH

Therapist Ronnie Kaye, in discussing the benefit of having to confront our mortality, notes that the Chinese character for "crisis" consists of two words, "danger" and "opportunity."[1] The crisis of cancer has the potential for changing our perspective, for we can use the experience as an opportunity to change and grow. We can decide to become better, to improve the quality of our lives, and, as LeShan expresses it, to sing our own songs.[2]

Growth means that we take control of our lives by searching for a lifestyle that is suited for us and then working toward living it. LeShan reminds us that we strengthen ourselves by working hard on our growth and by "moving closer to our potential."[3] Many couples we have interviewed who are experiencing cancer have re-evaluated their lives, deepened their relationships, and strengthened family ties. Others have dissolved destructive relationships, a positive step toward growth if such a relationship cannot be altered.

Lynn Gray's story of growth is told by Robert Shook in *Survivors: Living with Cancer*. After two mastectomies and several recurrences, Lynn's situation became critical when the cancer metastasized to her bones and kidneys. Fortunately, she responded to hormone therapy and her cancer was arrested. Knowing that there was no guarantee that it would not recur, Lynn returned to school to get a masters degree and began to make her life fulfilling by helping others. She has written a book, *Living with Cancer*; produced a cassette entitled *Mind over Matter*; founded Lifeline Institute; lectured; given workshops; and served on the Pennsylvania State Cancer Advisory Board. She said, "I can handle this life-threatening situation because my life is so fulfilling. I enjoy each day more than I ever have." The support of a loving spouse, children, and friends, and satisfying work and play in her life made dealing with cancer easier for Lynn.[4]

HELPING PATIENTS FIND MEANING IN LIFE

But what of cancer patients whose lives are not fulfilling like Lynn's? In working with these kinds of patients, LeShan has encountered those who simply have no will to fight because their lives have lost meaning. They don't feel living is worth the effort, and their bodies respond to that message. A practitioner of holism, LeShan works with them to help them find meaning so they can mobilize their immune systems against the cancer. Although they may not be able to defeat the cancer, they can achieve some measure of fulfillment and an improved quality of life. Advocates of the holistic approach believe that a positive social, emotional, spiritual, and nutritional environment can do a great deal to help the body's self-healing powers.[5]

LeShan has found that many persons have a hopeless attitude because they may have spent their lives being what others think they should be rather than what they want to be. For others, the necessity of making a living or caring for others has left no time to pursue their dreams and interests. The inner conflict from repressing these interests can result in loss of will and make it more difficult to handle discomfort and pain.

The problem is how to mobilize the self-healing powers of a person who has no goals or interests. For patients who wish to work with him, LeShan tries to discover why they feel despair. Emphasizing the positive, he explores with them what makes them feel best, what they have dreamed of becoming, what they would like to do if they had the time. Once he helps a patient identify and act on an interest, he has found that energy begins to improve.

An example is one of LeShan's patients, a lovable woman named Minnie, who had spent her life taking care of others. She was tired of being a caregiver but seemed to have no other compelling reason for living. Her condition was deteriorating. One day LeShan asked Minnie if she minded changing their appointment. She told him she didn't. When he saw her the next day, he apologized for the change and explained that a friend had gotten him a ticket at the last minute to attend the Danish Royal Ballet, which he thoroughly enjoyed. Much to his surprise, he discovered that Minnie also like ballet. He invited one of the leading ballerinas to visit with Minnie at the hospital. The young dancer graciously found time in her schedule and talked with Minnie for several hours. When LeShan asked how the visit had gone, the dancer told him they had a wonderful talk and she was amazed at Minnie's extensive knowledge of ballet.[6]

The outcome was that LeShan suggested Minnie write a history of ballet. He got books from the library, pencils and pads, and she undertook the enterprise with gusto. Her condition improved and the hospital staff complained that she was no longer an easy patient. LeShan knew his treatment was working when Minnie lost her complacence; she was too busy writing her history. Then a terrible heat wave turned the hospital into an inferno (in the days before there was air conditioning). Minnie succumbed to the cancer but not before she had begun to fulfill a lifelong dream of being immersed in ballet.

The life of Bernie Siegel, author of *Love, Medicine and Miracles*, also illustrates how a feeling of failure can be transformed into enthusiasm and growth.[7] His practice of surgery for over a decade had become painful. He went about his job as a mechanic would. Realizing that he was hiding his hurt by withdrawing into professional coldness when his patients needed him most, he had reached the point of despair. He was considering giving up surgery to enter psychiatry when several events began to change his thinking. First, a young cancer patient made him aware that he could be happier as a surgeon if he became more involved with patients. Then, a real change in his practice of medicine occurred when he attended a workshop given by the Simontons. During the session Siegel not only tried meditation but also met another young man, an advisor, who was sensitive to his feelings. The young man explained to Siegel that by changing himself, he could remain a surgeon and provide the support and guidance to his patients that he wanted to give them. That experience motivated him to start a therapy group that would help his patients mobilize their own resources against the disease. Bernie Siegel began treating patients as individuals and, in doing so, turned his life around.

TAKING STEPS TOWARD GROWTH

An important element in achieving growth and making positive changes is making a commitment to do so. Because spousal and familial support is so important to the woman with breast cancer, it is desirable that couples and families achieve growth together, at the same time respecting and nurturing one another's individual growth. For the patient and each family member a healthy balance should be found so that each one seeks the highest possible quality of life.[8]

It is difficult, but certainly not impossible, for one person to make changes without the cooperation of other family members. However, in a sensitive, flexible family the change of one member will influence the others; but for the most fulfilling change, there should be agreement on family goals. Children, even young ones, should be included in the commitment to growth. It cannot be overemphasized that children feel at fault when a parent is ill and especially responsible when a parent dies. Involving children in life-style changes gives them a sense of security and importance in the family unit.

Communication is essential in the commitment to growth. Family members show their respect for one another when they are open and truthful. To try to shield one another shows a lack of confidence in their ability to handle information and crises. Being excluded or patronized can weaken family relationships.

Beginning the Process of Growth

How does a person begin the process of growth? The first step is self-examination, whereby we consider how we would like to redirect our lives to make them more meaningful. LeShan suggests looking objectively at what peers seem to want and imagining what sort of life they will have if they attain their goals. By doing this we often realize that we would not like the kind of life that others pursue. Making comparisons can give us insight into the real goals that we have or would like to have.

Becoming well informed is another step toward growth. In treating and coping with cancer there are many decisions to make, which are often based on conflicting opinions from others. We can usually make a better decision if we have gathered as much information as we can; then we can weigh options in light of our own personal circumstances and feelings. Phyllis Loeff, a physician and cancer survivor about whom Robert Shook has written, believes that a patient who is not informed feels "dehumanized and depersonalized" when she is not able to talk knowledgeably with her physician.[9]

Another part of the process toward growth is to realize and believe in our own uniqueness. This acceptance of one's own value is a large part of finding meaning in life. As Barbara Hansen reminds us in *Picking Up the Pieces*, "each of us is a tiny piece in the mosaic of life" and we have something of value to give. However, we cannot give until we have acknowledged our own value. Hansen believes we find the foundation for our other resources "in our spiritual core."[10]

Closely related to our uniqueness is the necessity of resolving issues of low self-esteem and negative self-image. These issues are often deep-seated and of long standing. Often they are related to earlier experiences; our feelings of inadequacy are reinforced by the loss of a breast. Believing in our own uniqueness gives us the courage to take risks and try new things, which in turn improves our self-esteem. Because Phyllis Loeff had learned through her breast cancer how precious and fragile life can be, she developed "a certain zest for life" and felt more courageous about taking the risk of trying new things.[11]

Outcomes of Growth

From LeShan's point of view, to grow is to find and sing one's own song. As Phyllis Loeff did, Lynn Gray surmounted multiple recurrences and discouraging treatments to find a fulfilling life. She said, "I believe there's a high level of wellness which transcends all illness—a wellness of the spirit that is more important than wellness of the body. . . . If the spirit is healthy, the body cannot be defeated."[12]

Women and their families who have demonstrated the ability to turn the cancer crisis into growth have set goals for themselves. Fran Humphrey was always realistic about the seriousness of her cancer, but she went on making plans. She completed her masters degree and was preparing to work toward her doctorate, a goal she never achieved because the cancer stopped her. To the end, life was fulfilling for Fran.

In a story told by Dr. Richards, another cancer patient confessed that facing the possibility of cancer death motivated her to become more disciplined, self-confident, and resilient. Moreover, her relationship with her husband became more mature and satisfying. The emotional catharsis she underwent during her battle with cancer gave her initiative to put more quality into life. Out of her experience she gained a better ability to confront life's "harder tasks."[13]

Despite the hardships of coping with cancer, the experience has enriched the lives of many women and their families. It has made them examine their life-styles, cherish each day, and choose a more positive direction.

We need not wait for a life-threatening illness to make changes that will help us grow, but often the shock of facing our mortality gives us the incentive to do so. Dick and Beth Thornton are another example of turning the crisis of cancer into an opportunity for growth. As Norman Cousins wrote, "The ultimate tragedy is to die without discovering the possibilities of full growth."[14]

Having defined growth, we have explained the work of therapists and physicians who help people find meaning in their lives and regain their will to live. Steps that one takes to begin the process of growth result in "a wellness of spirit," discipline, self-confidence, resilience, and enrichment of life.

When death becomes imminent, how do families cope? In the following chapter we explore the effects of impending death on the marital relationship, Kübler-Ross's coping stages, the needs of the dying, and resources that may help the family cope. In addition, the importance of attending to practical matters and preparing those who will be left behind are reviewed. Finally, consideration is given to the effects on the bereaved spouse, young children, and adolescents, as well as the importance of communication during the death experience.

Chapter 16

Coping with Death

Earlier we talked about Fran Humphrey, who was affectionately called "The Energizer Bunny" because of her vitality. Despite all her enthusiasm for life, her indomitable spirit, her optimism and courage, Fran was not able to overcome the recurring tumors. While this book has been in progress, Fran has died.

Even at our first interview Fran was realistic about her cancer; but as her husband said, "she was never a victim of it." She went on with her life, living it fully, even when undergoing chemotherapy, bone marrow transplant, and other treatment regimens. She still had much to do: parents and a devoted husband to care for, clients to counsel, children and grandchildren to nurture. She had plans for writing a book and a doctoral degree she wanted to earn. Always accepting her setbacks with humor, she continued to set goals. But death came despite her fighting spirit. Her husband remarked, "she was so needed and so giving that there would never have been the right time for Fran to leave us." Sadly, cancer has no respect for the talented and the good. Sometimes it seems to rob us of those who are needed most.

FACING DEATH

When Ann Schneider had a second recurrence of her breast cancer, she became fearful that she might die. One morning just before Don was ready to leave for a meeting, Ann felt she had to talk with him and asked him if he could delay his meeting. Fortunately, Don could, and she was able to talk through her feelings with him. She was most concerned about how he would manage without her and wanted him to know that he should remarry.

Another couple, Beth and Dick Thornton, were also able to talk about Beth's impending death. Knowing that it was something they would have to accept, they prepared for it. One of their decisions, to have her body cremated, was very upsetting to her mother. While Beth worried about hurting her mother, Dick found a solution that was acceptable to his mother-in-law. He made all the arrangements for a memorial service. Beth was relieved of her concern for her mother; and when her condition worsened, Hospice volunteers enabled her to remain at home, where she died peacefully.

KÜBLER-ROSS'S COPING STAGES OF THE DYING

In recent years Elisabeth Kübler-Ross, therapists, and others have helped us understand the coping mechanisms of the dying person. In her book *On Death and Dying*, Kübler-Ross, who has worked with many patients who were dying of cancer, has identified five coping strategies.[1] These provide us with an approach to understanding death.

The first stage, denial, usually occurs when a person is diagnosed as having cancer and is told that the disease is very serious. Denial is more apt to occur when the information about a serious condition is given abruptly or prematurely to a patient without respect for her readiness for it.

Anger is a second stage. Families and health professionals need to be understanding and tolerant of the woman who is coping with anger, even when they may feel impatient and want to withdraw from her. The angry person should be loved and accepted just as the passive person is.

During a third stage, bargaining, the person may act childishly, making demands as a way of attempting to postpone the outcome. She makes promises to do things that she will carry out if she gets well.

When the ill person undergoes a fourth stage, depression, she may have many valid reasons for her feelings. The depression stage is difficult for the family, for they, too, are probably experiencing similar feelings just when the woman needs their support most. During this time, if the depression is not too severe, it may be important and helpful for the woman and family members to talk about their feelings.

When the woman and her family have been able to work through depression, they may come to the final stage, acceptance of death. Kübler-Ross has observed that at this point the family may need more assistance than the ill person.

Necessary throughout all these stages is the important element of hope—if not for cure, at least for comfort and support. This helps to sustain both the ill woman and the family.

Kübler-Ross's theoretical model of coping with death has met with considerable criticism. Her critics argue that there are many reactions to dying and that some people never face or accept their mortality. They also criticize her theory because it implies that these stages occur in a clearly identifiable sequence. It is true that some persons may not experience all the stages, nor will they occur in the order we have discussed. In fact, some persons may never go beyond one stage, such as denial or anger; others may regress and repeat stages. The process and length of grieving varies with each person.

Whether or not Kübler-Ross's theory accurately explains how we cope with death is not so important as the fact that her observations have been helpful. Because of her work, we have a better understanding of the experience of dying. More important, she has made it acceptable and therapeutic for family members to talk openly with one another and with the person facing death.

Talking enables the dying person to know and accept who she is, and in doing so, she may achieve a peaceful or "transcendent" death. LeShan has explained that we cannot say farewell to our lives "before fully accepting who we are. . . . We need to consider ourselves in the last days . . . as a part of a tapestry of life or symphony in which all the parts interact with each other and our life is an integrated, rich, and varicolored whole."[2]

Toward the end of her life, the great actress Helen Hayes wrote her autobiography, in which she visualized her life as a mosaic of many varicolored pieces reflecting "different worlds, events, people, places."[3] Miss Hayes enriched many lives through her acting and saw her own life as a part of a universal tapestry.

THE VALUE OF REVIEWING ONE'S LIFE

In her last years, after fighting to live through a severe heart attack, another great actress, Edith Evans, consented to allow Bryan Forbes to write her biography. In agreeing to have her life story recorded, she insisted that it be presented "not in soft touches of a picture, but in hard mosaic or tessellated pavement."[4]

In sharing information about her life, Forbes said that Miss Evans "rediscovered herself. . . . It was a unique experience for her—to look inwards and back . . . at the reflection of a young girl she had once known intimately and then grown apart from." Her biographer felt that he was the "go-between" as Edith Evans turned "the pages of a book she had once known by heart, refreshing the memory that fame had clouded." Forbes believed that the process of reviewing her life history was a source of satisfaction for her and may have actually prolonged Miss Evans's life.[5] This kind of sharing may help a dying person accept what her life is and has been.

Some women write journals in which they record experiences their family may not have been told. They also express feelings that they have not been able to verbalize. For example, Georgiana Morris of Texas, who has been fighting cancer for several years, is writing an account of her experiences. She calls it "My Wonder Book," a very appropriate title for a vivacious woman with a great sense of humor. When we talked, she was determined to keep up the fight against the cancer that began in her breast and had metastasized to other parts of her body.

When death becomes imminent, LeShan describes the "Dying Time" as "the last adventure." It is "the final integration of life when we see 'the whole' of our lives." The task, as he sees it, is to see our lives "as a pattern and a symphony in which the themes swell and recede." The importance of this final integration, he believes, cannot be overestimated.[6] Author Amy Harwell views the acceptance of one's death as coming to "a place of wholeness, completeness and peace."[7]

Achieving Acceptance

How do we come to this acceptance? Barbara Hansen, who has been a paraplegic for over thirty years as the result of an automobile accident, says that we have two choices. We may take the negative course and consider ourselves to be victims of circumstance. Our other choice is to take a positive attitude and focus on what we can do for ourselves and others.[8]

In coming to terms with one's own death, therapist Ronnie Kaye points out that although each of us will very likely feel sadness and loneliness, we possess "the internal resources to make peace with our own mortality."[9] Since Kaye's own breast cancer forced her to confront her death, she has counseled many women with breast cancer. She gives them a list of 10 "rights" she compiled and included in her book, and explores with them options for handling specific situations. In working with these women, Kaye has seen courage and joy as they make the most of the days that are left to them.

Meeting Important Needs

When we face the fact that our life may end soon, Viorst maintains that we have two important needs. We want to believe that we will endure through our work or our legacy, and we want to have some connection with a higher power.[10] Before a person can overcome her fear and fulfill these needs, she may have much work to do. She may have relationships to mend and deepen, persons to whom she wants to reach out, and important things in her life to remember and share. She may also have financial and legal affairs to put in order, and spiritual issues to resolve.

Kaye encourages women who have not grappled with issues related to the meaning of life and death to formulate beliefs that will comfort and sustain them. For those who accept this challenge, Kaye suggests that resources are available in books and people. There are close friends, family members, and spiritual leaders who are willing to talk with them and help resolve feelings of guilt.

PERSONAL ACCOUNTS

Like Jill Ireland, who did every positive thing that was suggested to help her conquer her breast cancer, Cynthia Ruether was doing the same. When Cynthia was told several years ago that her breast cancer was terminal, she became angry and found a physician who would give her hope. She took an aggressive approach to physical fitness and enjoyed several years of good health. However, another recurrence requiring chemotherapy made Cynthia fearful, and she wanted to talk about it.

She asked me to visit her in the hospital, where she shared her feelings and experiences with me. Among the things that she was doing to cope was visiting a therapist who helped her sustain hope and ease the physical discomfort of treatments. At the therapist's suggestion, she was visualizing her body as a shell in which her spirit resided, free from cancer. Cynthia also had body massages for relaxation and was working on her spiritual growth. She expressed her gratefulness for the constant support of her husband and her concerns for him. Several weeks after our visit, Cynthia lost her valiant fight.

Another person, Marvella Bayh, wife of former senator Birch Bayh, also exemplified courage. When she was first diagnosed with breast cancer, she decided she wanted to use her knowledge and public speaking ability to help other women who had the disease. Working with the American Cancer Society, she gave speeches to women's groups across the nation, granted interviews on television, and wrote her autobiography to inform women about breast cancer. She was feeling well and fulfilled by her work when she learned that her breast cancer had metastasized and was inoperable. She put her trust in God and kept going. Relying on new drugs to buy time, and reaching out to people who would give her hope and love, she continued her speaking appearances and interviews. She learned to "savor" life, to save her energy for what was important, and to deepen her spiritual commitment.[11]

When Walter Cronkite reported on the CBS evening news that Marvella Bayh had said she was dying, she immediately responded publicly: "I have *never, ever* said that I was dying of cancer. I am *living* with the knowledge that I have cancer. And my life is rather normal."[12]

Marvella Bayh died of cancer, but not until she had helped countless women and set an example of courage. In her last days she was sustained by her spiritual beliefs and the support of her devoted husband and son.

ATTENDING TO PRACTICAL MATTERS

When a person accepts her impending death, she can help the loved ones she is leaving behind by strengthening emotional bonds and by attending to legal, financial, and other practical matters. Making wills and the like are

168

Breast Cancer

not pleasant tasks at any time, but they can spare the bereaved a great deal of frustration and, sometimes, bitterness and family friction.

A woman and her spouse should attend to the making or updating of wills and trusts, the assignment of power of attorney, and the drafting of a living trust that specifies the extent to which she wishes life-sustaining support. She and her spouse should also appoint guardianships for any children who are under legal age, and designate the disposition of personal items. The location of keys to safety deposit boxes and important papers and other items should be recorded. Innumerable details such as these can be a source of inconvenience and distress to her surviving family members, unless a woman has left them explicit instructions.

As an example of the difficulties a surviving spouse can have, one of my closest friends, who had helped me through the death of my husband, died recently after several years of suffering. She left no instructions about the location or disposition of her personal possessions. Her spouse hunted everywhere for a piece of jewelry he had given her. It was finally found; and in the process of sorting through her things, he also discovered other mementos tucked away in unlikely places. How much easier it would have been for him had she kept a record or told him of her "hiding places."

George Humphrey told us that when Fran was first diagnosed with breast cancer, she insisted they see an attorney and get their legal and financial affairs in order. He hadn't wanted to deal with the possibility of her death, but she insisted. After she died he was very grateful for her foresight, which made the settlement of her estate a smooth transition for him. Waiting until a person is near death to make legal decisions and sign documents may result in costly and unpleasant legal entanglements that do not reflect the person's intentions or wishes.

As a guide, Beverly Kievman's book, *For Better or For Worse*, gives valuable information about the tasks left for the bereaved and ways to avoid some of the inconveniences they can cause. Whatever the dying person can do to lessen the burdens on her family will be an important part of her legacy. Kievman's book may be a helpful guide for you.

Many women with terminal cancer have not left a legacy that gained national recognition as Marvella Bayh did, but they have quietly and bravely continued to give to others until their death. Dottie Corcoran, administrator of a retirement and nursing home, continued to work until a week before she died. Beth Thornton demonstrated admirable courage to hundreds of friends as she fought to live a normal and full life, despite the limitations of her disease. Fran Humphrey counseled patients until the cancer necessitated hospitalization.

On my last visit with Fran in the hospital before her death, she shared with me a vision or dream she had experienced during her bone marrow transplant. With her husband's permission, I share it with you.

In this vision Fran found herself on a white horse, standing at the edge of a high rocky cliff overlooking a deep, barren valley. Looking down, she saw that the valley was filled with dry bones. Then she turned toward a bright light that shone from behind her to look upon an astounding golden city. Struck with awe, she gazed on its beauty. Then, a voice spoke to her: "Fran, are you ready to leave? Will you come with me to the golden city?" It was so beautiful, so enticing! Fran hesitated, then answered, "No, Lord, I still have some work that I must finish. I can't leave yet."

Fran lived for several months and during that time her husband, who had been so determined that she would survive, came to accept her impending death. Through her counseling she had already touched many lives in a positive way. Although there was a great deal more that Fran wanted to do, what seemed most important was to prepare her devoted partner to let her go. George Humphrey and I talked after Fran's death, and he told me she had done everything she could to make it easier for him. We have encountered other women who are preparing their loved ones and will leave a legacy of love, courage, and dignity.

Kübler-Ross has written, "It is my conviction that it is the intuitive, spiritual aspect of us humans—the inner voice—that gives us the 'knowing,' the peace, and the direction to go through the windstorms of life, not shattered but whole, joining in love and understanding."[13]

EFFECTS ON THE BEREAVED

In 1935, just a few days after Christmas, while British actress Edith Evans was in New York playing the role of Juliet's nurse in *Romeo and Juliet*, her beloved husband died in England. He had not been feeling well but there had been no diagnosis of cancer, so neither Edith Evans or her husband George Booth had any premonition that they would not see one another again. Had such a possibility occurred to her, she would never have gone to New York. When she received word of George's sudden death, she wired a message to her parents: "Too stunned to think." That message aptly describes the initial effect of death on a spouse.

Transportation being what it was in 1935, Miss Evans had to wait for a ship to sail home; and by the time she arrived in England, the burial had taken place and it was "all over." She said, "I nearly lost my reason during that time. Friends and family tried to be helpful, but friends can't wipe your mind clean, grief isn't something you can tidy up like dust on a mantlepiece."[14]

The loss that the spouse and other close family members feel is indescribable. Life suddenly takes a different direction, and because their lives have been very interdependent, the survivors suffer many losses. As Rando noted, the loss may recall "old issues" that will affect the "length and intensity" of the grieving period.[15]

Grieving is intensified by the many details concerning burial, estate settlement, and other matters that must be taken care of immediately. Emotionally and physically, the bereaved spouse may feel a loss of control. He may cry easily. He may be unable to think clearly, concentrate, or remember things. Tasks, however small, may become monumental. To make grief even more difficult, he may not get the support he needs. Others do not realize what it is like. They expect him to get on with life. As one woman said of a friend who had recently lost her husband, "I don't call her very often. She's just not fun to talk with anymore."

How the Bereaved Spouse Copes

If the progression of the cancer has been long and slow, as it was in Beth Thornton's case, both the patient and spouse have been on an emotional roller-coaster. If the couple has been understanding of what each is experiencing and have been able to work through the problems together, he may be better able to cope with his loss. Even so, the grieving process may be very difficult and lengthy.

Cohen and associates, who studied the family's adaptation to terminal illness and death of a parent, found that families were more likely to adjust well if they were able to talk and share information and decision making. When the deceased parent was the mother, who is usually the one who initiates talk about emotional issues, communication among surviving members was apt to be limited. Furthermore, after the death of the mother, members were more likely to have an increase in illness.[16]

The Positive Side of Loss

Barbara Hansen suggests that loss not only takes away but also gives us new values.[17] It helps us to appreciate the little things we have taken for granted. We become more aware of what we want from the rest of our lives.

In *Picking Up the Pieces*, Hansen outlines five steps for using our internal resources to change our attitudes and gain control over our lives. The first step is to realize that we are "unique and valuable" and have a place in the total pattern of life. Second, we can redefine our values and view of success. Third, we can focus our energy and time on the needs of others rather than our own pain. Fourth, we can live "in," rather than "for," the moment instead of fearing the future and lamenting the past. The final step is to discover new strength by investing in solitude.[18]

Having outlined the steps, Hansen gives specific ways for strengthening our internal resources, such as reading good books, scheduling quiet times, communicating with others, and believing in ourselves. Based on her own experiences after losing almost everything she had dreamed of having in life, Hansen's book is helpful, inspirational, and well worth reading.

Bereaved Young Children

Small children, as we know, are very frightened by separation from their parents. Kübler-Ross advocates that we deal with children "honestly and openly." The child who feels abandoned in some way by a parent is vulnerable and may develop "general mistrust," "fear" of close relationships, or feelings of "alienation" from the person he or she may blame for the separation. The child may also experience "deep grief" over the loss of love.[19]

Without emphasizing death, writers of children's literature in the early twentieth century imbedded the discussion of it in their main themes. *The Yearling* by M. K. Rawlings and *Charlotte's Web* by E. B. White illustrate how death was depicted as a part of life. In recent years the desire to cope more effectively with death has prompted the publication of many books to help children, as well as adults. Hannalore Wass and Charles Corr compiled an extensive listing in their publication *Helping Children Cope with Death: Guidelines and Resources.* Another source of titles exists in the references appearing in Richard Lonetto's book, *Children's Conceptions of Death.* See our Bibliography for publishers of these books.

Kübler-Ross believes future heartache can be prevented if bereaved children are encouraged to express and share their grief. They should also be allowed to take part in the care of an ill or dying family member. This gives them a sense of security and helps prepare them for losses in later life. I remember how lovingly the family of one of my high school friends helped with the care of their ill grandmother in their home. My friend has cared for her own mother and ill husband in the same manner.

Bereaved Adolescents

The grief that adolescents experience when death takes a parent, sibling, close family member, or friend can be extremely difficult to understand and resolve. Because teenagers already "have their hands full" in developing their individuality and drawing away from the family, the loss of a parent deprives them of a sense of security and makes them "different" from their peers.

The problems of grieving adolescents are not like those of a grieving adult. With the help of seventeen young people who had experienced the death of a parent, sibling, or close friend in their adolescent years, Gravelle and Haskins have written a book to explain adolescent bereavement. Adolescents vary greatly in their reactions. Whereas adults go through a phase of numbness, teenagers often do not experience their most intense pain for eight months or more following the loss. Teenagers often react with complete disbelief, whether the death is expected or happens suddenly. Initially some teenagers may seem to react abnormally. Their responses (such as laughter, acting crazy, physical illness, hysteria, and inattentiveness) are unexpected and sometime inappropriate.

When the shock wears off, adolescents often have some degree of depression that is apparent in eating, sleeping, and grooming habits. They may be able to function but have little feeling and are unable to cry, giving the impression that they are handling things well, almost too well. They may search and yearn for the deceased for months, even longer. Their feeling of loss increases; conflicting emotions may be overwhelming. Some make an effort to show no emotion, repressing their pain until later.

A "terrifying event" occurs when they return to school after the funeral. Suffering a loss of their former identity, they return to school "different" from their peers. When a parent has died, they may feel "like an orphan," less confident and less worthy.[20] Neither the bereaved nor their classmates know what to do or say. The stares, the whispering, the avoidance, the silence convey their confusion. The bereaved needs to know that classmates care and yet doesn't want to be treated differently. If a peer brings up the loss, the bereaved does not know what to say. If nothing is said, the grieving teenager feels classmates don't care.

Because the needs of bereaved parents are so acute and all-consuming, they are often not aware of the teenager's feelings. Furthermore, the parent's need for his children's help may inhibit the teenager's struggle for independence, thus increasing his or her emotional conflict.[21]

Friends and understanding adults outside the family can be very helpful to the grieving teenager. The adolescents who participated in the making of Gravelle and Haskins' book agreed that the efforts that others made were beneficial, especially if some gesture or acknowledgment of their loss came from peers. No matter how awkwardly it is expressed, that gesture reassures a bereaved teenager that a friend cares and that he still belongs to the group. Talking with someone who has been through the same experience relieves some of the pain. Adults should be considerate of a bereaved adolescent and give him or her the needed support.

EFFECTS OF DEATH ON FAMILY COMMUNICATION

Studies have documented the effects that a family's anxiety or fear of discussing death has upon their communication when a member has a terminal illness.[22] Their ability to talk openly in the face of death is affected by rules about permissible topics of conversation. Past patterns of interaction and the level of intimacy to which they are accustomed also determine their ability to talk openly about death.

Several sources of stress can account for the terminally ill person's avoidance of talk about dying. She may feel constrained and frustrated when members with whom she is close will not discuss it with her. Her loss of control over her life, the health care provider's obvious feelings of helplessness, and the reality of death can inhibit her efforts to talk.

Researchers suggest communication tasks that will facilitate a "good" death experience for a terminally ill person and her family. First, they should increase their knowledge of death. This can be acquired through books, professional and religious training, courses of study, past experience, and those who have coped with it. If they cannot overcome their anxiety about discussing it, they should seek therapy and/or training that will help them express their thoughts. If they cannot verbalize them, perhaps they can write them. They can surround the ill person with personal possessions, be there and listen when she wants to talk. They can encourage her to discuss her concerns, allowing her to set the agenda. Giving a dying person the opportunity to share her thoughts can help her to find "hope, meaning, purpose, and value in existence." It can also diminish her feelings of isolation and abandonment.[23]

Facing the death of a loved one and our own death is difficult. Thinking of it as Kübler-Ross has described it may be helpful. She has written that it is "the culmination of life, the graduation, the goodbye before another hello, the end before another beginning. Death is the great transition."[24]

For quick access and review, the next three chapters condense the survival guidelines that have been suggested throughout the book. Guidelines in Chapter 17 apply to the woman with breast cancer. Chapter 18 includes suggestions for the spouse/partner, the children, and other family members. Chapter 19 summarizes guidelines for friends.

Chapter 17

Survival Guidelines for the Woman with Breast Cancer

In each chapter we have presented explanations and suggestions to help you understand and cope with the various demands that breast cancer makes on you, your family members, friends, and health care team. For quicker access to guidelines we summarize them here according to the different problems to which they may apply. Recognizing that each individual is unique and will vary in reactions and challenges, we have included many suggestions from which you can select what may be appropriate for you and your family.

DETECTING SUSPICIOUS LUMPS

Before you detect a suspicious lump, you should be knowledgeable about the nature of the breasts and know your own breasts by being aware of changes that occur during menstruation, pregnancy, and menopause. You should also know the risk factors that could increase your chances of breast cancer: age, family history, race or national origin, menstrual history, pregnancies, hormonal factors, previous breast cancer, diet, and obesity.

You should have established the habit of BSE (breast self-examination) at least once a month. Before menopause, you should examine your breasts a week after the start of menstruation. After menopause, select your birthday or any easy date to remember. (See Appendix D for a specific procedure.)

You also should be having a yearly examination by your physician and a mammogram regularly. These regular mammograms should begin when you are age 39–40 to establish a basis (often referred to as a "baseline") for comparing future mammograms and detecting early changes in breast tissue. If you are age 40–49, have one every one to two years; every year, if over age 50. Make sure that you get a written report on the results of each of your mammograms.

Taking Action When a Lump Is Discovered

If you have pain in your breast or if you detect a lump, see a doctor immediately. The sooner cancer is detected the better are the chances of successful treatment and survival. Biopsy may be necessary for a diagnosis, whether the lump is benign or malignant.

RECEIVING THE DIAGNOSIS

The time between finding a lump and waiting to hear the diagnosis will be a difficult period for you. You will experience the fears associated with breast cancer; these fears will intensify if tests reveal that the lump is malignant. That is the time of most acute stress. Your ability to listen or think clearly will be impaired, so it is important that you have a friend or family member with you to take notes and ask questions when you see your physician.

Follow your intuition and be assertive if you feel uneasy about a physician's decision to wait and watch a lump or calcified area, or if the physician wants to schedule surgery immediately. Except in rare cases, you can safely wait for two weeks to a month. In any event, seek another opinion, a policy with which reputable physicians will agree. If yours does not, be more determined to acquire additional information. You can obtain this information from your local chapter of the American Cancer Society or a local hospital specializing in cancer treatment. Ask friends and relatives who have experienced breast cancer, or call the National Cancer Institute at 1–800–4–Cancer. The National Cancer Institute will send you current information on breast cancer and treatments. (See Resources, Appendix B.)

Release your emotions. Cry if you feel like doing so. Share your feelings with your spouse/partner and family. If you feel angry, channel that energy into positive action by attacking the problems that cancer has created for you. Solicit the help of your family in gathering information about cancer and treatment options so that you will be well informed when you talk with your physician.

Before seeing a surgeon make a list of your medical history, drugs you take, and questions you want answered. If you have learned about treatment options before seeing the surgeon, you will be better able to ask important questions. For example, if he or she should recommend a partial mastectomy or lumpectomy, there will be specific questions you should ask. See Appendix C for other questions you should ask of each physician you will see.

If you think you might consider reconstructive surgery, it is necessary to know that the surgical procedure will allow for that. Even if you are not sure about reconstruction, you should obtain information about it in the event that you change your mind later. Your physician should be able to supply you with written information that you can study later.

Because of the intensity of your emotional reactions to this disease, you will need time to read and discuss information about reconstruction with your family. You will want to consider the alternative of immediate and delayed reconstruction or none at all. (See Chapter 4 on Breast Reconstruction.) Ask the surgeon if you will be given explicit instructions for exercises to maintain arm and shoulder mobility.

Some doctors believe that the power of suggestion causes us to imagine or develop symptoms, and therefore they avoid giving too much information. Depending on your own desire for complete information, make clear how much you want to know and be persistent in getting it. Unless the type and stage of the cancer requires immediate surgery, you can take some time to make decisions.

Consider what other physicians you want on your team. Besides your surgeon you may need an oncologist, a pathologist, an oncology radiologist, and a plastic surgeon if you choose reconstructive surgery. If you plan to have immediate reconstruction, you should make an appointment with a plastic surgeon so that he or she can work with your surgeon. Choose medical professionals whom you like and who will answer your questions in clear and understandable language. You should have confidence in them. They should also have a belief system with which you feel comfortable.

In selecting an oncologist, you will have questions about procedures, types of drugs, how they are administered, their side effects (both short- and long-term), possible complications, and how the treatment will affect reconstruction if you have it. Other specific questions appear in Appendix C. Go to the library and check the drugs that may be used in your treatment. The *Physicians' Desk Reference* is one such source: it is a general guide to prescription drugs.[1] Your librarian may make other suggestions.

If you are going to have radiotherapy, ask if there will be a follow-up treatment and how it will be given. Ask about precautions you must take and what strange feelings you can expect. Question the radiologist about the possibility of permanent swelling and how long fatigue usually lasts. Also inquire about the effect on your skin and bones and how you should protect your skin. Other specific questions for the radiologist are listed in Appendix C.

Before receiving hormonal therapy, insist that you be given an estrogen-receptor test and request that you see the results. Should the test results be negative, this treatment will not be effective for you.

CHOOSING YOUR EMOTIONAL SUPPORT GROUP

Unless you are single or have little or no family, your most important emotional support is your spouse or partner. Be open about your special need for his support. For other support members select at least one positive role model and someone who can make you laugh. Tell them that you are going through a difficult time and will need their help. Explain that you want them to be sympathetic but that they should also encourage you to lead as normal a life as possible.

If you are single, widowed, or live alone, turn to friends for your support. Also, investigate support groups. Call the American Cancer Society for information.

BEFORE AND AFTER SURGERY

Prior to surgery adhere to a nutritional, low-fat diet and get exercise. Remember that your best defense against cancer is your own immune system. Look your best and prepare for your time in the hospital by assembling cosmetics, an attractive robe, and whatever will make you look and feel better as you begin your recovery.

Immediately after surgery you will feel drained of energy. The first anxious moment is feeling the flatness where your breast or breasts used to be. The next is seeing the scar and watching the reaction of your spouse/partner as he views it. Uppermost in your mind may be what this disfigurement will do to your marital and sexual life. You will be apprehensive about the resumption of sexual intimacy and how the loss of your breast(s) will affect that part of your life. If single, you may have the fear that you will never marry and have a family. You may have other anxieties, such as the possibility of recurrence, that will recede with time.

Initially, you may be glad to be rid of the cancer; the shock and denial that you experience at first will buy you time until you fully comprehend the reality of it. This may not come until you are at home and alone. In this stage of recovery it is important to share your feelings and fears with an understanding person, ideally your spouse or partner. Otherwise it should be a close friend, or someone who has been through the experience herself.

Let your family help you to become as self-sufficient as you can be. At the same time, encourage and show appreciation of their coping efforts. Be careful of being critical if their efforts do not measure up to your normal standards or expectations. They, too, are making adjustments.

USING ALL AVAILABLE RESOURCES

As your energy permits, take an active role in your own recovery. Continue to practice good health habits, draw upon your inner resources, attend support groups, and resume activities. To strengthen your inner resources and keep an optimistic attitude, read some of the inspiring stories of other women. Consider holistic approaches such as relaxation, imagery, meditation, and laughter. If adjustment is especially difficult for you, seek the help of a counselor or attend some of the community programs that are now being offered in many cities. (See Resources, Appendix B.)

REPAIRING AND ENRICHING RELATIONSHIPS

As we have seen in earlier chapters, the stress of illness can often impair what you thought were good or satisfactory relationships. If troubling issues between you and your spouse or partner and other family members have not been resolved and the breast cancer creates more tension, consider how you can begin to resolve them.

First, consider how and what you communicate to your loved ones. As you reflect, you may become aware of changes you can make in your way of talking with them. A change in your communication may, in turn, bring about changes in the way your family members talk with you and one another.

Be open with your children about your illness. You need not go into detail with younger children, but be honest with them because they will imagine the worst if you try to be secretive. Ask for their cooperation in helping with your needs and household chores until you are well enough to assume your duties again. Encourage them to talk about their interests and activities. Help them to express their feelings.

Although the fear of recurrence may dominate your thinking, express it and then try to set it aside. Men usually feel uncomfortable about discussing feelings and unpleasant experiences; they want to put what is past behind them and focus on the present. They also need relief from the many pressures in their lives. Making plans for activities together will turn your attention in a positive direction. Try to refocus your energy by doing something you have always wanted to do or learn, such as taking a class or starting a new hobby. Avoid letting your cancer become a regular topic of conversation. Above all, beware of taking on the identity of "a cancer patient." It will not be easy, but try to keep the disease in its place and continue with your normal roles as wife, mother, career woman, volunteer—whatever your particular roles are.

COMMUNICATING MORE EFFECTIVELY

If you realize you could make changes in your own way of talking with your spouse and other family members, seek to do so. Review the ways of approaching sensitive issues as discussed in the chapter on communication. Then initiate a discussion with your spouse (or entire family) in which you express your feelings about the ways in which you interact with one another. If blaming and criticism have become patterns, suggest that you as a family try to eliminate them. Open lines of communication by asking questions that do not evoke a "yes" or "no" answer, but word them so that they will encourage the other person to talk. Avoid words that label, accuse, blame, or criticize the other. Be aware of your tone of voice; it carries a message just as strongly as what you say. Remember, too, that nonverbal messages are often more powerful than words. By owning and expressing your feelings you can make your position clear to your family members and, one hopes, open the way for them to do the same. When they do, respect and value their feelings.

You demonstrate your caring when you give total attention to what a loved one is saying. Listen emphatically and respond nonjudgmentally to convey your understanding and support.

RECEIVING AND GIVING SUPPORT

The support you receive is probably the most important factor in your recovery from breast cancer. However, many people, especially if they have not been ill themselves, do not know how to give support. As psychologist Ronnie Kaye discovered, support will be more helpful if you let your family and friends know what your needs are. Follow Kaye's advice and tell family and friends what you need most.[2]

You can also "break the ice" and dispel the discomfort that some family members and friends may feel about your cancer by bringing up the topic yourself. Introduce some humor if you can. Realize that some persons may fail to give you support because they cannot cope with their feelings about cancer. Be understanding and forgiving. When family and friends offer to do things for you, accept their offers and let them know what their caring means to you. Remember that your attitudes and expectations can be a powerful force in helping you to recover.

LONG-TERM EFFECTS AND WELLNESS

Be prepared for new challenges when you have recuperated and return to a "new normal" life. For some of you this may be a time when your internal resources undergo the most severe test. Continue to make new friends, and make an effort to repair damaged relationships if they are important to you. When the situation is appropriate, try to dispel fears and myths with factual information about cancer. Accept the necessity of re-evaluating your goals and expectations.

Seek the help of individuals, agencies, and organizations that offer information about prostheses, clothing, looking attractive, understanding bills, filling out forms, dealing with the discriminating policies of employers and insurance companies. Find a support group where you can share your feelings as you accept the loss of your breast and learn to live with your fear of recurrence. Take seriously the warnings about injuries. As Rose Kushner advised, "Keep your calendar full."[3]

SEIZING THE OPPORTUNITY FOR GROWTH

Many of the guidelines already mentioned take you in the direction of growth. The cancer experience may cause you to re-evaluate your values and goals. In the process you will reflect on what would make your life more meaningful. It's a time to realize and believe in your uniqueness. It's an opportunity to deepen relationships, undertake new challenges, do what you have always yearned to do, and come to terms with what you want in life. Growth comes with a commitment to enrich your life.

FACING DEATH

Even though the survival rate for breast cancer is improving, some of you, despite all your effort and desire to live, may not be able to stop the cancer's growth. If you know or fear that death is imminent, you may have some very practical legal and financial matters to put in order, and some relationships to repair. It can be a time to say what you have not been able to express, or to make amends for utterances that you regret having made. It can be a time of reviewing and sharing your life with your family. You will be leaving a legacy that they, especially younger members, will cherish. It will help them know a part of you that you have never revealed and enable you to see your place in the tapestry of life. It will be a time when you can resolve spiritual issues and make peace with death. It can also be an opportunity to help those you will leave behind to accept your departure from their presence.

CONCLUSION

There are many guidelines for managing the experience of breast cancer that we have learned from professional care providers, researchers, and women who have lived it. There is no right way, for each of us is unique in our personality, experience, ways of coping, family heritage, and emotional makeup. Not all guidelines will appeal to you, but we hope you will find some of them helpful.

Chapter 18

Survival Guidelines for Spouse/Partner, Children, and Other Family Members

GUIDELINES FOR SPOUSE/PARTNER

Andy Murcia realized when his actress wife Ann Jillian was diagnosed with breast cancer in 1985 that there were no books or guidelines to address his needs. Murcia did have a close friend, Bob Stewart, who was going through the same turmoil and they could share their experiences. However, Mark Taylor, who gave us such a vivid account of his dilemma when Audrey lost her breast, could not find one person who would talk with him about it. Realizing that other husbands needed help, Murcia and Stewart decided to write a book giving men some direction when the woman they love has breast cancer.

As the spouse or partner, you will have many of the same emotional reactions that your loved one is experiencing. Because your reactions and behaviors are so important to her recovery and the functioning of your family unit, you will need to take control to maintain balance. Because you are the key person in her support system, the suggestions that will help you be supportive and maintain your other responsibilities are summarized in much the same order as those for the woman with breast cancer.

When She Finds a Suspicious Lump

You, too, will have an overwhelming emotional reaction to her discovery of a lump, but realize that she may be in a state of shock. Although some women prefer to take control, she may need for you to seek medical help and make some decisions. See that she makes an appointment with a doctor as soon as possible and arrange to accompany her if you can manage it. Both of you will be experiencing high anxiety. If you cannot be with her, see that another family member or friend can be. Ask that person to take notes, or ask the receptionist if the session with the doctor may be taped on a small recorder. While waiting for the appointment, give your wife or partner emotional support.

When the Lump Is Diagnosed as Cancer

If probable cancer is diagnosed, a biopsy may be suggested. Be aware that your spouse will probably be unable to focus on much of what the doctor tells her, answer his questions coherently, or remember what he says.

Seek a second opinion, particularly if the physician tells you she should "wait and see" or suggests that she see a surgeon at once. Most physicians will readily agree to your having a second opinion. If yours does not, you have more reason to do so. Search for a physician with whom each of you feels comfortable and confident.

When cancer is verified (probably by a biopsy), ask how advanced the cancer cells are and how far they have spread (the stage of the cancer). When surgery is recommended, take time to become well informed about the disease and available surgeons. Ask friends who have had the same diagnosis; check with the American Cancer Society and other sources for the names of surgeons. Together your wife and you can read information and jot down questions that you want answered before seeing a surgeon.

When you do see a surgeon, in the event that a mastectomy is recommended, ask questions about the surgical procedure, where the incision will be made, how much tissue will be removed, method of closure, how results will look, and what follow-up treatment will be required. Inquire about the normal length of the recuperative period and discuss how the surgical procedure will affect reconstructive surgery, should she want it. Ask for names of other patients who have gone through a similar experience with whom your wife or partner can talk.

Question the physician about the treatment options that he or she recommends for your wife's stage of the cancer. What are the side effects and long-term effects of the treatment? How will these affect reconstructive surgery? What preliminary tests such as bone scan, CT (computerized tomography) scan of the liver, and chest X ray will be done? Will the other breast be biopsied? Get recommendations for oncologists and plastic surgeons. (See Appendix C for questions to ask.)

While you are waiting for the surgery, be sensitive to your partner's emotional needs, and prepare children and other family members. Enlist their help in running the household and meeting their schedules and needs. When friends and neighbors offer assistance, accept it. Face your own feelings and try to keep a normal schedule.

If chemotherapy treatment is recommended, you will need to find an oncologist. Because he or she will be your wife's physician for the longest period of time, this person must be someone with whom both of you feel comfortable and confident. Ask questions about what drugs will be used, how they will be administered, how long treatment will be, what side effects (short- and long-term) of each drug and possible complications could occur. Ask how side effects will be managed and what your responsibilities during the treatment will be. Discuss effects on reconstruction. Inquire about anti-nausea drugs. (See Appendix C for questions to ask.)

If the physician recommends radiology treatment rather than chemotherapy, question the radiologist about the dangers of X ray. Ask how it is given, how dangers of overexposure and burns are minimized, and what precautions must be taken when radiotherapy has been used. You may have other questions also. (See Appendix C for questions to ask.)

Finding Emotional Support Groups

Unless your wife already has a good support system, help her to build one. Seek support for yourself as well. It is desirable to have more than one person to whom you can turn.

Before and After Surgery

If your spouse/partner is denying the cancer, realize that temporary denial can be a protective device until she can face the reality of her loss. Be sensitive to her emotional needs as well as those of your children and other family members. Show affection, if only nonverbally. Make thoughtful gestures that will assure your wife of your love.

Prepare for the time after surgery and be ready to make changes and eliminate stress as far as it is possible. Anticipate your first viewing of the scar. Because much of your wife's adjustment will depend on your reaction during that moment, visualize possible results and rehearse your reactions.

With so many demands being made on you, make an effort to get rest, nutritious meals, and exercise. If you feel anger, resentment, and a wish to get this experience over, "accept yourself and be gentle." Establish open and honest communication with your spouse. Honor her needs as much as you can without sacrificing your own integrity or that of other family members.

During Her Recuperation at Home

Include the family members in the care process. Explain their mother's needs and give children a part in helping her. At the same time, encourage and commend her for doing as much as she can to help herself. Realize that

she fatigues easily and will undergo mood changes, which may be caused
by medication. Remember that physical touch and closeness are important
to her.

Resuming Sexual Intimacy

You can be sure that your sexual intimacy is troubling your loved one and
perhaps you as well. Empathize with what she is feeling. She may be worrying that she is no longer attractive to you, and you may be fearful of
hurting her physically.

There is no easy way to approach the subject if you as a couple are not
comfortable with discussing it. Beverly Kievman suggests that you begin by
reading information about the effect of chronic illness on sexuality.[1] In fact,
one section of her book is particularly appropriate reading for you. To your
spouse, acknowledge your discomfort in talking about it but say that you
are bringing it up because it is important to your relationship. Talk about
your feelings and concerns honestly. If you cannot talk about it, an alternative is to talk with her physician or a trusted friend who could intercede
for you.

As She Returns to Wellness

Be understanding of her worry about recurrence. Help her to resume her
activities and social life gradually as her energy increases. Be optimistic and
supportive and make plans for future activities together. Reward health, not
illness. Don't give into demands that will make you develop a martyr feeling.
Remember that the most important thing you can do for your ill spouse is
to be willing to go through this experience with her.[2]

If Death Becomes Imminent

Knowing that your loved one cannot conquer the cancer changes the
color and quality of life. Each day becomes more precious, yet in the presence of acute pain and suffering it may seem interminable. If you can work
through your own feelings of denial, anger, guilt, and other intense emotions, you may come to acceptance and be able to help her. On the other
hand, if she has already reached a state of acceptance herself, she may help
you. Keep up warm and supportive relationships outside the family, and
obtain counseling if you cannot resolve difficulties. You and your family
members can increase your knowledge about death through reading and
utilizing other resources. Information on dying can help you come to terms
with your own feelings about death, develop psychological strength, and
enable you to understand your children's grieving.

Encourage your loved one to talk and reflect on her life and yours together. Help her to see what she has accomplished, the legacy she is leaving you and those whose life she has touched. Help her to resolve troubling issues and attend to practical matters such as wills and dispensation of her belongings, if you have not already done so. Make written instructions of her wishes. Learn where she has put away important items such as papers, family mementos, jewelry, and other treasured possessions. If she indicates a desire to do so, plan the kind of funeral service she would like.

Dealing with Your Loss

Before you can rebuild your life you must first allow yourself to grieve. While you are doing this, many practical details will demand your time and energy. If you have children, you will need to comfort and encourage them to express their grief. As each of you will go through the process of recovery in a different way, be especially sensitive to the needs of adolescents whose reactions may be difficult to understand and their grieving delayed.

GUIDELINES FOR CHILDREN

The effect of a death on children differs with their ages and developmental stages. Small children will probably feel frightened and abandoned, and they may blame themselves in some way for the death of their parent. They need to be included in the final rites, encouraged to share their grief, and treated with honesty, a great deal of love, and assurance.

The grieving of adolescents is more complex and difficult to understand. Their initial responses may seem abnormal. They may repress their emotions until the intensity of their loss surfaces some months later. Their parent's death has deprived them of a sense of security at a time when they are trying to draw away from that security. Don't try to make them a surrogate mother for younger children.

Because losing a parent makes adolescents "different," they do not know how to relate to their peers, who themselves feel awkward about how to behave toward a bereaved friend. The adolescent's struggle can be made easier if his or her friends make some gesture to acknowledge the death, letting him or her know that they care and that he or she still belongs to the group. Empathic adults and friends who will reach out to the grieving adolescent can often help them more than the immediate family.

It is important that attention be given to the grieving process of young children and adolescents. Their inability to cope satisfactorily may have serious adverse effects on relationships and behaviors in later life.

GUIDELINES FOR OTHER FAMILY MEMBERS

Parents, in-laws, and other close relatives have a need to be informed of a critical illness and the patient's needs and progress. How much information you will receive will be determined by the rules and traditions of each family. These can vary widely. Although you can give tremendous support and provide resources, you can also add to the stress of the situation. Some of you may abandon the ill woman. Others of you can be overprotective and, thus, add to the coping problems of the spouse/partner and children. When this happens, you should be made to realize that you are helping in a counterproductive manner. This will require honest but tactful communication. For example, if as the patient's mother you criticize and discourage your daughter's efforts to do things for herself, she or your son-in-law may say, "I understand that you want to be helpful, but the doctor has advised us that it is better for Mary to take care of these tasks herself. There are other things you can do that would be helpful to all of us." Then they should suggest specific things that you can do.

Some stress could be averted if the ill woman or her spouse can clarify their needs to you. This can be done when they inform you about the breast cancer and surgery. The ill person can make her wishes known to you and to friends before she enters the hospital. If she does not want visitors until she comes home, but prefers phone calls and cards, she can explain her reasons. On the other hand, she may want you to visit her often. By telling you her needs, she has possibly spared her spouse or partner a situation that could increase the strain he already feels.

If the patient is single or living alone, she can call upon the relatives and friends who will be most important and helpful in her recovery. Guidelines for friends appear in the next chapter.

Chapter 19

Guidelines for Friends

When Luci Shaw, a publisher in Illinois, heard Amy Harwell speak about cancer at an adult discussion group, she nodded in agreement with what Amy had to say about the importance of having loving friends. Having experienced the death of her husband from lung cancer only a year earlier, Luci Shaw was impressed with Amy Harwell's philosophy of cancer and friendship. She persuaded Harwell to put her thoughts into a book, which Shaw has published. *When Your Friend Gets Cancer* is invaluable to anyone who is at a loss about what to do when a friend has cancer.

Harwell's first entreaty to the person who learns that a friend has cancer is to reach out to her, "no matter how inadequate you feel."[1] As a friend you are a very significant person in the life of one who has cancer, particularly if she is single or alone. That is not to say you are any less important if your ill friend has a spouse and a family, for you are able to help her more objectively than close family members can.

Harwell outlined some simple suggestions. (1) Consider your attitudes about cancer and your friendship. If you believe cancer is punishment and a death sentence, you will not convey a hopeful message to your ill friend unless you can change your outlook. (2) When a friend has cancer, you should waste no time in reaching out to her. (3) Educate yourself on the jargon and emotional impact of the disease. (4) Help her by giving her encouragement, supporting her loved ones, making her surroundings more pleasant, and doing practical things for her. (5) Listen to her as she faces the changes cancer has made in her life, and assure her that you care. (6) Be there for her, especially if she asks you to help her deal with imminent death. Listen and help her with the decisions and issues she must resolve.[2]

As a friend, you want to show concern for the woman with breast cancer but don't know what to say. You may fear that you won't say or do the right thing. You may be afraid to bring up the cancer, but find that chatting about pleasantries and avoiding the issue on both your minds is superficial and stressful. Consequently, you may want to avoid your ill friend. One thing she needs is to know that your friendship has not changed.

Women with breast cancer and counselors have given us some guidelines for friends. First, as a genuine friend you should do something; for to do nothing conveys a message of not caring. Whether it is a card, flowers, or some other tangible gift such as a lipstick, nail polish, something to brighten her appearance, do something. If you want to visit the woman who is recuperating from breast cancer, do so because you care, knowing that somehow you will find the right words. It is less awkward to acknowledge the cancer immediately, saying "I'm so sorry about your cancer," than to try to be cheerful and ignore your friend's reason for being hospitalized. By saying you are sorry, you have "broken the ice" and lifted the women's burden of bringing up the subject herself. If she chooses not to talk about it, she will change the topic. However, she may welcome the opportunity of having someone like you who is willing to listen. If she does, listen attentively. Sharing your own feelings, even shedding tears, will be comforting because she knows you care.[3]

There are several things you should not say to her.[4] Don't say, "I know how you feel," or "You're lucky to have found the cancer so early." Don't try to cheer her up. Don't tell her about the women you have known who have died of breast cancer. Don't criticize her choice of physicians. Don't give her advice on how to cope with this disease.

If you want to be helpful, make a specific offer of what you can do for her. Tell her you will pick up her children after school, take dinner to her family on a specific evening, or drive her for treatments when they begin. Some women are reluctant to accept help, at least with the first offer and especially if it is the vague "Let me know if I can do anything to help." Offer again, if you really want to help, and be specific about what you will do.

Remember that your ill friend will need your friendship when she is recovering at home. She may need it even more then, for she will no longer be surrounded with professional caregivers. Give her your time then and make plans to do something together.

There are many ways to be helpful. Invite her to lunch or to dinner or ask her to spend a weekend with you. If she has a family, you can help by doing things for her family. A list of twenty-five practical tips for those wanting to help a seriously ill friend has been prepared by the Bethesda Pastoral Care Department and made available through Hospice of Cincinnati.[5] The suggestions appear in Appendix G. Among the practical tips are some that we have already suggested.

If you are the friend of someone who has breast cancer, or any illness for that matter, Amy Harwell's book is filled with suggestions of ways in which you can be helpful and show the person that she or he is important to you. For the single person, your friendship is what she needs most.

Epilogue

Our purpose in this book has been to give you information compiled from research studies and the testimonies of those who have experienced breast cancer, many of whom are living productive, satisfying lives. As Dr. David Spiegel has stated in his book *Living beyond Limits* (1993), it is possible that by learning better management of the stresses in their lives, people with serious illnesses will "allow their bodies to devote their fullest resources to fighting the illness."[1] The effectiveness of treatment methods such as visualizing the destruction of cancer cells or maintaining a "positive attitude" has not been proven. However, there is some evidence that these methods may help prolong the lives of those with chronic illness such as breast cancer. Moreover, the increased sense of control that we derive from managing our lives, relationships, and feelings is an important benefit of some psychological techniques. It is significant that Congress has directed $20 million of its appropriation to the National Cancer Institute toward cancer research that helps people cope with the disease.

Having shared our investigation into the effects of breast cancer and survival guidelines for women and their families, we leave you with the following parting thoughts. As frightening and traumatic as breast cancer is, and despite the changes it makes in your lives, it is not the automatic death sentence it is often thought to be. New treatments make possible longer and fulfilling lives, and new research holds the promise of finding ways to curb this disease.

Women with whom we have talked recounted its negative as well as its positive effects. One spouse said, "There really isn't anything good about the disease, but it does make you realize how much you love one another." Many said it had sharpened their appreciation of what they have.

Breast cancer can make you aware of the importance of having your health. You learn that when it is in jeopardy you can gather the fortitude and courage to survive no matter how much effort it takes. You realize you cannot take your health for granted but must make it your responsibility to protect it with proper diet, exercise, and an optimistic outlook, and by paying attention to your body's warning signs. This requires that you become knowledgeable about your body as well as assertive in pursuing the help that is now available.

You must seek the diagnosis and treatment of a medical team, basing your choices on your own information and on the competence of professionals and the confidence they instill in you. Your desire to live and the hope that your physicians impart are important to your recovery.

Breast cancer makes you aware of the need for supportive relationships within and beyond your family boundaries. The urgency of repairing and nurturing relationships becomes paramount. You realize the comfort of having someone to lean on when the going gets rough, and of their knowing that they can expect the same of you in their time of need. Erma Bombeck reminds us that it is fine to put up a front of bravery and optimism but that you should not exclude your loved ones from knowing what you are feeling and experiencing.[2] By respecting the individual needs, goals, and experiences of your loved ones, you find that sharing your feelings honestly and empathically heals and strengthens your bonds. You learn the importance of having a family member or friend who will listen without judging or advising when you need to talk, and of becoming a good listener yourself.

Yes, you will indulge in moments of self-pity, but you still want to be treated as an adult, not as an ill person or a child. Reaching out to one another for support, you will be sustained by hope, make plans for the future, laugh together, and cherish each day. By pulling together you can surmount life's inevitable challenges.

You come to realize that the negative thoughts that communicate your shortcomings and self-doubts prevent you from reaching your potential. You learn that life is too dear to cling to an old image, so you discard it for new insight into who you can become. You dispense with trivialities and direct your energy to the worthwhile things that give your life a sense of purpose and meaning. You realize that the pursuit of some of your goals inhibits the deepening of relationships, the cultivation of your inner resources, and the fulfillment of long-held yearnings. You learn that each day is precious; and instead of the long-term goals that you tend to postpone, you set smaller ones that can be accomplished today. Your cancer experience teaches you to accept what you cannot change and to savor the moments you have now. Remembering that the "little things" often make a real difference in someone else's life, you become more compassionate and more understanding.

Marvella Bayh left a legacy of what it is to turn the cancer experience into spiritual and emotional growth. As it did for her, "cancer makes you get your priorities in order."[3] The late Clare Boothe Luce, who had tremendous curiosity and zest for life even as her health was failing, said that she looked forward to the dawning of each new day with anticipation of being a part of its drama. And she was . . . to the end of a fulfilling life.

Appendix A

Suggested Readings

The following readings have been especially meaningful and helpful to us in writing this book. We think some of them will be the same for you. There are many we have omitted but we recommend these as informative, interesting, and often uplifting reading.

Bayh, Marvella. *A Personal Journey.* New York: Harcourt Brace Jovanovich, 1979. The wife of former senator Birch Bayh takes us through her long, courageous battle with breast cancer. Her remarkable drive to overcome it and help others enabled her to turn breast cancer into a meaningful experience and a peaceful death.

Brinker, Nancy, with Catherine McEvily Harris. *The Race Is Run One Step at a Time: Everywoman's Guide to Taking Charge of Breast Cancer.* New York: Simon & Schuster, 1990. After losing her sister to breast cancer, Nancy Brinker established the Susan G. Komen Breast Cancer Foundation in her sister's memory. Then Nancy discovered a lump in her own breast. In telling her story of treatment and recovery, she stresses the importance of taking control and finding a good medical team. She offers vital information in a concise, comprehensive manner. A valuable resource list includes phone numbers of regional support organizations.

Bruning, Nancy. *Coping with Chemotherapy: How to Take Care of Yourself While Chemotherapy Takes Care of You.* Garden City, NY: Doubleday, 1985. Writing from personal experience and consultations with over fifty chemotherapy experts, Bruning explains types of chemotherapy, side effects, emotional aspects, and sources of support. She emphasizes the whole person. There are new medications since this book was written, but it is a helpful book to those having chemotherapy.

Cousins, Norman. *Anatomy of an Illness.* New York: W. W. Norton, 1979. Cousins explains his theory of the mind–body connection in fighting disease. When he was diagnosed with a serious disease, he became a partner with his physician in undertaking to tame his illness. He became the first influential spokesman for the holistic approach, with laughter having an essential function, and he set out to find scientific support for his belief.

Cousins, Norman. *Head First: The Biology of Hope.* New York: W. W. Norton, 1979. Invited to join the UCLA staff to do research on positive emotions, he began to document his hunches. He observed that a sensitive physician has the ability to invoke the patient's own defenses against disease, and that emotions and states of mind make a real difference.

Dreher, Henry. *Your Defense against Cancer.* New York: Harper & Row, 1988. This guide explains cancer and its risk factors, and gives steps for preventive action. Dreher takes a holistic approach with chapters on diet, life-style, and psychological factors.

Felder, Leonard. *When a Loved One Is Ill: How to Take Better Care of Your Loved One, Your Family, and Yourself.* New York: Penguin Books, 1991. The author writes in the hope that he can help readers turn the crisis of a loved one's illness into a meaningful, loving experience. He helps the caretaker know what to say, how to deal with guilt, and how to take care of one's self.

Gravelle, Karen, and Charles Haskins. *Teenagers Face to Face with Bereavement.* Englewood Cliffs, NJ: Julian Messner, 1989. The authors have compiled the experiences of bereaved teenagers whose behavior often masks the turmoil they are experiencing. A helpful book for understanding and helping teenagers to cope with grief.

Hansen, Barbara. *Picking Up the Pieces: Healing Ourselves after Personal Loss.* Dallas: Taylor, 1990. A car accident left Barbara Hansen paralyzed. From her struggle with the grief of her losses, she explains how she has put her life together to become a productive, charitable, and happy person. It is an inspirational story of a courageous woman.

Harwell, Amy, and Kristine Tomasik. *When Your Friend Gets Cancer: How You Can Help.* Wheaton, IL: Harold Shaw, 1987. A practical and inspiring book, this should be read by anyone who has a friend with breast cancer or any other illness. It explains the importance of your friendship and what to do and say.

Holleb, A. I., ed. *The American Cancer Society Cancer Book: Prevention, Detection, Diagnosis, Treatment, Rehabilitation, Cure.* Garden City, NY: Doubleday, 1986. A survey of all types of cancer with chapters on new insights and attitudes, steps you can take to prevent cancer, and how to live with it. There are specific chapters on breast cancer and pain. Look for an updated edition.

Kaye, Ronnie. *Spinning Straw into Gold: Your Emotional Recovery from Breast Cancer.* New York: Simon & Schuster, 1991. Offering a candid and compassionate discussion of her own emotional recovery from breast cancer and a recurrence, Kaye now counsels women suffering the same trauma. For dealing with fear read her Chapter 3, " . . . And Do You Have a Teddy Bear?" She lists precautions to prevent infections.

Kievman, Beverly, with Susie Blackmun. *For Better or For Worse: A Couple's Guide to Dealing with Chronic Illness.* Chicago: Contemporary Books, 1989. In dealing with her husband's diabetes, Kievman experienced problems that are the same for any chronic illness. She candidly discusses and offers solutions for every challenge that arises in relationships, medical costs, and legal matters A very helpful book written by a woman and others who have experienced all of it.

Kübler-Ross, Elisabeth. *On Death and Dying*. New York: Macmillan, 1969. This book opened the way for a new understanding of the grief process of the dying and those they leave. It gives insight into the emotional and life changes that the bereaved experience. Helpful for understanding interaction of family members during this time.

Kübler-Ross, Elisabeth. *Death: The Final Stage of Growth*. Englewood Cliffs, NJ: Prentice-Hall, 1975. For an understanding of the compassion of Kübler-Ross, read the chapters "Death as a Part of My Own Personal Life" and "Omega." The remainder of the book explains how other cultures view death, important information for professional caregivers.

Lerner, Harriet Goldhor. *The Dance of Anger*. New York: Harper & Row, 1985. Because anger often accompanies the breast cancer experience, this book can give insight into handling the emotion.

Lerner, Harriet Goldhor. *The Dance of Intimacy*. New York: Harper & Row, 1989. In long-term relationships, we are often challenged by too much distance, too much intensity, or too much pain. A staff psychologist at the Menninger Clinic, Lerner explains how we can make changes in relationships.

LeShan, Lawrence. *Cancer as a Turning Point: A Handbook for People with Cancer, Their Families, and Health Professionals*. New York: E. P. Dutton, 1989. A psychotherapist, LeShan helps people with cancer to direct their lives so that they will have as many satisfying, good moments as possible. He tries to build an understanding of the kind of life that would be most fulfilling for the person and, in turn, would help them with coping and recovery.

Love, Susan, with Karen Lindsey. *Dr. Susan Love's Breast Book* Reading, MA: Addison-Wesley, 1990. This is an authoritative book on all aspects of the breast, its diseases, and treatments by a well-known medical expert. It is a book every woman should read.

McAllister, R. M., S. T. Horowitz, and R. V. Gilden. *Cancer*. New York: Basic Books, 1993. A physician, biochemist, and scientist have collaborated in presenting findings on diagnosis and treatment of the ten most common cancers. Good if you want in-depth information. Includes a listing of cancer centers as well as clinical, basic, and consortium centers in the United States.

Murcia, Andy, and Bob Stewart. *Man to Man: When the Woman You Love Has Breast Cancer*. New York: St. Martin's Press, 1989. When his wife Ann Jillian got breast cancer, Murcia found nothing to help him deal with his feelings and problems. He turned to his friend, whose wife also had breast cancer. Together they wrote this book to help other men in the same situation. Candid and conversational.

Napier, Augustus Y. *The Fragile Bond*. New York: Harper & Row, 1988. A therapist, Napier gives insight into how we balance family loyalty and personal growth and create a family life that is better and happier than the one in which we grew up. Chapters 16, 17, and 18 are especially pertinent for troubled relationships.

Nessim, Susan, and Judith Ellis. *Cancervive: The Challenge of Life after Cancer*. Boston: Houghton Mifflin, 1991. Nessim, whose cancer occurred in her late teens, encountered many problems after her recovery. When she learned that others were having similar problems, she founded Cancervive, a support group for survivors. This book is based on the experiences of members of Cancervive and the advice of experts. It contains information for handling everything from the practical problems of insurance to writing resumes. (See Appendix B for address of Cancervive.)

Parker, J. H., and R. B. Parker. *Three Weeks in Spring.* Boston: Houghton Mifflin, 1978. This is a chronicle of the Parkers' experience from the time Joan found a lump through the next six weeks of diagnosis through initial recovery. Each discloses their feelings and thoughts on issues that are of greatest concern to a couple. Candid, humorous, enlightening, it is a good book for a couple to read together to open lines of communication.

Rosenbaum, E. H. *Living with Cancer.* New York: Praeger Publishers, 1975. A caring physician, Dr. Rosenbaum encourages families to seek open communication with their physicians and others on the health care team. The major part of the book consists of the stories of individual patients. Rosenbaum also explains therapies and treatments.

Siegel, Bernie S. *Love, Medicine and Miracles.* New York: Harper & Row, 1986. As a surgeon, Siegel realized he had to change his attitude toward his profession to overcome the despair he was feeling. A seminar with the Simontons changed his approach to patients. This book discusses his new attitude and the exceptional patients he treated. He offers exercises in relaxation and visualization.

Spiegel, David. *Living beyond Limits.* New York: Random House, 1993. A Stanford University psychiatrist, Spiegel provides guidelines for living with cancer. Pointing out the dangers of putting too much faith in promises of holistic methods, he integrates them with medical treatment. He is an advocate of support groups.

Appendix B

Resources

SUPPORT GROUPS AND INFORMATION SOURCES

Albert Einstein Medical Center Breast Cancer Program

Staffed by nurses who answer questions regarding mastectomy, lumpectomy, or reconstruction, this program serves the metropolitan area of Philadelphia and the surrounding eastern areas (New Jersey, Delaware and Pennsylvania). Call 1 (800) Einstein (the last letter in Einstein is dropped when the number is dialed).

> Klein Building, Room 101
> 5401 Old York Road
> Philadelphia, PA 19141

American Cancer Society (ACS)

Call your local unit for information and materials on breast cancer and referrals to other resources in your area as well as doctors for second opinions. ACS also has the Cancer Response System: 1 (800) 227–2345; call for a free breast cancer packet and/or *Cancer Facts and Figures*, which is issued annually. The national office address is:

> 3340 Peachtree Road, NE
> Atlanta, GA 30026
> (404) 320–3333

American Council of Life Insurance

For information on questions about insurance, write:

> American Council of Life Insurance
> 1001 Pennsylvania Avenue, NW
> Washington, DC 20004

American Society of Plastic and Reconstructive Surgeons

Will provide information on reconstructive surgery and a list of certified reconstructive surgeons by geographical area.

> American Society of Plastic and Reconstructive Surgeons
> 444 East Algonquin Road
> Arlington Heights, IL 60005
> (708) 228–9900

Batesville Management Services

A business and educational resource for funeral service as well as health care, counseling, and support groups. Audiovisual programs and pamphlets on children and death, grief support, widows and widowers, and coping with grief are available. For information on these materials, call or write:

> Batesville Management Services
> 1069 State Route 46E
> Batesville, IN 47006–9989
> 1 (800) 622–8373 (United States)
> 1 (800) 446–2504 (Canada)

Cancer Care, Inc.

This social service agency provides professional counseling to patients with advanced stages of cancer and their families. It also provides helpful materials such as the booklet "What about Me?" for the teenaged children of patients with cancer. The booklet is available at Cincinnati's Cancer Family Care, which is patterned after Cancer Care, Inc. Call or write the national office for information about local organizations:

> Cancer Care, Inc.
> 1180 Avenue of the Americas
> New York, NY 10036
> (212) 221–3300

Cancer Information Service

Administered by the National Cancer Institute, this service supplies information and answers questions about cancer and cancer-related resources (prevention, detection, local medical facilities, financial aid). Write:

> Office of Cancer Communication
> National Cancer Institute
> Bldg. 31, Rm. 10 & 18
> Bethesda, MD 20205

Cancervive

A support service for those who have survived cancer, started by Susan Nessim and a friend who realized the need for a support group. If you would like to start a chapter, contact:

Cancervive, Inc.
6500 Wilshire Boulevard, Suite 500
Los Angeles, CA 90048

CanSurmount

Carefully trained volunteers, who have had cancer, visit with patients and their families to provide support and education. For information call your local chapter or write to the national headquarters of the American Cancer Society at the number and address listed above.

Community Cancer Information Center (CCIC)

This organization in Ohio represents a joint effort of the Hamilton County Unit of the American Cancer Society and the Barrett Center to provide educational material and to make referrals to support and service groups providing educational, financial, and nutritional help. It is located at the University of Cincinnati Medical Center.

Barrett Cancer Center
234 Goodman Avenue
Cincinnati, OH 45267
(513) 558–3200

Coping Magazine

For a catalog on books/videos/audios offered by this magazine, write:

Coping Catalog
2019 North Carothers
Franklin, TN 37064

Encore Program

A program offered by the YWCA, this provides discussion and rehabilitation for women who have had breast cancer. Contact your local Y or write:

YWCA Encore Program
YWCA National Headquarters
624 Ninth Street, NW
Washington, DC 20001
(202) 628–3636
Fax: (202) 783–7123

Federal Drug Administration (FDA)

For information concerning problems with breast implants or for information about reconstructive surgery, call the FDA: 1 (800) 638–6725. For informational material on breast implants or to report problems with devices, call the same number.

Food and Drug Administration
5600 Fishers Lane
Rockville, MD 20857

Health Insurance Association of America (HIAA)

This organization responds to questions concerning insurance covering breast cancer prevention and treatment. Write:

Health Insurance Association of America
Fulfillment Department
PO Box 41455
Washington, DC 20018

I Can Cope

Designated as a national program by the American Cancer Society, *I Can Cope* focuses on educational and psychological needs of persons with cancer. Contact your local American Cancer Society or the ACS Cancer Response System at the address and phone number listed above.

Look Good, Feel Better

This national program, sponsored by the American Cancer Society; the Cosmetic, Toiletry, and Fragrance Association; and the National Cosmetology Association Foundation, is for patients undergoing chemotherapy and radiation treatments. Workshops given by volunteer certified hairdressers and makeup artists help women feel better by improving their appearance. Call your local office of the American Cancer Society or the national office for information.

National Alliance of Breast Cancer Organizations (NABCO)

A national clearinghouse of information about breast cancer and an advocate for legislative concerns. Individuals and organizations may join this information network. For information, write:

National Alliance of Breast Cancer Organizations
1180 Avenue of the Americas, Second Floor
New York, NY 10036

National Cancer Institute

This organization deals with difficult questions about the treatment of cancer. It calls Consensus Conferences of clinical investigators, supporting professionals and patients. It evaluates available scientific information, consolidates it and makes recommendations about what ought to be done in practice. It stimulates research and analysis that may be useful in finding the cause and cure of breast cancer. It also supports a number of cancer centers countrywide that investigate new methods of diagnosis and treatment.

National Center Institute
Bethesda, MD 20892
1 (800) 4–Cancer

National Hospice Organization

This organization provides service for the patient who is terminally ill. Call your local organization or contact:

National Hospice Organization
1901 N. Moore Street, Suite 901
Arlington, VA 22209
(703) 243–5900

Physician Data Query (PDQ)

A computer system that includes current treatments as well as a directory of doctors and hospitals that have cancer programs. You will need to go through a physician to use this.

Reach to Recovery

Sponsored by the American Cancer Society, this group consists of trained volunteers who help patients with physical, emotional, and cosmetic needs. Call your local American Cancer Society office or the national office for information:

> American Cancer Society Tower Place
> 3340 Peachtree Road, NE
> Atlanta, GA 30026
> (404) 320–3333

Susan G. Koman Breast Cancer Foundation

Will provide information on screening, breast self-examination, and other related topics. The booklet "Caring for Your Breasts" is available in English, Spanish, and Braille; so are names of accredited mammography facilities. Write:

> Susan G. Koman Breast Cancer Foundation
> 6820 LBJ Freeway, Suite 130
> Dallas, TX 75240

Wellness Community Support Groups

This support organization offers companionship, recovery skills, and advice. The philosophy of this group is humor. It exists in Santa Monica, South Bay Cities, San Diego, Knoxville, Chicago, Orange County, Pasadena, San Francisco, greater Cincinnati, Westlake Village, Boston, Baltimore, Philadelphia, and greater St. Louis. For information, call your local American Cancer Society or (310) 314–2555.

Y-ME

This national nonprofit organization for breast cancer information and support sponsors monthly meetings in the Chicago area and states where chapters exist. It provides a toll-free line for information, referrals, and emotional support.

> Y-ME National Breast Cancer Organization
> 212 West Van Buren
> Chicago, IL 60607
> (800) 221–2141 (9 A.M. to 5 P.M. CST)

Appendix C

Questions to Ask Doctors

QUESTIONS TO ASK THE PHYSICIAN WHEN YOU FIND A LUMP

1. Do I need a mammogram? (If he says "yes," ask him if he will call you with the results. If he recommends a biopsy instead of a mammogram, ask him how and when that will be done.)
2. If you draw fluid out of the lump, will it be examined for cancer cells?
3. How soon can I know the results?
4. If it is normal, should the lump be checked regularly? If so, how often?
5. If the lump is cancerous, should I see a surgeon? If so, would you give me the names of several surgeons you recommend?

QUESTIONS TO ASK THE PHYSICIAN WHEN CANCER CELLS ARE FOUND

1. What are my alternatives for treatment (i.e., surgery, chemotherapy, radiation)?
2. Please explain the surgical procedure. Exactly what will you be removing? How will I look?
3. How many lymph nodes and glands will you be removing, and why should they be removed?
4. How many days will I be in the hospital?
5. What are the side effects of each type of treatment?
6. Does research show advantages of one type of treatment over the other? How does the mastectomy compare to the lumpectomy/radiation procedure?
7. Do you recommend chemotherapy after a mastectomy?

8. Should I expect a recurrence of cancer or a cure?

9. If I choose mastectomy surgery, when may I have reconstruction done?

10. Please give me the names of two plastic surgeons and two oncologists (or radiologists) with whom you work well.

11. Please give me the names of agencies and support groups that are involved with breast cancer.

12. How much time do I have to make a decision?

13. Do you have an associate registered nurse who works with you?

14. Whom may I call for further information if I need it?

15. What is the cost of this surgery?

QUESTIONS TO ASK THE PLASTIC SURGEON

1. What are the various methods of breast reconstruction?

2. What are the advantages and disadvantages of each procedure?

3. Which technique best fits my need?

4. What are the possible complications and side effects?

5. How many surgeries will be required?

6. What type of anesthesia is necessary for each surgery?

7. How long will I be in the hospital for each surgery?

8. What are the physical limitations and length of recovery for each?

9. How long will the entire procedure take?

10. Will the reconstructed breast match my other breast?

11. May I see photographs of your successful and unsuccessful results?

12. How many reconstructions do you perform a year, especially the procedure we decide upon for me?

13. Are you a certified plastic surgeon?

14. Will the reconstruction interfere with detecting recurrences?

15. What is the cost of the complete process of reconstruction?

16. How much of the cost will be covered by insurance?

17. Will you refer me to two or three of your patients who have been through this type of surgery?

QUESTIONS TO ASK AN ONCOLOGIST BEFORE CHEMOTHERAPY TREATMENT

1. How do we decide whether I need chemotherapy?

2. How does chemotherapy work?

3. How and where is it given?

4. How often would I be getting treatments?

5. What are the possible side effects?

6. Will it make me nauseous? If it does, what medications are there to relieve it and any other side effects?

7. Will I lose my hair? Will I gain weight with these drugs?

8. How long will the treatments be necessary?

9. Will I be able to continue my work while receiving treatments?

10. Can you give me the names of any of your patients who have had this treatment?

11. What is the cost of these treatments? How much is covered by insurance?

QUESTIONS TO ASK A RADIOLOGIST BEFORE RECEIVING RADIATION

1. What does radiation therapy do?

2. How safe is it?

3. What are the risks and side effects?

4. How often and where will the treatments occur?

5. Please describe the procedure.

6. Will I be hospitalized? How long will it take?

7. What precautions are taken to insure that I do not receive too much?

8. Will I be radioactive?

9. What precautions must I take after having radiation?

10. Will I be able to work while receiving it?

11. If I have radiation therapy, will I be able to have reconstruction in the future? If not, why not?

12. What will be the cost of this treatment? How much is covered by insurance?

QUESTIONS TO ASK IF HORMONE THERAPY IS RECOMMENDED

1. How does hormone therapy work?

2. What are hormone receptor tests?

3. Have you given me hormone receptor tests yet? If so, may I see the results? Would you explain what they mean? If my tests haven't been done yet, when will they be?

4. Why do you recommend hormone therapy for me?

5. How is it administered?

6. How long will it be continued?

7. What are the side effects?

8. Would you give me names of two or three of your patients who have had this treatment?

Appendix D

Procedures for Detecting Breast Cancer

The three procedures for detecting early breast cancer are breast self-examination (BSE), a physical examination by a doctor or a nurse, and a mammogram.

BREAST SELF-EXAMINATION

Check your breasts each month at the same time: five to seven days after the start of your menstrual period. After menopause, select any day of the month (such as the date of your birthday).

Look for changes in your breasts by observing them in a mirror. Feel for changes in your breasts while showering. Also check them while lying on your bed. Place a rolled towel under one shoulder, raise your arm overhead. Using the pads of your fingers of the other hand, begin at the top of your breast and move around the breast in circles from the outside toward the nipple so that you feel the entire breast. Check under the arm as well. Repeat the procedure on the other breast.

PHYSICAL EXAMINATION

Once a year see a doctor or nurse for a check of your breasts. Report any pain or changes in your breasts.

MAMMOGRAM

The mammogram takes an X ray of the breast. You will disrobe to the waist so that each breast can be squeezed between the two flat plates and X-rayed to detect problems inside the breast.

Your first mammogram should be taken by age 39–40. From age 40 to 49, have a mammogram every two years. Over age 50, have one every year.

Appendix E

Precautions for Avoiding Lymphedema

Because infection is your greatest danger when you have had surgical removal of a tumor and adjacent lymph nodes and vessels, it is necessary to protect and avoid injury in the arm closest to the treatment of your breast cancer. When lymphatic flow is obstructed, the fluid that accumulates creates a condition favorable for the growth of bacteria. This eventually leads to infection. To prevent and treat early infections, the following precautions should always be taken:

In working around your house and garden

- Take care in using sharp objects such as kitchen knives, scissors, needles, and pins.

- Avoid carrying heavy objects.

- Do not work above your head. For chores requiring overhead work, use an extension pole.

- Wear rubber gloves while doing dishes, housework, or any chores that can result in minor injuries.

- Wear gloves at all times when doing any gardening.

- Take care when handling plants, such as roses, that are prickly or have thorns.

- Be cautious in using sharp or pointed tools.

- Treat an insect bite or sting at once by cleaning the skin thoroughly and seeking medical attention.

Adapted from S.R.J. Thiadens, *Lymphedema: An Information Booklet*, 3rd edition, San Francisco, 1993, p. 4, and an unidentified list of instructions.

In personal care

• Limit your salt intake, fats, alcohol, and smoking.

• Maintain your ideal weight through a regular, well-balanced diet. Drink adequate fluids.

• Keep skin clean and dry by using hypoallergenic soaps and deodorants.

• Take care when cutting and filing nails. Avoid cutting cuticles.

• Use an electric razor rather than a safety razor.

• Do not wear tight jewelry or elastic bands around affected fingers or arms.

• Elevate the affected arm when possible.

When engaging in physical activity

• Avoid overexertion and activities that require vigorous or repetitive movements, such as rubbing, scrubbing, pushing, or pulling. Avoid sports such as racquetball and tennis.

• Consult your therapist about activities that will not aggravate the limb. Beneficial exercises are walking and swimming. Avoid swinging the arm when walking.

• Avoid extreme temperature changes, such as in bathing, sunning, using a hot tub or sauna.

• Avoid lifting or carrying heavy objects, such as suitcases or heavy handbags, especially those with shoulder straps.

• Wear sunscreen, avoid overexposure, and keep the affected limb protected from the sun.

Medical Care

• Do not allow your blood pressure to be taken or have injections or blood drawn in the affected arm.

• Request a lightweight prosthesis if yours is heavy and puts too much pressure on the lymph nodes above the collar bone.

• Carry a prescription for antibiotics when you travel. If traveling out of the country, carry your medication with you.

• Watch for any or all signs of infection: redness, increased swelling, heat, and pain.

• Contact a physician immediately if you suffer an injury to the affected limb, or if you suspect an infection.

Appendix F

Bill of Rights for Cancer Patients and Family Members

For Cancer Patients

I have the right to be told the truth about my disease.

I have the right to feel badly if I receive bad news.

I have the right to talk to my doctor and my family about my cancer. And I have the right to privacy in refusing to talk with others about it if that is my choice.

I have the right to be treated as a person and not merely as a "patient" while I am sick. The fact that I am sick does not give others the right to make decisions for me.

I have the right to think about other things besides my cancer. I do not have to allow cancer to control every detail of my life.

I have the right to ask others for help in the things I cannot do for myself, within reason.

I always have the right to hope—for a full cure, a longer life, or a happier life here and now.

I have the right and it is OK to be angry with people I love. My anger does not mean I have stopped loving them.

I have the right to cope with my cancer in my own way, and my family has the right to cope with it in theirs. Our ways may be different, but that is OK.

I have the right to be free of pain if that is my choice.

Printed with permission of Cancer Family Care, Inc., Cincinnati, Ohio.

For Family Members

I have the right to enjoy my own good health without feeling guilty. It is not my fault that someone I love has cancer.

I have the right to choose whom I will talk to about the cancer. If I hurt others' feelings because they are asking too many questions, it is not my fault.

I have the right to know what is going on in our family, even if I am a child. I have the right to be told the truth about the cancer in words I can understand.

I have the right to disagree with the patient even if he or she has cancer. I can feel angry with someone and not always feel guilty, because sickness does not stop someone from being a real person.

I have the right to feel what I feel now, not what someone else says I "should" feel.

I have the right to look after my own needs, even if they do not seem as great as the patient's. I am permitted to take "time out" from the cancer without feeling disloyal.

I have the right to get outside help for the patient if I cannot manage all the responsibilities of home care myself.

I have the right to get help for myself, even if others in my family choose not to get help.

Appendix G

Twenty-five Practical Tips You Can Use to Help Those Facing Serious Illness

1. Don't avoid me. Be the friend . . . the loved one you've always been.

2. Touch me. A simple squeeze of my hand tells me you still care.

3. Call and tell me you're bringing over my favorite dish. Bring food in disposable containers so I won't worry about returning them.

4. Watch my children while I take a little time to be alone with my loved one. My children also may need a little vacation from my illness.

5. Cry with me when I cry and laugh with me when I laugh. Don't be afraid to share these emotions with me. Pain isolates. Help me reconnect with others.

6. Take me out for a pleasure trip, but know my limitations.

7. Call for my shopping list and make a special delivery to my home.

8. Before you visit, call to let me know, but don't be afraid to visit. I need you. I can get lonely.

9. Help me celebrate holidays (and life) by decorating my hospital room or home by bringing me flowers or other natural treasures.

10. Help my family. Invite them out. Take them places. I am sick, but they may be suffering also. Offer to come stay with me to give my loved ones a break.

11. Be creative! Bring me a book of thoughts, taped music, a poster for my wall, cookies to share with my family and friends.

12. Let's talk about it. Maybe I need to talk about my illness. Find out by asking me: "Do you feel like talking about it?"

13. Don't always feel we have to talk. Sitting quietly together is fine.

Condensed from a brochure compiled by St. Anthony's Hospital in Alton, Illinois. Prepared by the Bethesda Pastoral Care Department and made available through Hospice in Cincinnati. Printed with permission of Hospice of Cincinnati, Inc., Cincinnati, Ohio.

14. Can you take me and or my children somewhere? I may need transportation to a treatment . . . to the store . . . or to my physician.

15. Help me feel good about my looks. Tell me I look good, considering my illness.

16. Please include me in decision making. I've been robbed of so many things. Please don't deny me a chance to make decisions in my family or in my life.

17. Talk to me of the future. Tomorrow, next week, next year. Hope is so important to me.

18. Bring me a positive attitude. It's catching. Help me respect reality.

19. What's in the news? Magazines, photos, newspapers, and verbal reports keep me from feeling the world is passing me by.

20. Could you help me with some cleaning? During my illness my family and I still face dirty clothes, dirty dishes, and a dirty house.

21. Water my flowers.

22. Just send a card to let me know you care.

23. Pray for me and share your faith with me.

24. Tell me how you'd like to help me and when I agree, please do so.

25. Tell me about support groups so I can share with others.

Notes

CHAPTER 1

1. S. M. Love with K. Lindsey, *Dr. Susan Love's Breast Book* (Reading, MA: Wesley Publ., 1990), p. 176.

2. P. Preece, M. Baum, and R. Mansel, "Importance of Mastalgia in Operable Breast Cancer," *British Medical Journal* 284 (1982): 1299–1300; Love with Lindsey, *Breast Book*, p. 94.

3. J. N. Wolfe, "Breast Cancer Screening: A Brief Historical Review," *Breast Cancer Research & Treatment* 18 (1991): S89.

4. Love with Lindsey, *Breast Book*, pp. 22, 110 111.

5. Love with Lindsey, *Breast Book*, p. 22.

6. *Cancer Facts & Figures—1994*, (Atlanta: American Cancer Society, 1994), p. 110.

7. Love with Lindsey, *Breast Book*, pp. 177–178.

8. R. Dodd, "Radiation Detection and Diagnosis of Breast Cancer," *Cancer* 47 (1981): 1768.

9. *Cancer Facts & Figures—1994*, p. 110.

10. E. F. Scanlon and P. Strax, "Breast Cancer," in A. I. Holleb, ed., *The American Cancer Society Cancer Book* (Garden City, NY: Doubleday, 1986), pp. 304–305.

11. Love with Lindsey, *Breast Book*, p. 189.

12. E. E. Kim, D. A. Podoloff, et al., "Magnetic Resonance Imaging, Positron Emission Tomography, and Radioimmunoscintography of Breast Cancer," *Cancer* 45 (1993): 501.

13. D.G.R. Evans, L. D. Burnell, et al., "Perception of Risk in Women with a Family History of Breast Cancer," *British Journal of Cancer* 67 (1993): 612.

14. Love with Lindsey, *Breast Book*, p. 144.

15. V. G. Vogel and A. C. Yeomans, "Evaluation of Risk and Preventive Approaches to Breast Cancer," *Cancer Bulletin* 45 (1993): 489.

16. H. T. Lynch, W. A. Albano, et al., "Genetics, Biomarkers and Control of Breast Cancer: A Review," *Cancer Genetics and Cytogenetics* 13 (1984): 43–92; H. T. Lynch and J. F. Lynch, "Breast Cancer Genetics in an Oncology Clinic: 328 Consecutive Patients," *Cancer Genetics and Cytogenetics* 22 (1986): 371; R. C. Go, M. C. King, et al., "Genetic Epidemiology of Breast Cancer and Associated Cancers in High-Risk Families. I. Segregation Analysis," *Journal of the National Cancer Institute* 71 (September 1983): 455–461; D. E. Anderson and M. D. Badzioch, "Risk of Familial Cancer," *Cancer* 56 (1985): 386.

17. M. C. King, S. Rowell, and S. M. Love, "Inherited Breast and Ovarian Cancer—What Are the Risks? What Are the Choices?" *Journal of the American Medical Association* 269 (1993): 1975–1980.

18. V. G. Vogel and A. C. Yeomans, "Evaluation of Risk," p. 489.

19. J. H. Harris, M. Morrow, and G. Bonadonna, "Cancer of the Breast," in V. T. DeVita, J. S. Hellman, and S. A. Rosenberg, eds., *Cancer: Principles and Practices of Oncology*, vol. 1, 4th ed. (Philadelphia: Lippincott, 1993), pp. 1266–1267; J. M. Black and E. Matassarin-Jacobs, *Luckman and Sorensen's Medical-Surgical Nursing, A Psychologic Approach* (Philadelphia: W. B. Saunders, 1993), pp. 2174–2175; Scanlon and Strax, "Breast Cancer," pp. 198–300.

20. M. E. Stefanek and P. Wilcox, "First Degree Relations of Breast Cancer Patients: Screening Practices and Provision of Risk Information," *Cancer Detection and Prevention* 15 (1991): 379–385.

21. T. Bernay, S. Porrath, et al., "The Impact of Breast Cancer Screening on Feminine Identity: Implications for Patient Education," *Breast, Diseases of the Breast* 9 (1982): 2–3.

22. I. C. Bennett, D. A. Robert, J. M. Osborne, and C. A. Baker, "Discomfort during Mammography: A Survey of Women Attending a Breast Screening Center," *Breast Disease* 7 (1994): 35–41.

23. L. Garfinkel, "Evaluating Cancer Statistics," *CA—A Cancer Journal for Clinicians* 44 (1994): 5–6; C. C. Boring, T. S. Squires, T. Tong, and S. Montgomery, "Cancer Statistics, 1994," *CA—A Cancer Journal for Clinicians* 44 (1994): 5–6.

24. *Cancer Facts & Figures*, p. 10.

CHAPTER 2

1. B. E. Meyerowitz, R. L. Heinrich, and C. C. Schag, "A Competency-Based Approach to Coping," in T. G. Burish and L. A. Bradley, eds., *Chronic Disease: Research and Applications* (New York: Academic Press, 1983), p. 142.

2. M. Clark, H. Morris, P. King, et al., "Living with Cancer: 'Learning to Survive,' " *Newsweek* (April 8, 1985): 73.

3. P. Gagnon, M. J. Massie, and J. C. Holland, "The Woman with Breast Cancer: Psychosocial Considerations," *Cancer Bulletin* 45 (1993): 538.

4. J. L. Katz, H. Weiner, T. F. Gallagher, and L. Hellman, "Stress, Distress and Ego Defenses: Psychoendocrine Response to Impending Breast Tumor Biopsy," *Archives of General Psychiatry* 23 (1970): 131–142.

5. R. S. Lazarus and S. Folkman, *Stress, Appraisal, and Coping* (New York: Springer Publ., 1984), p. 150.

6. J. Polivy, "Psychological Effects of Mastectomy on a Woman's Feminine Self-Concept," *Journal of Nervous and Mental Disease* 164 (1977): 86.

7. R. H. Moos and V. D. Tsu, "The Crisis of Physical Illness: An Overview," in R. H. Moos, ed., *Coping with Physical Illness* (New York: Plenum Press, 1977), p. 7.

8. S. E. Singletary, M. A. Schusterman, and M. D. McNeese, "Breast Conservation vs. Breast Reconstruction," *Cancer Bulletin* 45 (1993): 512–513.

9. L. J. Fallowfield, A. Hall, G. P. Maguire, and M. Baum, "Psychological Outcomes and Different Treatment Policies in Women with Early Breast Cancer outside a Clinical Trial," *British Medical Journal* 301 (1990): 575–580.

10. K. M. Foley, "Cancer and Pain," in A. I. Holleb, ed., *The American Cancer Society Cancer Book* (New York: Doubleday, 1986), p. 235.

11. S. Simonton and R. L. Shook, *The Healing Family: The Simonton Approach for Families Facing Illness* (New York: Bantam Books, 1984), p. 220.

12. S. M. Love with K. Lindsey, *Dr. Susan Love's Breast Book* (Reading, MA: Addison-Wesley Publ., 1990), pp. 93–94, 213.

13. J. C. Holland and L. O. Cullen, "New Insights and Attitudes," in A. I. Holleb, ed., *The American Cancer Society Cancer Book* (New York: Doubleday, 1980), p. 11.

14. L. Freeman and H. L. Strean, *Guilt, Letting Go* (New York: John Wiley & Sons, 1986), p. 81.

15. H. G. Lerner, *The Dance of Intimacy* (New York: Harper & Row, 1989), pp. 66–67.

16. L. Felder, *When a Loved One Is Ill: How to Take Better Care of Your Loved One, Your Family and Yourself* (New York: New American Library, 1990), p. 180.

17. I. Sullivan, "Cancer Curriculum for Well Siblings of Pediatric Cancer Patients," in A. Blitzer et al., eds., *Communicating with Cancer Patients and Their Families* (Philadelphia: Charles Press, 1990), p. 91.

18. Felder, *When a Loved One Is Ill*, pp. 183–200.

19. M. Watson, S. Greer, L. Rowden, et al., "Relationships between Emotional Control, Adjustment to Cancer, and Depression and Anxiety in Breast Cancer Patients," *Psychological Medicine* 21 (1991): 51–57.

20. Love with Lindsey, *Breast Book*, p. 365.

21. P. Gagnon, M. J. Massie, and J. C. Holland, "The Woman with Breast Cancer: Psychosocial Considerations," *Cancer Bulletin* 45 (1993): 539.

CHAPTER 3

1. K. Arms and P. S. Camp, *Biology*, 3rd ed. (Philadelphia: Saunders, 1988); R. M. McAllister, S. T. Horowitz, and R. V. Gilden, *Cancer* (New York: Basic Books, 1993), Chs. 1–5; M. Dollinger, E. H. Rosenbaum, and Greg Cable, *Everyone's Guide to Cancer Therapy* (Kansas City: Andrews and McMeel, 1991), pp. 1–7; N. Bruning, *Coping with Chemotherapy* (Garden City, NY: Doubleday, 1985), pp. 5–10.

2. F. A. Holmes and A. B. Deisseroth, "Genetic and Molecular Approaches to the Use of Autologous Stem Cells to Enhance the Therapeutic Index of Chemotherapy for Breast Cancer," *Cancer Bulletin* 45 (1993): 151.

3. S. M. Love with K. Lindsey, *Dr. Susan Love's Breast Book* (Reading, MA: Addison-Wesley, 1990), p. 209; B. Fisher, "Laboratory and Clinical Research in

Breast Cancer—A Personal Adventure. The David Karnofsky Memorial Lecture," *Cancer Research* 40 (1980): 3864–3874; J. Gershon-Cohen, S. M. Berger, and H. S. Klickstein, "Roentgenography of Breast Cancer Moderating Concept of 'Biological Determinism,' " *Cancer* 16 (1963): 961–964.

4. Love with Lindsey, *Breast Book*, p. 115.

5. Love with Lindsey, *Breast Book*, p. 22.

6. J. E. Brody, "The Value and Limits of Mammography," *New York Times* (September 22, 1988): Y24.

7. J. H. Harris, M. Morrow, and G. Bonadonna, "Cancer of the Breast," in V. T. DeVita, J. S. Hellman, and S. A. Rosenberg, eds., *Cancer Principles and Practices of Oncology*, vol. 1, 4th ed. (Philadelphia: Lippincott, 1993), p. 1273.

8. E. R. Frykberg and K. I. Bland, "Noninvasive Carcinoma of the Breast," *Cancer Bulletin* 45 (1993): 506.

9. E. F. Scanlon and P. Strax, "Breast Cancer," in A. I. Holleb, ed., *The American Cancer Society Cancer Book* (Garden City, NY: Doubleday, 1986), p. 317.

10. Harris, Morrow, and Bonadonna, "Cancer of the Breast," pp. 1272–1273; J. M. Black and E. Matassarin-Jacobs, *Luckman and Sorensen's Medical-Surgical Nursing, A Psychologic Approach*. (Philadelphia: W. B. Saunders, 1993), p. 2176.

11. Scanlon and Strax, "Breast Cancer," pp. 319–320.

12. G. A. Staerkel, "Fine-Needle Aspiration: Technique and Application in the Evaluation of Malignancies," *Cancer Bulletin* 45 (1993): 8–9.

13. Love with Lindsey, *Breast Book*, p. 132.

14. S. H. Parker, J. D. Lovin, W. E. Jobe, et al., "Nonpalpable Breast Lesions: Stereotactic Automated Large Core Biopsies," *Radiology* 180 (1990): 406.

15. P. Gagnon, M. J. Massie, and J. C. Holland, "The Woman with Breast Cancer: Psychosocial Considerations," *Cancer Bulletin* 45 (1993): 541.

16. Love with Lindsey, *Breast Book*, pp. 150–151; L. J. Humphrey, "Subcutaneous Mastectomy Is Not a Prophylaxis against Carcinoma of the Breast: Opinion or Knowledge?" *American Journal of Surgery* 145 (1983): 311.

17. V. G. Vogel and A. C. Yeomans, "Evaluation of Risk and Preventive Approaches to Breast Cancer," *Cancer Bulletin* 45 (1993): 492.

18. Black and Matassarin-Jacobs, *Luckman and Sorensen's*, p. 2179.

19. B. Fisher, C. Redmond, R. Poisson, et al., "Eight-Year Results of a Randomized Clinical Trial Comparing Total Mastectomy and Lumpectomy with or without Irradiation in the Treatment of Breast Cancer," *New England Journal of Medicine* 320 (March 30, 1989): 822–828; A. Recht, J. L. Connolly, S. J. Schnitt, et al., "Conservative Surgery and Primary Radiation Therapy for Early Breast Cancer: Results, Controversies and Unresolved Problems," *Seminars in Oncology* 13 (1986): 446.

20. Black and Matassarin-Jacobs, *Luckman and Sorensen's*, p. 2181.

21. A. U. Buzdar and G. N. Hortobagyi, "Recent Developments and New Directions in Adjuvant Therapy for Breast Cancer," *Cancer Bulletin* 45 (1993): 523.

22. Black and Matassarin-Jacobs, *Luckman and Sorensen's*, p. 2181.

23. N. Bruning, *Coping with Chemotherapy* (Garden City, NY: Doubleday, 1985), p. 23.

24. Scanlon and Strax, "Breast Cancer," p. 330.

25. W. H. Redd and M. A. Andrykowski, "Behavioral Intervention in Cancer

Treatment: Controlling Aversion Reactions to Chemotherapy," *Journal of Consulting Clinical Psychology* 50 (1982): 1025.

26. Cheryl Hilton, "New Drug Offers Relief from Chemotherapy Nausea," *University Currents* 2 (University of Cincinnati, May 21, 1993): 5.

27. Scanlon and Strax, "Breast Cancer," p. 330.

28. Love with Lindsey, *Breast Book*, p. 327.

29. R. R. Love, "Tamoxifen Therapy in Primary Breast Cancer: Biology, Efficacy, and Side Effects," *Journal of Clinical Oncology* 7 (1983): 803–815.

30. Love, "Tamoxifen Therapy," p. 803; Black and Matassarin-Jacobs, *Luckman and Sorensen's*, p. 2181.

31. H. N. Brown and M. J. Kelly, "Stages of Bone Marrow Transplantation, A Psychiatric Perspective," in R. H. Moos and J. A. Shaefer, eds., *Coping with Physical Illness 2: New Perspectives* (New York: Plenum, 1984), pp. 241–252; Black and Matassarin-Jacobs, *Luckman and Sorensen's* pp. 1363–1364.

32. G. N. Hortobagyi and S. E. Singletary, "Spectrum of Breast Cancer," *Cancer Bulletin* 45 (1993): 471–472.

CHAPTER 4

1. J. Bostwick III, "Reconstruction after Mastectomy," *Surgical Clinics of North America* 70 (October 1990): 1125–1140.

2. S. E. Singletary, M. A. Schusterman, and M. D. McNeese, "Breast Conservation vs. Breast Reconstruction," *Cancer Bulletin* 45 (1993): 515.

3. S. M. Love with K. Lindsey, *Dr. Susan Love's Breast Book* (Reading, MA: Addison-Wesley Publ., 1990), pp. 350–355.

4. Love with Lindsey, *Breast Book*, p. 357.

5. Singletary et al., "Breast Conservation," p. 515.

6. L. A. Stevens, M. H. McGrath, et al., "The Psychological Impact of Immediate Breast Reconstruction for Women with Early Breast Cancer," *Plastic and Reconstructive Surgery* (April 1984): 623.

7. Singletary et al., "Breast Reconstruction," p. 513.

8. *Breast Implant Resource Guide* (Arlington Heights, IL: American Society of Plastic and Reconstructive Surgeons, May 1992).

9. *Breast Implant Resource Guide*, 1992.

10. Love with Lindsey, *Breast Book*, p. 189.

11. FDA Update, "Bio-Dimentional Silicone Breast Implant OK'd," *Coping* 7 (January/February, 1993): 26.

12. W. S. Schain, D. K. Wellisch, et al., "The Sooner the Better: A Study of Psychological Factors in Women Undergoing Immediate versus Delayed Breast Reconstruction," *American Journal of Psychiatry* 142 (1985): 140.

13. A. Murcia and B. Stewart, *Man to Man: When the Woman You Love Has Breast Cancer* (New York: St. Martin's Press, 1989), p. 186.

CHAPTER 5

1. J. S. Smuts, *Holism and Evolution* (London: MacMillan & Co., 1927).

2. N. Cousins, *Anatomy of an Illness* (New York: Norton, 1989), pp. 119–120.

3. N. Cousins, *Head First: The Biology of Hope* (New York: E. P. Dutton, 1989), pp. 86–87.

4. H. Steven Greer, T. Morris, and K. W. Pettingale, "Psychological Response to Breast Cancer: Effect on Outcome," *Lancet* 2 (1979): 787.

5. Cousins, *Head First*, p. 269.

6. B. Inglis and R. West, eds., *The Alternate Health Guide* (New York: Knopf, 1983), p. 268.

7. H. Benson and M. Z. Klipper, *The Relaxation Response* (New York: William Morrow, 1975), p. 109.

8. J. Kiecolt-Glaser, R. Glaser, et al., "Modulation of Cellular Immunity in Medical Students," *Journal of Behavioral Medicine* 9 (1986): 19.

9. O. C. Simonton, S. Matthews-Simonton, and J. Creighton, *Getting Well Again* (Los Angeles: Tarcher, 1978), p. 7.

10. B. S. Siegel, *Love, Medicine and Miracles* (New York: Harper & Row, 1986), pp. 85–86.

11. Simonton et al., *Getting Well Again*, p. 133.

12. J. Achterberg, *Imagery in Healing* (Boston: New Science Library, 1985), p. 3.

13. A. Montagu, *Touching: The Human Significance of Skin* (New York: Harper & Row, 1971), pp. 404–406.

14. S. M. Love with K. Lindsey, *Dr. Susan Love's Breast Book* (Reading, MA: Addison-Wesley, 1990), pp. 335–336.

15. W. A. Nolen, *Healing: A Doctor in Search of a Miracle* (New York: Random House, 1974), pp. 307–308.

16. R. T. Chlebowski, et al., "Adjuvant Dietary Fat Intake Reduction in Post-menopausal Breast Cancer Patient Management," *Breast Cancer Research and Treatment* 20 (1991): 81–84; L. Holm, E. Nordevang, et al., "Dietary Intervention as Adjuvant Therapy in Breast Cancer Patients—A Feasibility Study," *Breast Cancer Research and Treatment* 16 (1990): 103–109.

17. A. Schatzkin, P. Greenwald, et al., "The Dietary Fat–Breast Cancer Hypothesis Is Alive," *Journal of the American Medical Association* 261 (1989): 3284–3287; N. F. Boyd, M. L. Cousins, S. E. Bayliss, et al., "Diet and Breast Disease: Evidence for the Feasibility of a Clinical Trial Involving a Major Reduction in Dietary Fat," in T. G. Burish, S. M. Levy, and B. E. Meyerowitz, eds., *Cancer, Nutrition, and Eating Behaviors: A Biobehavioral Perspective* (Hillsdale, NJ: Laurence Earlbaum Assoc., 1985), p. 167.

18. B.L.G. Morgan, *Nutrition Prescriptions: Strategies for Preventing and Treating 40 Common Diseases* (New York: Crown, 1987), pp. 60–64.

19. D. M. Wolfrom, A. R. Rao, and C. W. Welsch, "Caffeine Inhibits Development of Benign Mammary Gland Tumors in Carcinogen-Treated Female Sprague-Dawley Rats," *Breast Cancer Research & Treatment* 19 (1991): 269–275.

20. J. Steinberg and P. J. Goodwin, "Alcohol and Breast Cancer Risk—Putting the Controversy into Perspective," *Breast Cancer Research & Treatment* 19 (1991): 221–231; A. Schatzkin, D. Y. Jones, R. N. Hoover, et al., "Alcohol Consumption and Breast Cancer in the Epidemiologic Follow-Up Study of the First National Health and Nutrition Examination Survey," *New England Journal of Medicine* 316 (1987): 1169–1173; P. Veer, F. Kok, R. Herman, and F. Sturmans, "Alcohol Dose: Frequency and Age at First Exposure in Relation to the Risk of Breast Cancer," *International Journal of Epidemiology* 18 (1989): 511–517.

21. K. R. Pelletier, *Holistic Medicines: From Stress to Optimum Health* (New York: Delacorte Press, 1979), App. A, p. 218.

22. Morgan, *Nutrition Prescription*, pp. 61–65; Dreher, *Your Defense Against Cancer* (New York: Harper & Row, 1985), pp. 105, 122–136.

23. Simonton et al., *Getting Well Again*, p. 209.

24. N. Brinker with C. M. Harris, *The Race Is Run One Step at a Time: Everywoman's Guide to Taking Charge of Breast Cancer* (New York: Simon & Schuster, 1990), pp. 144–145.

25. D. B. Ardell, *The History and Future of Wellness* (Dubuque, IA: Kendall Hunt, 1985).

26. P. Pearsall, *Superimmunity* (New York: McGraw-Hill, 1987), Chs. 4–7.

27. Cousins, *Head First*, pp. 132–134.

28. Pearsall, *Superimmunity*, p. 307.

29. N. Cousins, *The Healing Heart* (New York: Norton, 1983), p. 234.

30. H. J. Bennett, ed., *The Best of Medical Humor* (Philadelphia: Hanley & Belfus, 1991), pp. xv–xvi.

31. B. Felson, *Humor in Medicine . . . and Other Topics* (Cincinnati: RHA Inc., 1989), p. 2.

32. M. B. Panos and J. Heimlich, *Homeopathic Medicine at Home* (Los Angeles: Tarcher, 1980), pp. 9–11; M. Kaufman, *Homeopathy in America* (Baltimore: Johns Hopkins Press, 1971).

33. Brinker with Harris, *One Step at a Time*, pp. 126–127.

34. C. Isley, "The Fatal Choice: Cancer Quackery," *R.N. Magazine* (September 1974): 56.

35. L. LeShan, *Cancer as a Turning Point* (New York: E. P. Dutton, 1989), pp. 330.

36. P. C. Roud, *Making Miracles: An Exploration into Dynamics of Self* (New York: Warners, 1990), p. 69.

37. D. Spiegel, *Living beyond Limits* (New York: Random House, 1993).

38. Love with Lindsey, *Breast Book*, p. 343.

CHAPTER 6

1. E. M. Nuehring and W. E. Barr, "Mastectomy: Impact on Patients and Families," *Health and Social Work* 5 (1980): 56; R. F. Klein, A. Dean, and M. D. Bogdonoff, "The Impact of Illness upon the Spouse," *Journal of Chronic Disease* 20 (1967): 246.

2. C. B. Wortman and C. Dunkel-Schetter, "Interpersonal Relationships and Cancer: A Theoretical Analysis," *Journal of Social Issues* 35 (1979): 122; P. Gagnon, M. J. Massie, and J. C. Holland, "The Woman with Breast Cancer: Psychosocial Considerations," *Cancer Bulletin* 45 (1993): 540; D. K. Wellisch, "The Psychologic Impact of Breast Cancer on Relationships," *Seminars in Oncology Nursing* 3 (1985): 195–196.

3. C. A. Moetzinger and L. G. Dauber, "The Management of the Patient with Breast Cancer," *Cancer Nursing* (August 1982): 290.

4. S. B. Westlake and F. E. Selder, "Breast Cancer: Living with Uncertainty," in A. Blitzer, A. H. Kutscher, et al., eds., *Communicating with Cancer Patients and Their Families* (Philadelphia: Charles Press, 1990), p. 131.

5. Wortman and Dunkel-Schetter, "Interpersonal Relationships," pp. 131–134.

6. R. Klein, "A Crisis to Grow on," *Cancer* 28 (1971): 1664.

7. C. Garfield, "Impact of Death on the Health Care Professional," in H. Feifel, ed., *New Meanings of Death* (New York: McGraw-Hill, 1977), p. 148.

8. E. Gottheil, W. C. McGurn, and O. Pollack, "Awareness and Disengagement in Cancer Patients," *American Journal of Psychiatry* 136 (May 1979): 632–636.

9. S. C. Klagsbrun, "Communications in the Treatment of Cancer," *American Journal of Nursing* 71 (May 1971): 945.

10. Wortman and Dunkel-Schetter, "Interpersonal Relationships," p. 133; R. A. Kalish, "Dying and Preparing for Death: A View of Families," in H. Feifel, ed., *New Meanings of Death* (New York: McGraw-Hill, 1977), p. 230.

11. K. R. Jamison, D. K. Wellisch, and R. O. Pasnau, "Psychological Aspects of Mastectomy: I. The Woman's Perspective," *American Journal of Psychiatry* 135 (April 1978): 432–436.

12. N. Grandstaff, "The Impact of Breast Cancer on the Family," *Frontiers in Radiation Therapy Oncology* 11 (1976): 155.

13. R. R. Lichtman, S. E. Taylor, and J. V. Wood, "Social Support and Marital Adjustment after Breast Cancer," *Journal of Psychosocial Oncology* 5 (1987): 56–57.

14. Wortman and Dunkel-Schetter, "Interpersonal Relationships," pp. 137–149.

15. E. H. Rosenbaum, *Living with Cancer* (New York: Praeger, 1975), pp. 4–20, 24.

16. D. K. Wellisch, K. R. Jamison, and R. O. Pasnau, "Psychosocial Aspects of Mastectomy: II. The Man's Perspective," *American Journal of Psychiatry* 135 (May 1978): 543–546; P. Maguire, "The Repercussions of Mastectomy on the Family," *International Journal of Family Psychiatry* 1 (1981): 485–503; L. Baider and A. K. De-Nour, "Couples' Reactions and Adjustment to Mastectomy: A Preliminary Report," *International Journal of Psychiatry in Medicine* 14 (1984): 265–276; L. L. Northouse and M. A. Swain, "Adjustment of Patients and Husbands to the Initial Impact of Breast Cancer," *Nursing Research* 36 (July/August 1987): 221–225.

17. Grandstaff, "Impact of Breast Cancer," p. 147.

18. E. Kubler-Ross, *On Death and Dying* (New York: MacMillan, 1969).

19. Grandstaff, "Impact of Breast Cancer," p. 148.

20. Maguire, "Repercussions," p. 492.

21. L. R. Derogatis, "Breast and Gynecologic Cancers," *Frontiers in Radiation Therapy Oncology* 14 (1980): 1–11.

22. Grandstaff, "Impact," p. 154.

23. R. Renneker and M. Cutler, "Psychological Problems of Adjustment to Cancer of the Breast," *Journal of the American Medical Association* 148 (March 1, 1952): 835.

24. A. Murcia and B. Stewart, *Man to Man: When the Woman You Love Has Breast Cancer* (New York: St. Martin's Press, 1989), p. 170.

25. Murcia and Stewart, *Man to Man*, pp. 168, 171.

26. L. Leiber, M. M. Plumb, et al., "The Communication of Affection between Cancer Patients and Their Spouses," *Psychosomatic Medicine* 38 (1976): 379.

27. Jamison, et al., "Psychological Aspects," p. 433.

28. C. C. Gates, "Husbands of Mastectomy Patients," *Patient Counseling and Health Education* 1–2 (1980): 38.

29. S. Kent, "Coping with the Sexual Identity Crises after Mastectomy," *Geri-*

atrics 30 (1975): 145; M. H. Witkin, "Psychosexual Counseling of the Mastectomy Patient," *Journal of Sex and Marital Therapy* 4 (1978): 20–28; Derogatis, "Breast and Gynecologic Cancers," p. 1.

30. A. J. Wabrek and C. J. Wabrek, "Mastectomy: Sexual Implications," *Primary Care* 3 (1976): 805.

31. J. H. Parker and R. B. Parker, *Three Weeks in Spring* (Boston: Houghton Mifflin, 1978), p. 169.

32. P. Fobair and N. L. Mages, "Psychosocial Morbidity among Cancer Patient Survivors," in P. Ahmed, ed., *Living and Dying with Cancer* (New York: Elsevier, 1981), pp. 300–301.

33. M. H. Witkin, "Sex Therapy and Mastectomy," *Journal of Sex and Marital Therapy* 1 (1975): 290–304.

34. Grandstaff, "Impact of Breast Cancer," p. 155; M. A. Lamb and N. F. Woods, "Sexuality and the Cancer Patient," *Cancer Nursing* (April 1981): 140.

35. G. P. Maguire, E. G. Lee, D. J. Bevington, et al., "Psychiatric Problems in the First Year after Mastectomy," *British Medical Journal* 1 (April 1978): 964.

36. N. F. Woods and J. L. Earp, "Women with Cured Breast Cancer: A Study of Mastectomy Patients in North Carolina," *Nursing Research* 27 (1978): 284.

37. Lichtman, et al., "Social Support," p. 61.

38. N. Stinnett and J. DeFrain, *Secrets of Strong Families* (Boston: Little, Brown & Co., 1985), pp. 8, 14.

39. Lichtman, et al., "Social Support," p. 52.

40. T. I. Rubin with E. Rubin, *Compassion and Self-Hate: An Alternative to Despair* (New York: David McKay, 1975), pp. 142–143.

41. R. L. Heinrich, C. C. Schag, and P. A. Ganz, "Living with Cancer: The Cancer Inventory of Problem Situations," *Journal of Clinical Psychology* 40 (1984): 979.

42. L. R. Schover, "The Impact of Breast Cancer on Sexuality, Body Image, and Intimate Relationships," *CA—A Cancer Journal for Clinicians* 41 (March/April 1991): 118–119.

43. J. K. Kiecolt-Glaser, L. D. Fisher, et al., "Marital Quality, Marital Disruption, and Immune Function," *Psychosomatic Medicine* 49 (1987): 13.

44. S. Kennedy, J. K. Kiecolt-Glaser, and R. Glaser, "Immunological Consequences of Acute and Chronic Stressors: Mediating Role of Interpersonal Relationships," *British Journal of Medical Psychology* 61 (1988): 83.

CHAPTER 7

1. J. M. Farrow, D. K. Cash, and G. Simmons, "Communicating with Cancer Patients and Their Families," in A. Blitzer, A. K. Kutscher, et al., eds., *Communicating with Cancer Patients and Their Families* (Philadelphia: Charles Press, 1990), p. 14.

2. E. H. Olsen, "The Impact of Serious Illness on the Family System," *Postgraduate Medicine* 47 (1970): 172; E. J. Anthony, "The Impact of Mental and Physical Illness on Family Life," *American Journal of Psychiatry* 127 (August 1970): 141.

3. C. M. Parkes, "The Emotional Impact of Cancer on Patients and Their Families," *Journal of Laryngology and Otology* 89 (1975): 1271.

4. B. Kievman with S. Blackmun, *For Better or For Worse: A Couple's Guide to Dealing with Chronic Illness* (Chicago: Contemporary Books, 1989), p. 50.

5. N. Grandstaff, "The Impact of Breast Cancer on the Family," *Frontiers in Radiation Therapy and Oncology* 11 (1976): 152.

6. R. Klein, "A Crisis to Grow On," *Cancer* 28 (1971): 1663.

7. Kievman with Blackmun, *For Better or For Worse*, p. 54.

8. L. LeShan, *Cancer as a Turning Point*, Rev. ed. (New York: Penguin, 1994), p. 9.

9. Klein, "A Crisis to Grow On," p. 1663.

10. E. S. Ellison, "Cancer and the Family Experiences of Children and Adolescents," in A. Blitzer, A. H. Kutscher, et al., eds., *Communicating with Cancer Patients and Their Families* (Philadelphia: Charles Press, 1990), p. 119.

11. D. K. Wellisch, "Family Relationships of the Mastectomy Patient: Interactions with the Spouse and Children," *Israel Journal of Medical Science* 17 (1981): 995; M. M. Cohen and D. K. Wellisch, "Living in Limbo: Psychosocial Intervention in Families with a Cancer Patient," *American Journal of Psychotherapy* 32 (October 1978): 565.

12. D. K. Wellisch, "Adolescent Acting Out When a Parent Has Cancer," *International Journal of Family Therapy* 1 (Fall 1979): 232–233; A. L. Cullinan, "Social Context of Breast Cancer within the Family," in A. Blitzer, A. H. Kutscher, et al., eds., *Communicating with Cancer Patients and Their Families* (Philadelphia: Charles Press, 1990), p. 145.

13. Grandstaff, "Impact," p. 153.

14. R. Lichtman, "Close Relationships after Breast Cancer" (Doctoral diss., U. of California, 1982), *Diss. Abst. International* 43, 3411B.

15. J. Viorst, *Necessary Losses* (New York: Ballantine Books, 1987), p. 167.

16. Grandstaff, "Impact," p. 153.

CHAPTER 8

1. E. G. Stolar, "Coping with Mastectomy: Issues for Social Work," *Health and Social Work* 7 (February 1982): 31; F. T. Gallo, "Counseling the Breast Cancer Patient," *Family Therapy* 4 (1977): 250.

2. J. Zanca, "Making Decisions about Breast Reconstruction," *Cancer Nursing News* 11 (Winter 1993): 3.

3. Zanca, "Making Decisions," p. 3.

4. Zanca, "Making Decisions," p. 3.

5. S. Dyck and K. Wright, "Family Perceptions: The Role of the Nurse throughout an Adult's Cancer Experience," *Oncology Nursing Forum* 12 (1985): 54–55.

6. R. Klein, "A Crisis to Grow On," *Cancer* 28 (1971): 1663.

7. M. J. Asken, "Psychoemotional Aspects of Mastectomy: A Review of Recent Literature," *American Journal of Psychiatry* 132 (January 1975): 58.

8. Richard Hillier, "Terminal Care—The Doctor's Anxieties," *Cancer Care* 5 (July 1988): 9–10.

9. P. A. Fritz, E. M. Wilcox, et al., "Research Topics in Health Care: The Kingdoms of Conflict," paper delivered at Speech Communication Association of Ohio (October 1, 1981), pp. 1–17.

10. T. G. Addington, *Communication and Cancer* (Fayetteville, AR: Cornerstone Group, 1991), p. 1.

11. Seminar on Communication and Cancer, presented by Hospice of Cincinnati, Cancer Family Care, and the American Cancer Society, Cincinnati, Ohio, September 15, 1993.

12. E. H. Rosenbaum, *Living with Cancer* (New York: Praeger, 1975), p. 24.

CHAPTER 9

1. L. LeShan, *Cancer as a Turning Point*, Rev. ed. (New York: Penguin, 1994), pp. 83–84.

2. F. Cournos, "Psychosocial Interventions with Cancer Patients and Their Families," in A. Blitzer, et al., *Communicating with Cancer Patients and Their Families* (Philadelphia: Charles Press, 1990), p. 45.

3. R. J. Burke and T. Weir, "Husband–Wife Helping Relationships as Moderator of Experienced Stress: The 'Mental Hygiene' Function in Marriage," in H. I. McCubbin, A. E. Cauble, and J. M. Patterson, eds., *Family Stress, Coping and Social Support* (Springfield, IL: Charles C. Thomas, 1983), p. 227.

4. J. A. Vettese, "Family Stress and Mediation in Cancer," in P. Ahmed, eds., *Living and Dying with Cancer* (New York: Elsevier, 1981), p. 277.

5. A. Y. Napier, *The Fragile Bond* (New York: Harper & Row, 1988), p. 162.

6. W. A. Nolen, *Crisis Time!* (New York: Dodd, Mead and Co., 1984), pp. 49–50.

7. S. W. Littlejohn, *Theories of Human Communication*, 2d ed. (Belmont, CA: Wadsworth, 1983), pp. 161–191.

8. A. L. Scoresby, *The Marriage Dialogue* (Reading, MA: Addison-Wesley, 1977), p. 110.

9. M. Frank-Stromberg and P. Wright, "Ambulatory Cancer Patients' Perceptions of the Physical and Psychosocial Changes in Their Lives Since the Diagnosis of Cancer," *Cancer Nursing* 7 (1984): 124.

10. S. M. Simonton with R. Shook, *The Healing Family* (New York: Bantam Books, 1984), p. 4, 85.

11. LeShan, *Cancer as a Turning Point*, p. 73.

12. E. H. Rosenbaum, *Living with Cancer* (New York: Praeger, 1975), pp. 11, 101.

13. Rosenbaum, *Living with Cancer*, p. 101.

14. A. P. Bochner and C. W. Kelly, "Interpersonal Competence: Rationale, Philosophy and Implementation of a Conceptual Framework," *Speech Teacher* 23 (November 1974): 289.

15. H. Lee, *To Kill a Mockingbird* (New York: Warner Books, 1960), p. 34.

16. R. F. Verderber and K. S. Verderber, *Interact: Using Interpersonal Communication Skills*, 6th ed. (Belmont, CA: Wadsworth, 1992), p. 233.

17. Napier, *Fragile Bond*, pp. 349–354.

18. O. C. Simonton, S. Matthews-Simonton, and J. Creighton, *Getting Well Again* (Los Angeles: J. P. Tarcher, 1978), p. 236.

19. Simonton with Shook, *Healing Family*, p. 93.

20. J. Viorst, *Necessary Losses* (New York: Ballantine Books, 1987), pp. 265–266.

21. J. D. Feezel and P. E. Shepherd, "Cross Generational Coping with Interpersonal Relationship Loss," *Western Journal of Speech Communication* 51 (Summer 1987): 324.

22. L. Baider and A. K. De-Nour, "Couples' Reactions and Adjustment to Mastectomy: A Preliminary Report," *International Journal of Psychiatry in Medicine* 14 (1984): 275.

23. Simonton et al., *Getting Well Again*, p. 232.

24. B. Kievman with S. Blackmun, *For Better or For Worse: A Couple's Guide to Dealing with Chronic Illness* (Chicago: Contemporary Books, 1989), pp. 34–35; S. Greer and T. Morris, "Psychological Attributes of Women Who Develop Breast Cancer: A Controlled Study," *Journal of Psychosomatic Research* 19 (1975): 150; Simonton with Shook, *Healing Family*, p. 87.

25. Bruno Klopfer, "Psychological Variables in Human Cancer," *Journal of Projective Techniques* 21 (1957): 336.

26. Simonton with Shook, *Healing Family*, p. 90.

27. Simonton with Shook, *Healing Family*, p. 86.

28. Simonton with Shook, *Healing Family*, p. 92.

29. C. T. Brown and P. W. Keller, *Monologue to Dialogue*, 2d ed. (Englewood Cliffs, NJ: Prentice-Hall, 1979), p. 175.

30. A. W. Combs and D. L. Avila, *Helping Relationships*, 3d ed. (Boston: Allyn and Bacon, 1985), p. 137.

31. S. Kent, "Coping with Sexual Identity Crises after Mastectomy," *Geriatrics* 30 (1975): 145–146.

32. Simonton with Shook, *Healing Family*, p. 182.

33. J. Parker and R. Parker, *Three Weeks in Spring* (Boston: Houghton Mifflin, 1978), p. 180.

34. Kievman with Blackmun, *For Better or For Worse*, p. 98.

35. S. Miller, E. Nunnally, and D. B. Wackman, *Couple Communication I: Talking Together* (Sydney: Family Life Movement of Australia, 1980).

36. Kievman with Blackmun, *For Better or For Worse*, p. 95.

37. Simonton with Shook, *Healing Family*, p. 96.

38. Kievman with Blackmun, *For Better or For Worse*, p. 54.

39. Simonton with Shook, *Healing Family*, p. 97.

CHAPTER 10

1. B. J. Loveys and K. Klaich, "Breast Cancer: Demands of Illness," *Oncology Nursing Forum* 18 (1991): 77–78.

2. D. K. Olson, H. I. McCubbin, et al., *Families: What Makes Them Work* (Beverly Hills, CA: Sage, 1983), p. 140.

3. A. D. Weisman and H. J. Sobel, "Coping with Cancer through Self-Instruction: A Hypothesis," *Journal of Human Stress* 5 (March 1979): 4.

4. R. H. Moos and J. A. Schaefer, "The Crisis of Physical Illness: An Overview and Conceptual Approach," in R. H. Moos and J. A. Schaefer, eds., *Coping with Physical Illness 2: New Perspectives* (New York: Plenum, 1984), p. 14.

5. L. I. Pearlin and C. Schooler, "The Structure of Coping," *Journal of Health and Social Behavior* 19 (1978): 2.

6. Olson, McCubbin, et al., *Families*, pp. 207–212.

7. H. I. McCubbin and J. M. Patterson, "Family Transitions: Adaptation to Stress," in H. I. McCubbin and C. R. Figley, eds., *Stress and the Family, Vol. I. Coping with Normative Transitions* (New York: Brunner/Mazel, 1983), p. 15.

8. M. G. MacVicar and P. Archbold, "A Framework for Family Assessment in Chronic Illness," *Nursing Forum* 15 (1976): 181.

9. R. S. Lazarus and S. Folkman, *Stress, Appraisal, and Coping* (New York: Springer, 1984), p. 159.

10. Lazarus and Folkman, *Stress*, pp. 56, 159–162.

11. B. K. Breitbart, "Factors That Contribute to Control and Hopefulness," in A. Blitzer, A. H. Kutscher, et al., eds., *Communicating with Cancer Patients and Their Families* (Philadelphia: Charles Press, 1990), pp. 27–29.

12. J. L. Johnson and P. A. Norby, "We Can Weekend: A Program for Cancer Families," *Cancer Nursing* 4 (February 1981): 23–28.

13. Lazarus and Folkman, *Stress*, p. 165.

14. Olson, McCubbin, et al., *Families*, pp. 215–216.

15. K. M. Galvin and B. J. Brommel, *Family Communication: Cohesion and Change*, 2d ed. (Glenview, IL: Scott, Foresman, 1986), p. 176.

16. H. G. Lerner, *The Dance of Intimacy* (New York: Harper & Row, 1989), p. 103.

17. A. Y. Napier, *The Fragile Bond* (New York: Harper & Row, 1988), pp. 37–41.

18. Lazarus and Folkman, *Stress*, p. 134.

19. Olson, McCubbin, et al., *Families*, p. 145.

20. Pearlin and Schooler, "Structure of Coping," p. 10.

21. H. I. McCubbin, B. Dahl, et al., "Coping Repertoires of Families Adapting to Prolonged War-Induced Separation," *Journal of Marriage and the Family* 38 (1976): 470.

22. S. Cobb, "Social Support as a Moderator of Life Stress," *Psychosomatic Medicine* 38 (1976): 300–314; J. Cassel, "The Contribution of the Social Environment to Host Resistance," *American Journal of Epidemiology* 104 (1976): 121.

23. Lazarus and Folkman, *Stress*, pp. 35–38.

24. Z. J. Lipowski, "Physical Illness, the Individual and the Coping Process," *International Journal of Psychiatry in Medicine* 1 (1970—1971): 98.

25. O. C. Simonton, S. Matthew-Simonton, and J. Creighton, *Getting Well Again* (Los Angeles: J. P. Tarcher, 1978), pp. 126–139.

26. S. M. Simonton with R. L. Shook, *The Healing Family* (New York: Bantam Books, 1984), pp. 33–38.

27. S. Thorne, "The Family Cancer Experience," *Cancer Nursing* 8 (October 1985): 289.

28. B. Kievman with S. Blackmun, *For Better or For Worse: A Couple's Guide to Dealing with Chronic Illness* (Chicago/New York: Contemporary Books, 1989), pp. 8–10.

29. T. I. Rubin and E. Rubin, *Compassion and Self-Hate: An Alternative to Despair* (New York: David McKay, 1975), pp. 223–224.

30. A. Bandura, "Self Efficacy: Toward a Unifying Theory of Behavior Change," *Psychological Review* 84 (1977): 191–215.

CHAPTER 11

1. C. Ervin, "Psychologic Adjustment to Mastectomy," *Medical Aspects of Human Sexuality* 7 (1973): 42–61.

2. R. Zemore and L. F. Shepel, "Effects of Breast Cancer and Mastectomy on Emotional Support," *Social Science and Medicine* 28 (1989): 19.

3. D. K. Wellisch, "The Psychologic Impact of Breast Cancer on Relationships," *Seminars in Oncology Nursing* 1 (August 1985): 196; L. Leiber, M. M. Plumb, M. L. Gerstanzang, and J. D. Holland, "The Communication of Affection between Cancer Patients and Their Spouses," *Psychosomatic Medicine* 38 (1976): 384.

4. R. Kaye, *Spinning Straw into Gold* (New York: Simon & Schuster, 1991), p. 163.

5. S. Cobb, "Social Support as a Moderator of Life Stress," *Psychosomatic Medicine* 38 (1976): 300.

6. Ervin, "Psychologic Adjustment," p. 53.

7. Leiber, Plumb, et al., "Communication of Affection," 386.

8. L. David, "A Brave Family Faces Up to Breast Cancer," in R. H. Moos and K. D. Tsu, eds., *Coping with Physical Illness* (New York: Plenum, 1977), pp. 73–79. Reprinted in abridged form in *Today's Health* 50 (June 1972): 78.

9. Kaye, *Spinning Straw*, p. 164.

10. O. C. Simonton, S. Matthews-Simonton, and J. Creighton, *Getting Well Again* (Los Angeles, J. P. Tarcher, 1978), p. 231.

11. N. Brinker with C. M. Harris, *The Race Is Run One Step at a Time* (New York: Simon & Schuster, 1990), p. 47.

12. Simonton et al., *Getting Well Again*, p. 232.

13. Simonton et al., *Getting Well Again*, pp. 232–233.

14. Kaye, *Spinning Straw*, pp. 142–145.

15. M. B. Maxwell, "The Use of Social Networks to Help Cancer Patients Maximize Support," *Cancer Nursing* 5 (August 1982): 279.

16. A. Murcia and Bob Stewart, *Man to Man: When the Woman You Love Has Breast Cancer* (New York: St. Martin's Press, 1989), Chs. 8 and 9.

17. M. Rutter, "Stress, Coping and Development: Some Issues and Some Questions," *Journal of Child Psychology and Psychiatric Medicine* 22 (1981): 343.

18. J. Parker and J. Parker, *Three Weeks in Spring* (Boston: Houghton Mifflin, 1978), p. 146.

19. A. Harwell with K. Tomasik, *When Your Friend Gets Cancer* (Wheaton, IL: Harold Shaw Publ., 1987), p. 7.

20. B. Kievman with S. Blackmun, *For Better or For Worse: A Couple's Guide to Dealing with Chronic Illness* (Chicago/New York: Contemporary Books, 1989), p. 83.

21. Harwell with Tomasik, *When Your Friend Gets Cancer*, p. 9.

22. B. D. Blumberg, P. Ahmed, et al., "Living with Cancer: An Overview," in P. Ahmed, ed., *Living and Dying with Cancer* (New York: Elsevier, 1981), p. 14.

23. Harwell with Tomasik, *When Your Friend Gets Cancer*, pp. 10–11.

CHAPTER 12

1. R. Kaye, *Spinning Straw into Gold* (New York: Simon & Schuster, 1991), p. 85–86; N. Brinker with C. M. Harris, *The Race Is Run One Step at a Time* (New York: Simon & Schuster, 1990), p. 139.

2. M. Huntington, "Weight Gain in Patients Receiving Adjuvent Chemotherapy for Carcinoma of the Breast," *Cancer* 56 (1985): 474.

3. Brinker with Harris, *One Step at a Time*, pp. 137–138.

4. American Cancer Society, Cincinnati, Ohio (August 5, 1993).

5. Cosmetic, Toiletry, and Fragrance Association Foundation, " 'The Look Good . . . Feel Better' Cosmetic Program," in M. Dollinger, E. H. Rosenbaum, and G. Cable, eds., *Everyone's Guide to Cancer Therapy* (Kansas City: Andrews and McMeel, 1991), pp. 153–155.

6. M. B. Crocker, "Outside Help: Cancer Patients Get a New Look," *Cincinnati Enquirer* ("Tempo," E, August 4, 1993): 1–2.

CHAPTER 13

1. S. Nessim and J. Ellis, *Cancervive: The Challenge of Life after Cancer* (Boston: Houghton Mifflin, 1991), pp. 116–117.

2. L. Felder, *When a Loved One Is Ill: How to Take Better Care of Your Loved One, Your Family and Yourself* (New York: New American Library, 1990), pp. 48–175.

CHAPTER 14

1. S. Nessim and J. Ellis, *Cancervive: The Challenge of Life after Cancer* (Boston: Houghton Mifflin, 1991), pp. 12–15.

2. J. Ireland, *Life Wish* (Boston: Little, Brown, 1987), p. 41.

3. E. M. Nuehring and W. E. Barr, "Mastectomy: Impact on Patient and Families," *Health and Social Work* 5 (1980): 54–55.

4. O. C. Simonton, S. Matthews-Simonton, and J. Creighton, *Getting Well Again* (Los Angeles: J. P. Tarcher, 1978), p. 238.

5. J. M. Worden and H. J. Sobel, "Ego Strength and Psychosocial Adaptation to Cancer," *Psychosomatic Medicine* 40 (1978): 585–592.

6. D. K. Wellisch, F. I. Fawzy, J. Landsverk, et al., "Evaluation of Psychosocial Problems of the Home-Bound Cancer Patient: The Relationship of Disease and the Sociodemographic Variables of Patients to Family Problems," *Journal of Psychosocial Oncology* 1 (1983): 1–15.

7. J. R. Bloom, R. D. Ross, and G. Burnell, "The Effect of Social Support on Patient Adjustment after Breast Surgery," *Patient Counseling and Health Education* 1 (1978): 57.

8. Nuehring and Barr, "Mastectomy," pp. 52, 56.

9. H. G. Lerner, *The Dance of Intimacy* (New York: Harper & Row, 1989), pp. 5–10.

10. Nessim and Ellis, *Cancervive*, p. 31.

11. Nessim and Ellis, *Cancervive*, pp. 37–38.

12. Y. Hirshaut and P. I. Pressman, *Breast Cancer: The Complete Guide* (New York: Bantam, 1992), pp. 212–219.

13. Nessim and Ellis, *Cancervive*, pp. 178–179.

14. Simonton et al., *Getting Well Again*, p. 96.

15. J. Vettese, "Family Stress and Mediation in Cancer," in P. Ahmed, ed., *Living and Dying with Cancer* (New York: Elsevier, 1981), p. 277.

16. P. Schoenung, "Raising Self-Esteem Crucial after Mastectomy," *Prime Times* (Cincinnati Deaconess Hospital, November 1991), p. 9.

17. N. Brinker with C. M. Harris, *The Race Is Run One Step at a Time* (New York: Simon & Schuster, 1990), pp. 58–59.

18. K. R. Jamison, D. K. Wellisch, and R. O. Pasnau, "Psychosocial Aspects of Mastectomy: I. The Woman's Perspective," *American Journal of Psychiatry* 135 (April 1978): 433.

19. A. J. Wabrek and C. J. Wabrek, "Mastectomy: Sexual Implications," *Primary Care* 3 (December 1976): 804.

20. Brinker with Harris, *One Step at a Time*, p. 162.

21. Brinker with Harris, *One Step at a Time*, p. 55.

CHAPTER 15

1. R. Kaye, *Spinning Straw into Gold* (New York: Simon & Schuster, 1991), p. 179.

2. L. LeShan, *Cancer as a Turning Point*, Rev. ed. (New York: Penguin, 1994), pp. 1–47, 135.

3. LeShan, *Cancer*, p. 207.

4. R. L. Shook, *Survivors: Living with Cancer* (New York: Harper & Row, 1983), p. 35.

5. LeShan, *Cancer*, p. 133.

6. LeShan, *Cancer*, p. 53–56.

7. B. S. Siegel, *Love, Medicine and Miracles* (New York: Harper & Row, 1986), pp. 13–22.

8. S. M. Simonton with R. L. Shook, *The Healing Family* (New York: Bantam Books, 1984), p. 101.

9. Shook, *Survivors*, p. 94.

10. B. Hansen, *Picking Up the Pieces* (Dallas: Taylor Publ., 1990), pp. 57, 65–66.

11. Shook, *Survivors*, p. 98.

12. Shook, *Survivors*, pp. 40–41.

13. D. Richards, *The Topic of Cancer: When the Killing Has to Stop* (New York: Pergamon Press, 1982), p. 81.

14. N. Cousins, *Head First* (New York: E. P. Dutton, 1989), p. 25.

CHAPTER 16

1. E. Kübler-Ross, *On Death and Dying* (New York: Macmillan, 1969), Chs. 3–7.

2. L. LeShan, *Cancer as the Turning Point* (New York: E. P. Dutton, 1989), p. 157.

3. H. Hayes with K. Hatch, *My Life in Three Acts* (New York: Harcourt Brace Jovanovich, 1990), p. 8.

4. B. Forbes, *Dame Edith Evans, Ned's Girl* (Boston: Little, Brown, 1977), p. xiii.

5. Forbes, *Dame Edith Evans*, p. xvi.

6. LeShan, *Cancer*, pp. 158, 183.

7. A. Harwell with K. Tomasik, *When Your Friend Gets Cancer* (Wheaton, IL: Harold Shaw Publ., 1987), p. 68.

8. B. Hansen, *Picking Up the Pieces* (Dallas: Taylor Publ., 1990), pp. 83, 102.

9. R. Kaye, *Spinning Straw into Gold* (New York: Simon & Schuster, 1991), p. 22.

10. J. Viorst, *Necessary Losses* (New York: Ballantine Books, 1987), pp. 320–321, 333.

11. M. Bayh with M. L. Katz, *A Personal Journey* (New York: Harcourt Brace Jovanovich, 1979), p. 27.

12. Bayh, *Personal Journey*, Epilogue. Also in *Washington Post* (April 26, 1979).

13. E. Kübler-Ross, *On Children and Death* (New York: Macmillan, 1983), p. xviii.

14. Forbes, *Dame Edith Evans*, pp. 164–165.

15. T. A. Rando, *Grieving: How to Go On Living When Someone You Love Dies* (Lexington, MA: D. C. Heath, 1988), p. 16.

16. P. Cohen, I. M. Dizenhuz, and C. Winget, "Family Adaptation to Terminal Illness and Death of a Parent," *Social Casework* 58 (April 1977): 224.

17. Hansen, *Picking Up the Pieces*, p. 83.

18. Hansen, *Picking Up the Pieces*, pp. 59–60.

19. Kübler-Ross, *On Children and Death*, pp. 82, 84.

20. K. Gravelle and C. Haskins, *Teenagers Face to Face with Bereavement* (Englewood Cliffs, NJ: Julian Messner, 1989), pp. 35, 40.

21. Gravelle and Haskins, *Teenagers*, pp. 89–90.

22. M.J.A. Nimocks, L. Webb, and J. R. Connell, "Communication and the Terminally Ill: A Theoretical Model," *Death Studies* 11 (1987): 323–344.

23. Nimocks et al., "Communication," p. 339.

24. Kübler-Ross, *On Children and Death*, p. xvii.

CHAPTER 17

1. *Physician's Desk Reference* (Oradell, NJ: Medical Economics Data, 1994).

2. R. Kaye, *Spinning Straw into Gold* (New York: Simon & Schuster, 1991), p. 163.

3. N. Brinker with C. M. Harris, *The Race Is Run One Step at a Time* (New York: Simon & Schuster, 1990), p. 55.

CHAPTER 18

1. B. Kievman with S. Blackmun, *For Better or For Worse* (Chicago/New York: Contemporary Books, 1989), p. 101.

2. O. C. Simonton, S. Matthews-Simonton, and J. Creighton, *Getting Well Again* (Los Angeles: J. P. Tarcher, 1978), p. 232.

CHAPTER 19

1. A. Harwell with K. Tomasik, *When Your Friend Gets Cancer* (Wheaton, IL: Harold Shaw Publ., 1987), p. xi.

2. Harwell with Tomasik, *When Your Friend Gets Cancer*, pp. xiii–xiv.

3. G. Photopolus and B. Photopolus, "What to Say to Someone Who Is Really Sick," *Looking Forward* 6 (Cincinnati, Good Samaritan Hospital, Fall 1993), p. 6.

4. D. Callan, "When Your Friend Has Cancer," *CFC Newsletter* 10 (Cincinnati, December 1988), p. 3.

5. "25 Practical Tips You Can Use to Help Those Facing Serious Illness" (Brochure available through Hospice of Cincinnati, by permission of St. Anthony's Hospital, Alton, IL).

EPILOGUE

1. D. Spiegel, *Living beyond Limits* (New York: Random House, 1993), p. 274.

2. E. Bombeck, Television interview (Spring 1994).

3. M. Bayh with M. L. Katz, *A Personal Journey* (New York: Harcourt Brace Jovanovich, 1979), p. 245.

Glossary

adjuvant therapy—The use of anticancer drugs and/or radiation in conjunction with surgery as treatment to prevent the spread or recurrence of cancer.

alopecia—Hair loss, commonly caused by some drugs used in chemotherapy.

analgesic—An agent that relieves pain without causing loss of consciousness.

androgen—Male sex hormones that produce male characteristics.

antioncogenes—Tumor-suppressor genes that act as "brakes" for undesirable cell growth. They are important in about 50 percent of breast cancers.

areola—A circular area of a different-colored pigment surrounding the nipple of the breast.

aspiration—The withdrawal of fluid from a mass by means of inserting a needle.

autoimmune disorders—Disorders directed against the body's own tissue.

axilla—The space between the upper lateral part of the chest and medial side of the arm, including the armpit and a large number of lymph nodes.

axillary dissection—A cutting or separation of axilla.

benign tumors—A mass or group of abnormal cells that are adjacent to normal cells that may function like normal cells but remain localized.

bilateral surgery—Removal of both breasts.

biofeedback—The act of voluntarily controlling the body functions (such as heart rate) that are not normally under conscious control.

biological response modifiers—Protein molecules, such as interferon and interleukin-2, used in treating cancer.

biopsy—A surgical procedure in which a section of tissue is removed for testing. There are several types of biopsies: fine-needle, "tru-cut," incisional, and excisional.

bone marrow rescue, or transplant—A process in which cancer-free bone marrow is taken from the patient to be infused intravenously into the patient at a later time.

calcifications—Small deposits of calcium salts in the breast tissue that can be seen by a mammogram.

capsular contracture—Shrinking of fibrous membrane.

carcinogen—A cancer-causing agent.

carcinogenesis—A multistep process that begins with a series of specific changes, or mutations, in the DNA of a single cell.

carcinoma—A tumor that appears in the breast and other organs, the most common category of cancer.

CAT scan (computerized axial tomography)—A method of examining the body in cross-sectional slices.

chemotherapy—The treatment of a disease by chemical agents.

chromosome—A structure in the nucleus of a cell that contains the linear thread of DNA, which transmits genetic information.

clinical—Refers to actual observation and treatment of patients, as in a clinic or at the bedside.

comedocarcinomas—Cancer that grows into a duct, causing the duct to become enlarged. It is less likely to spread beyond the breast than other cancers.

cyst—A sac that contains a liquid or semi-solid material.

cytoplasm—A gel-like fluid containing chemical substances that are required for the cell's metabolism.

cytotoxic—Pertaining to antibodies or drugs used in chemotherapy that kill cells.

displacement—The act of transferring an emotion to an inappropriate object or person, such as displacing one's anger toward a person by kicking the dog.

DNA (deoxyribonucleic acid)—A set of proteins in the nucleus of a cell, having the shape of a double helix or spiral, which directs the cell to make an exact copy of itself. It also directs the synthesis of the proteins that carry out the functions of living organisms.

dysplasia—Alteration in size, shape, and organization of adult cells.

ego strength—One's overall capacity for adapting to life changes and stresses and the ability to cope with and master challenging situations.

empathy—The ability to detect, understand, and share another person's feelings. It differs from sympathy, which is a similarity of feelings or compassion or pity.

enzymes—Proteins that speed up and control the rate of chemical reactions that take place in living things.

epidemiology—The field of medicine concerned with specific causes of outbreaks of diseases.

estrogen—The females sex hormones produced by the ovaries, adrenal glands, placenta, and fat. Used to give relief in cancer of the breast after menopause or in treatment of osteoporosis.

estrogen-receptor test—A test to determine a tumor's sensitivity to hormones. If a test is negative, hormone treatments will be of no avail.

excision—Removal, as of an organ or tumor, by cutting off or out.

fibroadenoma—Benign fibrous tumor of the breast that usually forms in early years of menstruation.

fibrocystic disease—A term used to describe an overgrowth of fibrous tissues of the breast, a benign condition.

gynecologist—A physician who specializes in treating diseases of the female reproductive system.

holism—An approach to treatment that includes treating the whole person, not just the affected area.

homeopathy—A method of therapy believed to stimulate the immune system by using small doses of drugs to produce symptoms in healthy people that are similar to those of a disease being treated.

hormone—A chemical substance produced by the glands in the body that affects other tissues.

hormone therapy—The use of drugs to block or halt the production of hormones.

immunotherapy—A treatment aimed at strengthening the body's immune system. Interferon, which is manufactured by cells to inhibit viruses, is a major component of this treatment.

implant—Material inserted or grafted into the body.

in situ—Refers to non-invasive tumors that have not grown into neighboring tissue.

interferon—A protein molecule, referred to as a biological modifier, that enables cells to resist infection by a virus.

interleukin-2—A protein molecule that triggers killer cells to attack cancer cells, seen as foreign bodies.

invasive ductal cancer—Cancers that are hard to the touch and spread rapidly to the lymph nodes. About 70 percent of breast cancers are of this type.

iridium implant—Radioactive iridium needles for internal radiation are implanted to eliminate residual cancer cells.

laetrile—A product of the bitter almond plant, also found in the soft kernel of peaches, cherries, and other sources, that is believed to be helpful in treating cancer. Its effectiveness is very controversial and its use is illegal in the United States.

lesions—Also referred to as neoplasms and displasia, these are a precancerous condition of abnormal cell development in which cells are altered in shape, size, and organization.

leukemia—A type of cancer that occurs in bone marrow.

leukocytes—The cells that produce white blood cells and leukemias.

lobular and ductal carcinomas in situ—These appear as small areas of calcification on a mammogram. It is difficult to predict which ones will become invasive.

lumpectomy—The surgical removal of a lump and a small area of tissue that is around it.

lupus erythematosus—A skin condition implying local degeneration. Discoid is a superficial inflammation generally forming lesions over nose and cheeks. Systemic is a generalized disorder of connective tissue.

lymphedema—A swelling of the arm that can follow removal of lymph nodes under the arm.

lymphomas—A general term applied to any neoplastic disorder of the lymphoid tissue, including Hodgkin's Disease.

malignant—Cancerous.

mammotest (or stereotactic needle-core biopsy)—A procedure that helps in locating lumps and placing the biopsy needle.

mastalgia—Pain that occurs in the mammary glands or breast gland.

mastectomy—The removal or excision of a breast.

medullary carcinoma—Cancer that grows within the duct in capsule form, not as apt to metastasize as other cancers.

metastases—The plural of metastasis.

metastasis—The dislodging of cancer cells and moving to distant sites to establish subcolonies of cancer cells.

micrometastasis—Microscopic spread of tumor cells, not yet detectable.

modified compression technique—A technique used for screening the breasts of women who have implants.

monoclonal antibodies—Protein produced by the white blood cells to destroy a virus or other intruder that enters the body.

MRI (Magnetic resonance imaging)—A method of detection by exposing a patient to a magnetic field that records a picture.

mucinous carcinoma—A form of ductal cancer that may grow quite large without metastasizing.

mutation—A change in form, quality, or some other characteristic in genetic material.

myocutaneous flap—A person's own tissue and muscle used in reconstruction of the breast.

neoadjuvant chemotherapy—Chemotherapy given before surgical removal of cancer.

neoplasm—Any new or abnormal growth.

oncogenes—Small pieces of genetic material capable of infecting animal cells and producing tumors.

oncologist—A physician who studies and treats tumors.

oophorectomy—The removal of an ovary or ovaries.

osteoporosis—A softening of the bones, seen most commonly in the elderly.

palliation—The act of relieving a symptom but not removing the cause.

palpate—To examine or feel by the hand.

palpation—The act of feeling with the hand.

pathologist—An expert in examining tissue and diagnosing disease.

phlebitis—Inflammation of the vein, frequently resulting in formation of a vascular obstruction, causing swelling, stiffness, and pain.

PNI (psychoneuroimmunology)—An approach to the mental, emotional, and spiritual aspects of cancer. It encompasses various techniques for treating cancer as well as alleviating pain and other side effects.

prognosis—The possible or probable outcome of a disease or treatment.

projection—An unconscious process of attributing one's ideas or impulses to others, especially when the ideas are undesirable.

prosthesis—An artificial substitute for an absent body part, such as a breast prosthesis.

protocol—Research designed to test a hypothesis, often a specific treatment of disease under controlled conditions.

protooncogenes—A family of genes that promote growth; they are normal genes.

pseudolump—Breast tissue that feels like a lump that may appear during pregnancy or lactation; when examined it proves to be normal tissue.

psychotherapist—One who treats a person by use of mental effects such as suggestion, re-education, reassurance, and support.

PTSD (post-traumatic stress disorder)—A term describing the stress that occurs to a woman who has survived breast cancer but who often encounters stigma, physical and emotional and discriminatory aftereffects.

quadrantectomy—Removal of approximately one-quarter of the breast that contains a lump and surrounding tissue.

radioisotope—A chemical element that is radioactive. It has an unstable nucleus that gives it the property of decay by one or more processes. It is important for diagnostic and therapeutic use.

radiologist—A specialist in the use of radiology.

radiotherapy—The use of cobalt or radiant energy in diagnosis and treatment of disease. It involves directing a beam of ionizing radiation in the area of malignant tissue to interfere with cell division.

sarcomas—A type of cancer that develops in connective tissue.

scleroderma—A chronic disorder of the dermis.

selenium—A nonmetallic element resembling sulphur, found in food.

staging—A term describing the stages of a cancerous growth; stages are determined according to an elaborate scale.

stoicism-fatalism—Stoicism describes a reaction of calm to pain, suffering, and misfortune. This is often based on the belief (fatalism) that all events are determined by fate and are, therefore, inevitable.

target-zone pain—Pain that can be pinpointed; it does not occur cyclically.

thermography—A test using an infrared camera to find "hot spots" or tumors. Its accuracy is not dependable.

tissue expander—A plastic bag having a tube with a valve that is inserted under the woman's pectoralis muscle. In reconstructive surgery it is injected with a saline solution to stretch the skin before a permanent implant is inserted.

trauma—An injury.

tubular ductal cancer—A tube-shaped cancer, which rarely occurs.

tumor—An abnormal mass of tissue that may be either malignant or benign.

tumor-suppressing genes—A family of genes that retard growth. A series of alterations in these genes makes possible the controlled growth of a single cell into a mass of cancer tissue or leukemia.

tylectomy—Removal of the tumor mass only, leaving the rest of the breast intact.

ultrasound—The use of high-frequency sound to detect breast abnormalities. Accurate equipment is needed for routine usage.

ultrasound guided aspiration—A process by which a mass that has been detected by mammogram is examined before inserting a needle to aspirate it.

Bibliography

Achterberg, Jeanne. *Imagery in Healing: Shamanism and Modern Medicine.* Boston: New Science Library, 1985.

Addington, Thomas G. *Communication and Cancer.* Fayetteville, AR: Cornerstone Group, 1991.

Ahmed, Paul, ed. *Living and Dying with Cancer.* New York: Elsevier, 1981.

Akehurst, A. C. "Postmastectomy Morale." *Lancet* 2 (1972): 181–82.

Ames, B. N. "Dietary Carcinogens and Anticarcinogens." *Science* 217 (1983): 1256–64.

Anderson, B., and F. Wolf. "Chronic Physical Illness and Sexual Behavior: Psychological Issues." *Journal of Consulting and Clinical Psychology* 54 (1986): 168–75.

Anderson, David. "Breast Cancer in Families." *Cancer* 40 (1977): 1855–60.

Anderson, D. E., and M. D. Badzioch. "Risk of Familial Cancer." *Cancer* 56 (1985): 383–87.

Anthony, E. J. "The Impact of Mental and Physical Illness on Family Life." *American Journal of Psychiatry* 127 (August 1970): 138–46.

Antonovsky, A. *Health, Stress and Coping.* San Francisco: Jossey Bass, 1979.

Antonucci, T. C., and J. S. Jackson. "Physical Health and Self-Esteem." *Family and Community Health* 6 (1983): 1–9.

Ardell, D. B. *The History and Future of Wellness.* Dubuque, IA: Kendall Hunt, 1985.

Arms, K., and P. S. Camp. *Biology*, 3d ed. Philadelphia: Saunders, 1988.

Ashcroft, J. J., S. J. Leinster, and P. D. Slade. "Breast Cancer—Patient Choice of Treatment: Preliminary Communication." *Journal of the Royal Society of Medicine* 78 (1985): 43–46.

Asken, M. J. "Psychoemotional Aspects of Mastectomy: A Review of Recent Literature." *American Journal of Psychiatry* 132 (1975): 56–59.

Bahnson, C. B. "Psychologic and Emotional Issues in Cancer: The Psychotherapeutic Care of the Cancer Patient." *Seminars in Oncology* 2 (1975): 293–309.

Baider, Lea, and A. K. DeNour. "Couples' Reactions and Adjustment to Mastec-
    tomy: A Preliminary Report." *International Journal of Psychiatry in Medicine*
    14 (1984): 265–76.
Baider, Lea, S. Rizel, and A. Kaplan De-Dour. "Comparison of Couples' Adjustment
    to Less Mutilating and Highly Mutilating Breast Cancer Surgery." *General
    Hospital Psychiatry* 8 (July 1986): 251–57.
Bain, Alastair. "The Capacity of Families to Cope with Transitions: A Theoretical
    Essay." *Human Relations* 31 (1978): 675–88.
Bandura, A. "Self-Efficacy: Toward a Unifying Theory of Behavior Change." *Psy-
    chological Review* 84 (1977): 191–215.
Barbour, T. "I Traveled the Mastectomy Road." *Supervisor Nurse* 6 (1975): 40–43.
Bard, Morton, and A. M. Sutherland. "Psychological Impact of Cancer and Its Treat-
    ment; IV Adaptation to Radical Mastectomy." *Cancer* 8 (1955): 656–72.
Bartimus, Ted. "Friends for Life, in Life, to Life: Women Bound by Pain of Cancer."
    Cincinnati Enquirer (February 24, 1991): Sec. G, p. 144.
Baudry, F., and A. Weiner. "The Family of the Surgical Patient." *Surgery* 63 (1968):
    416–22.
Bayh, Marvella, with M. L. Kotz. *A Personal Journey*. New York: Harcourt Brace
    Jovanovich, 1979.
Bennett, H. J., ed. *The Best of Medical Humor*. Philadelphia: Hanley & Belfus, 1991.
Bennett, I. C., D. A. Robert, J. M. Osborne, and C. A. Baker. "Discomfort during
    Mammography: A Survey of Women Attending a Breast Screening Center."
    Breast Disease 7 (1994): 35–41.
Benson, Herbert and M. Z. Klipper. *The Relaxation Response*. New York: William
    Morrow, 1975.
Berger, Karen, and John Bostwick III. *A Woman's Decision: Breast Care, Treatment
    and Reconstruction*. St. Louis: C. V. Mosby, 1984.
Bernay, Toni, Saar Porrath, J. M. Golding-Mather, and Joan Murray. "The Impact
    of Breast Cancer Screening on Feminine Identity: Implications for Patient
    Education." *Breast, Diseases of the Breast* 8 (January/March 1982): 2–5.
Bernstein, I. L., and M. M. Webster. "Learned Food Aversions: A Consequence of
    Cancer Chemotherapy," in T. G. Burish, S. M. Levy, and B. E. Meyerowitz,
    eds., *Cancer, Nutrition and Eating Behavior: A Biobehavioral Perspective*.
    Hillsdale, NJ: Lawrence Earlbaum, 1985, pp. 103–16.
Black, J. M., and E. Matassarin-Jacobs. *Luckman and Sorenson's Medical-Surgical
    Nursing, A Psychologic Approach*. Philadelphia: W. B. Saunders, 1993.
Blitzer, Andrew, A. H. Kutscher, S. C. Klagsbrun, R. DeBellis, F. E. Selder, I. B.
    Seeland, and M. Siegel, eds. *Communicating with Cancer Patients and Their
    Families*. Philadelphia: Charles Press, 1990.
Bloch, R. A. "Ten Commandments for Fighting Cancer." *Coping: Living with Can-
    cer* 7 (1993): 25.
Bloom, J. "Social Support, Accommodation to Stress and Adjustment to Cancer."
    Social Science & Medicine 16 (1982): 1329–38.
Bloom, J. R., R. D. Ross, and G. Burnell. "The Effect of Social Support on Patient
    Adjustment after Breast Surgery." *Patient Counseling & Health Education* 1
    (1978): 50–59.
Blumberg, B. D., P. Ahmed, M. Flaherty, J. Lewis, and J. Shea. "Living with Cancer:

An Overview," in P. Ahmed, ed., *Living and Dying with Cancer*. New York: Elsevier, 1981.

Blumberg, B. D., P. R. Kerns, and M. J. Lewis. "Adult Cancer Patient Education: An Overview." *Journal of Psychosocial Oncology* 1 (Summer 1983): 19–39.

Blumberg, Barbara, Mara Flaherty, and Jane Lewis, eds. *Coping with Cancer*. Bethesda, MD: U.S. Department of Health & Human Services, National Cancer Institute, 1980.

Bochner, A. P., and C. W. Kelly. "Interpersonal Competence: Rationale, Philosophy and Implementation of a Conceptual Framework." *Speech Teacher* 23 (November 1974): 279–301.

Boettcher, R. D. "Interspousal Empathy, Marital Satisfaction, and Marriage Counseling." *Journal of Social Service Research* 1 (Fall 1977): 105–13.

Bond, Senga. "Communicating with Families of Cancer Patients—1. The Relatives and Doctors." *Nursing Times* 78 (1982): 962–65.

———. "Relatively Speaking—2. Communicating with Families of Cancer Patients: The Nurse." *Nursing Times* 78 (June 1982): 1027–29.

Boring, C. C., T. S. Squires, T. Tong, and S. Montgomery. "Cancer Statistics, 1994." *CA—A Cancer Journal for Clinicians* 44 (1994): 9–11.

Bostick, J., III. "Breast Reconstruction after Mastectomy." *Surgical Clinics of North America* 70 (October 1990): 1125–40.

Boyd, N. F., M. L. Cousins, E. E. Bayliss, E. B. Fish, et al. "Diet and Breast Disease: Evidence for the Feasibility of a Clinical Trial Involving a Major Reduction in Dietary Fat," in T. G. Burish, S. M. Levy, B. E. Meyerowitz, et al., eds., *Cancer, Nutrition and Eating Behavior: A Biobehavioral Perspective*. Hillsdale, NJ: Lawrence Earlbaum, 1985, pp. 165–86.

Brammer, L. M. *The Helping Relationship: Process and Skills*, 2d ed. Englewood Cliffs, NJ: Prentice-Hall, 1979.

Bransfield, D. D. "Breast Cancer and Sexual Functioning: A Review of the Literature and Implications for Future Research." *International Journal of Psychiatry in Medicine* 12 (1982–1983): 197–211.

Breast Implant Resource Guide. Arlington Heights, IL: American Society of Plastic Reconstructive Surgeons, May 1992.

Brietbart, B. K. "Factors That Contribute to Control and Hopefulness," in A. Blitzer et al., eds., *Communicating with Cancer Patients and Their Families*. Philadelphia: Charles Press, 1990, pp. 26–32.

Brinker, Nancy, with C. M. Harris. *The Race Is Run One Step at a Time: Everywoman's Guide to Taking Charge of Breast Cancer*. New York: Simon & Schuster, 1990.

Brody, Jane E. "The Value and Limits of Mammography." *New York Times* (September 22, 1988): Y24, Personal Health Section.

Brown, C. T., and P. W. Keller. *Monologue to Dialogue*. Englewood Cliffs, NJ: Prentice-Hall, 1979.

Brown, H. N., and M. J. Kelly. "Stages of Bone Marrow Transplantation: A Psychiatric Perspective," in R. H. Moos, and J. A. Schaefer, eds., *Coping with Physical Illness 2: New Perspectives*. New York: Plenum, 1984, pp. 241–52.

Bruning, Nancy. *Coping with Chemotherapy*. Garden City, NY: Doubleday, 1985.

Brunner, S., and B. Langfeldt, eds. *Advances in Breast Cancer Detection*. New York: Springer-Verlag, 1990.

Buell, P. "Changing Incidence of Breast Cancer in Japanese-American Women." *Journal of National Cancer Institute* 5 (1973): 1479–83.

Burdick, D. "Rehabilitation of the Breast Cancer Patient." *Cancer* 36 (1975): 645–48.

Burish, T. G., and J. N. Lyles. "Coping with Adverse Effects of Cancer Treatments," in T. G. Burish and L. A. Bradley, eds., *Coping with Chronic Disease: Research and Applications.* New York: Academic Press, 1983, pp. 159–89.

Burish, T. G., and L. A. Bradley. "Coping with Chronic Disease: Definitions and Issues," in T. G. Burish and L. A. Bradley, eds., *Coping with Chronic Disease: Research and Applications.* New York: Academic Press, 1983, pp. 3–11.

Burish, T. G., W. H. Redd, and M. P. Carey. "Conditioned Nausea and Vomiting in Cancer Chemotherapy: Treatment Approaches," in T. G. Burish, S. Levy, and B. E. Meyerowitz, eds., *Cancer, Nutrition, and Eating Behaviors: A Biobehavioral Perspective.* Hillsdale, NJ: Lawrence Earlbaum, 1985, pp. 205–24.

Burke, R. J., and T. Weir. "Husband-Wife Helping Relationships: The 'Mental Hygiene' Function in Marriage." *Psychological Reports* 40 (1977): 911–25.

———. "Marital Helping Relationships: The Moderator between Stress and Well-Being." *Journal of Psychology* 95 (1977): 121–30.

Buzdar, A. U., and G. N. Hortobagyi. "Recent Developments and New Directions in Adjuvant Therapy for Breast Cancer." *Cancer Bulletin* 45 (1993): 523–27.

Byrd, B. F. "Sex after Mastectomy." *Medical Aspects of Human Sexuality* 9 (1975): 53–54.

Callan, David. "When Your Friend Has Cancer." *Cancer Family Care Newsletter* 10 (December 1988): 3.

Cancer Facts and Figures—1992. Atlanta: American Cancer Society.

Cancer Facts and Figures—1994. Atlanta: American Cancer Society.

Carkhuff, R. R., and D. H. Berenson and R. M. Pierce. *The Skills of Teaching: Interpersonal Skills.* Amherst, MA: Human Resources Development Press, 1977.

Carroll, Rose Mary. "Stress and Cancer: Etiological Significance and Implications." *Cancer Nursing* 4 (December 1981): 467–73.

Cassel, J. "The Contribution of the Social Environment to Host Resistance." *American Journal of Epidemiology* 104 (1976): 107–23.

Charlesworth, E. A., and R. G. Nathan. *Stress Management: A Comprehensive Guide to Wellness.* New York: Atheneum, 1984.

Chekryn, Joanne. "Cancer Recurrence: Personal Meaning, Communication, and Marital Adjustment." *Cancer Nursing* 7 (December 1984): 491–98.

Chlebowski, R. T., et al. "Adjuvant Dietary Fat Intake Reduction in Postmenopausal Breast Cancer Patient Management." *Breast Cancer Research and Treatment* 20 (1991): 73–84.

Christ, G. H. "A Psychosocial Assessment Framework for Cancer Patients and Their Families." *Health and Social Work* 8 (1983): 59–64.

Clark, M., H. Morris, P. King, P. Abramson, M. Gosnell, M. Hager, B. Burgower, and J. Huck. "Living with Cancer: Learning to Survive." *Newsweek* (April 8, 1985): 64–77.

Cobb, S. "Social Support and Health through the Life Course," in R. M. White, ed., *Aging from Birth to Death: Interdisciplinary Perspective.* Boulder: Westview Press, 1979.

————. "Social Support as a Moderator of Life Stress." *Psychosomatic Medicine* 38 (1976): 300–14.

Cobb, S., and C. Erbe. "Social Support for the Cancer Patient." *Forum on Medicine* 1 (1978): 24–29.

Cobliner, S. G. "Psychological Factors in Gynecological or Breast Malignancies." *Hospital Physician* 10 (1977): 38–42.

Cohen, M. M. "Psychosocial Morbidity in Cancer: A Clinical Perspective," in M. M. Cohen et al., eds., *Psychosocial Dimensions of Cancer: A Discussion of Research Issues.* New York: Raven Press, 1980.

Cohen, M. M., and D. K. Wellisch, "Living in Limbo: Psychosocial Intervention in Families with a Cancer Patient." *American Journal of Psychotherapy* 32 (1978): 561–71.

Cohen, Pauline, I. M. Dizenhuz, and C. Winget. "Family Adaptation to Terminal Illness and Death of a Parent." *Social Casework* 58 (April 1977): 222–28.

Combs, A. W., and D. L. Avila. *Helping Relationships: Basic Concepts for the Helping Professions,* 3d ed. Boston: Allyn & Bacon, 1985.

Cournos, Francine. "Psychosocial Interventions with Cancer Patients and Their Families," in A. Blitzer et al., eds., *Communicating with Cancer Patients and Their Families.* Philadelphia: Charles Press, 1990, pp. 45–48.

Cousins, Norman. *Anatomy of an Illness.* New York: Norton, 1979.

————. *Head First: The Biology of Hope.* New York: E. P. Dutton, 1989.

————. *The Healing Heart: Antidotes to Panic and Helplessness.* New York: Norton, 1983.

Craytor, J. K. "Effects of Carcinoma of the Breast on Individual and Family," in D. P. Hymovich and M. U. Barnard, eds., *Family Health Care V, II. Developmental and Situational Crises.* New York: McGraw Hill, 1979, pp. 315–36.

Creech, R. H. "The Psychologic Support of the Cancer Patient: A Medical Oncologist's View." *Seminar in Oncology* 2 (1976): 285–309.

Crocker, M. B. "Outside Help: Cancer Patients Get a New Look." *Cincinnati Enquirer* ("Tempo," E, August 4, 1993): 1–2.

Croog, S. H., A. Lipson, and S. Levine. "Help Patterns in Severe Illnesses: The Roles of Kin Network, Non-Family Resources, and Institutions." *Journal of Marriage and the Family* 34 (1972): 32–41.

Cullinan, A. L. "Social Context of Breast Cancer within the Family," in A. Blitzer et al., eds., *Communicating with Cancer Patients and Their Families.* Philadelphia: Charles Press, 1990, pp. 134–49.

Cuniberti, Betty. "The Fight of Heather Farr's Life." *Golf Digest* (July 1992): 81–90.

David, Lester. "A Brave Family Faces Up to Breast Cancer," in R. H. Moos and V. D. Tsu, eds., *Coping with Physical Illness.* New York: Plenum, 1977, pp. 73–79. Reprinted in abridged form in *Today's Health* 50 (June 1972): 18–21.

Dean, C., F. Chetty, and A. O. Forrest. "Effects of Immediate Breast Reconstruction on Psychological Morbidity after Mastectomy." *Lancet* 1 (1983): 459–62.

Degner, L. F., C. Gow, and L. A. Thompson. "Critical Nursing Behaviors in Care for the Dying." *Cancer Nursing* 14 (1991): 246–53.

Deliman, Tracy, and J. S. Smolowe, eds. *Holistic Medicine: Harmony of Body, Mind, Spirit.* Reston, VA: Reston Publ., 1982.

Derdiarian, Anayis. "Informational Needs of Recently Diagnosed Cancer Patients: A Theoretical Framework, Part I." *Cancer Nursing* 10 (1987): 107–15.

———. "Informational Needs of Recently Diagnosed Cancer Patients, Part II. Methods and Description." *Cancer Nursing* 10 (1987): 156–63.

Derogatis, L. R. "Breast and Gynecologic Cancers: Their Unique Impact on Body Image and Sexual Identity in Women." *Frontiers in Radiation and Therapeutic Oncology* 14 (1980): 1–11.

Derogatis, L. R., and S. M. Kourlesis. "An Approach to Evaluation of Sexual Problems in the Cancer Patient." *CA—A Cancer Journal for Clinicians* 31 (1981): 46–50.

Dervin, Brenda, Sylvia Harlock, Rita Atwood, and Carol Garzona. "The Human Side of Information: An Exploration in a Health Communication Context," in D. Nimmo, ed., *Communication Yearbook 4*. New Brunswick, NJ: International Communication Association, 1980.

DeVita, V. T., J. S. Hellman, and S. A. Rosenberg, eds. *Cancer: Principles and Practices of Oncology*, 4th ed. Philadelphia: J. B. Lippincott, 1993.

DiMatteo, M., and R. Hays. "Social Support and Serious Illness," in B. Gottlieb, ed., *Social Networks and Social Support*. Beverly Hills: Sage, 1981.

Di Salvo, V. S., J. K. Larsen, and D. K. Backus. "The Health Care Communicator: An Identification of Skills and Problems." *Communication Education* 35 (July 1986): 231–42.

Dodd, R. "Radiation Detection and Diagnosis of Breast Cancer." *Cancer* 47 (1981): 1766–69.

Dohrenwend, B. S., and B. P. Dohrenwend. "Life Stress and Illness: Formulation of the Issues," in R. S. Lazarus, ed., *Stressful Life Events and Their Contexts*. New York: Prodist, 1981, pp. 1–27.

Dollinger, Malin, E. H. Rosenbaum, and C. Benz. "Breast," in M. Dollinger, E. H. Rosenbaum, and G. Cable, eds., *Everyone's Guide to Cancer Therapy*. Kansas City: Andrews and McMeel, 1991, pp. 241–64.

Dow, Karen H. "Developments in Diagnosis and Staging." *Seminars in Oncology Nursing* 7 (1991): 166–74.

Downie, P. A. "Rehabilitation of the Patient after Mastectomy." *Nursing Mirror* 140 (1975): 58–59.

Dracup, K. A., and C. S. Breu. "Using Nursing Research Findings to Meet the Needs of Grieving Spouses." *Nursing Research* 27 (1978): 212–16.

Dreher, Henry. *Your Defense against Cancer*. New York: Harper & Row, 1985.

Driever, M. J., and R. McCorkle. "Patient Concerns at 3 and 6 Months Postdiagnosis." *Cancer Nursing* 7 (June 1984): 235–41.

Dunkel-Schetter, C., and C. Wortman. "The Interpersonal Dynamics of Cancer: Problems in Social Relationships and Their Impact on the Patient," in H. S. Frieman and M. R. DiMatteo, eds., *Interpersonal Issues in Health Care*. New York: Academic Press, 1982, pp. 69–100.

Dyck, Stella, and K. Wright. "Family Perceptions: The Role of the Nurse Throughout an Adult's Cancer Experience." *Oncology Nursing Forum* 12 (1985): 53–56.

Early Breast Cancer Trialist Collaborative Group. "Effects of Adjuvant Tamoxifen and of Cytotoxic Therapy on Mortality in Early Breast Cancer: An Overview of 61 Randomized Trials among 28,896 Women." *New England Journal of Medicine* 319 (1988): 1681.

Eddy, D. M., V. Hasselblad, W. McGivhey, and W. Hendee. "Mammography Screening in Women under Age 50 Years." *Journal of American Medical Association* 259 (March 11, 1988): 1512–19.

Edstrom, Susan, and M. W. Miller. "Preparing the Family to Care for the Cancer Patient at Home: A Home Care Course." *Cancer Nursing* 4 (1981): 49–52.

Egan, G. *The Skilled Helper*. Monterey, CA: Brooks Cole, 1986.

Ellison, E. S. "Cancer and the Family: Experiences of Children and Adolescents," in A. Blitzer et al., eds., *Communicating with Cancer Patients and Their Families*. Philadelphia: Charles Press, 1990, pp. 115–24.

Engleman, S. R., and Ray Craddick. "The Symbolic Relationship of Breast Cancer Patients to Their Cancer, Cure, Physician and Themselves." *Psychotherapy and Psychosomatics* 41 (March 1984): 68–76.

Ervin, C. E., Jr. "Psychologic Adjustment to Mastectomy." *Medical Aspects of Human Sexuality* 7 (1973): 42–61.

Evans, D.G.R., L. D. Burnell, P. Hopwood, et al. "Perceptions of Risk in Women with a Family History of Breast Cancer." *British Journal of Cancer* 67 (1993): 612–14.

Fallowfield, L. J., A. Hall, G. P. Maguire, and M. Baum. "Psychological Outcomes and Different Treatment Policies in Women with Early Breast Cancer outside a Clinical Trial." *British Medical Journal* 301 (1990): 575–80.

Farrow, J. M., D. K. Cash, and G. Simmons. "Communicating with Cancer Patients and Their Families," in A. Blitzer et al., eds., *Communicating with Cancer Patients and Their Families*. Philadelphia: Charles Press, 1990, pp. 1–17.

FDA Update. "Bio-Dimensional Silicone Breast Implant OK'd." *Coping* 7 (January/ February 1993): 26.

Feezel, J. D., and P. E. Shepherd. "Cross-Generational Coping with Interpersonal Relationship Loss." *Western Journal of Speech Communication* 51 (Summer 1987): 317–27.

Felder, Leonard. *When a Loved One Is Ill: How to Take Better Care of Your Loved One, Your Family, and Yourself*. New York: New American Library, 1990.

Felson, B. *Humor in Medicine . . . and Other Topics*. Cincinnati: RHA, 1989.

Felton, B. J., and T. A. Revenson. "Coping with Chronic Illness: A Study of Illness Controllability and the Influence of Coping Strategies on Psychological Adjustment." *Journal of Consulting and Clinical Psychology* 52 (1984): 343–53.

Fisher, Bernard. "Laboratory and Clinical Research in Breast Cancer—A Personal Adventure. The David Karnofsky Memorial Lecture." *Cancer Research* 40 (1980): 3863–74.

Fisher, B., C. Redmond, P. Poisson, R. Margolese, et al. "Eight-Year Results of a Randomized Clinical Trial Comparing Total Mastectomy and Lumpectomy with or without Radiation in Treatment of Breast Cancer." *New England Journal of Medicine* 320 (1989): 822–28.

Fisher, S. G. "The Psychosexual Effects of Cancer and Cancer Treatment." *Oncology Nursing Forum* 10 (1983): 63–68.

Fobair, Pat, and N. L. Mages. "Psychosocial Morbidity among Cancer Patient Survivors," in P. Ahmed, ed., *Living and Dying with Cancer*. New York: Elsevier, 1981, pp. 287–304.

Foley, K. M. "Cancer and Pain," in A. I. Holleb, ed., *The American Cancer Society Cancer Book*. Garden City, NY: Doubleday, 1986, pp. 225–37.

Forbes, Bryan. *Dame Edith Evans, Ned's Girl*. Boston: Little, Brown, 1977.

Fortune, Ellen. "A Nursing Approach to Body Image and Sexuality Adaptation in the Mastectomy Patient." *Sexuality and Disability* 2 (1979): 47–53.

Fowles, John, and Daniel Martin. "Toward a Holistic Approach to Carcinogenesis," in A. M. de la Pena, ed., *The Psychobiology of Cancer*. New York: Praeger, 1983, pp. 1–16.

Frank-Stromberg, Marilyn, and Penny Wright. "Ambulatory Cancer Patients' Perception of the Physical and Psychosocial Changes in Their Lives since the Diagnosis of Cancer." *Cancer Nursing* 7 (1984): 117–29.

Freeman, Lucy, and H. L. Strean. *Guilt: Letting Go*. New York: John Wiley & Sons, 1986.

Freidenbergs, Ingrid, G. Wayne, M. Hibbard, L. Levine, C. Wolf, and L. Diller. "Psychosocial Aspects of Living with Cancer: A Review of the Literature." *International Journal of Psychiatry in Medicine* 11 (1981–1982): 303–29.

Freireich, E. J. "Experimental Treatments and Research." *American Cancer Society Cancer Book*. Garden City, NY: Doubleday, 1986, pp. 151–70.

Fritz, P. A., M. Wilcox, C. G. Russell, and J. R. Wilcox. "Research Topics in Health Care: The Kingdom of Conflict." Paper Presented at Speech Communication Association, Columbus, Ohio, 1982.

Frykberg, E. R., and K. I. Bland. "Noninvasive Carcinoma of the Breast." *Cancer Bulletin* 45 (1993): 506–11.

Funch, D. P., and J. Marshall. "The Role of Stress, Social Support and Age in Survival from Breast Cancer." *Journal of Psychosomatic Research* 27 (1983): 77–83.

Gaffney, E. V., A. T. Sharmanov, W. E. Moody, et al. "Hormone Receptor Assays and Their Value in Breast Cancer Therapy." *Cancer Biotherapy* 8 (1993): 17–28.

Gagnon, Pierre, M. J. Massie, and J. C. Holland. "The Woman with Breast Cancer: Psychosocial Considerations," *Cancer Bulletin* 45 (1993): 538–42.

Gallo, Frank T. "Counseling the Breast Cancer Patient." *Family Therapy* 15 (1977): 247–53.

Galvin, K. M., and B. J. Brommel. *Family Communications: Cohesion and Change*, 2d ed. Glenview, IL: Scott, Foresman, 1986.

Garfield, C. A. "Impact of Death on the Health-Care Professional," in H. Feifel, ed., *New Meanings of Death*. New York: McGraw-Hill, 1977, pp. 143–52.

Garfinkel, Lawrence. "Evaluating Cancer Statistics." *CA—A Cancer Journal for Clinicians* 49 (January/February 1994): 5–6.

Gates, C. C. "Husbands of Mastectomy Patients." *Patient Counseling and Health Education* 1–2 (1980): 38–41.

Gazda, G. M., and T. D. Evans. "Empathy as a Skill," in R. C. McKay, J. R. Hughes, and E. J. Carver, eds., *Empathy in the Helping Relationship*. New York: Springer, 1990, pp. 65–77.

Georgiade, G. S., N. G. Georgiade, K. S. McCarty, B. J. Ferguson, and H. F. Seigler. "Modified Radical Mastectomy with Immediate Reconstruction for Carcinoma of the Breast." *Annals of Surgery* 193 (May 1981): 565–73.

Gershon-Cohen, J., S. M. Berger, and H. S. Klickstein. "Roentgenography of Breast

Cancer Moderating Concept of 'Biological Predeterminism.'" *Cancer* 16 (1963): 961–64.

Giacquinta, Barbara. "Helping Families Face the Crisis of Cancer." *American Journal of Nursing* 77 (1977): 1585–88.

Given, Barbara A., and C. W. Given. "Creating a Climate for Compliance." *Cancer Nursing* 7 (April 1984): 139–47.

Glenn, B. L., and L. A. Moore. "Relationship of Self-Concept, Health, Locus of Control, and Perceived Treatment Options to the Practice of Breast Self-examination." *Cancer Nursing* 13 (1990): 361–65.

Go, R. C., M. C. King, J. E. Bailey-Wilson, et al. "Genetic Epidemiology of Breast Cancer and Associated Cancer in High Risk Families I. Segregation Analysis." *Journal of the National Cancer Institute* 71 (1983): 455–61.

Goodwin, J., W. C. Hunt, C. R. Key, and J. M. Samet. "The Effects of Marital Status on Stage, Treatment and Survival of Cancer Patients." *Journal of the American Medical Association* 258 (December 4, 1987): 3215–30.

Gordon, W. A., I. Freidenbergs, L. Diller, M. Hibbard, C. Wolf, L. Levine, R. Lipkins, O. Ezrach, and D. Lucido. "Efficacy of Psychosocial Intervention with Cancer Patients." *Journal of Consulting and Clinical Psychology* 48 (1980): 743–59.

Gore, S. "Stress-Buffering Function of Social Support: The Significance of Context," in B. Gottlieb, ed., *Social Networks and Social Support.* Beverly Hills: Sage, 1981, pp. 43–68.

Gottheil, Edward, W. C. McGurn, and Otto Pollak. "Awareness and Disengagement in Cancer Patients." *American Journal of Psychiatry* 136 (May 1979): 632–35.

Grandstaff, N. W. "The Impact of Breast Cancer on the Family." *Frontiers in Radiation Therapy Oncology* 11 (1976): 146–56.

Gravelle, Karen, and Charles Haskins. *Teenagers Face to Face with Bereavement.* Englewood Cliffs, NJ: Julian Messner, 1989.

Gray-Price, Hilarie, and Susan Szczesny. "Crisis Intervention with Families of Cancer Patients: A Developmental Approach." *Topics in Clinical Nursing* 7 (1985): 58–70.

Green, E., and A. Green. "Beyond Feedback," in B. Englis and R. West, eds., *The Alternative Health Guide.* New York: Knopf, 1983.

Greenblatt, M. "The Grieving Spouse." *American Journal of Psychiatry* 135 (1978): 45–47.

Greer, H. S., Tina Morris, and K. W. Pettingale. "Psychological Response to Breast Cancer: Effect on Outcome." *Lancet* 2 (1979): 785–87.

Greer, S. "Psychological Enquiry: A Contribution to Cancer Research." *Psychological Medicine* 9 (1979): 81–89.

Greer, S., and Tina Morris. "Psychological Attributes of Women Who Develop Breast Cancer: A Controlled Study." *Journal of Psychosomatic Research* 19 (1975): 147–53.

Gruber, B. L., N. R. Hall, S. P. Hersh, and P. Dubois. "Immune System and Psychologic Changes in Metastatic Cancer Patients while Using Ritualized Relaxation and Guided Imagery: A Pilot Study." *Scandinavian Journal of Behavior Therapy* 17 (1988): 25–46.

Grunberg, N. E. "Specific Taste Preferences: An Alternative Explanation for Eating

Changes in Cancer Patients," in B. E. Meyerowitz, S. Levy, and T. Burish, eds., *Cancer, Nutrition and Eating Behavior: A Behavioral Perspective*. Hillsdale, NJ: Lawrence Earlbaum, 1985, pp. 43–61.

Hagopian, G. A., and J. H. Rubenstein. "Effects of Telephone Call Intervention on Patients' Well-Being in a Radiation Department." *Cancer Nursing* 13 (December 1990): 339–44.

Hampe, S. "Needs of the Grieving Spouse in a Hospital Setting." *Nursing Research* 24 (1975): 113–20.

Hansen, Barbara. *Picking Up the Pieces*. Dallas: Taylor, 1990.

Harris, J. H., M. Morrow, and G. Bonadonna. "Cancer of the Breast," in V. T. DeVita, J. S. Hellman, and S. A. Rosenberg, eds., *Cancer: Principles and Practices of Oncology I*, 4th ed. Philadelphia: Lippincott, 1993, pp. 1264–1332.

Harris, J. R., J. L. Connolly, S. J. Schnitt, et al. "The Use of Pathological Features in Selecting the Extent of Surgical Resection Necessary for Breast Cancer Patients Treated by Primary Radiation Therapy." *Annals of Surgery* 201 (1985): 164–69.

Harvey, E. B., C. Schairer, L. A. Brinton, R. N. Hoover, and J. F. Fraumeni. "Alcohol Consumption and Breast Cancer." *Journal of the National Cancer Institute* 78 (1987): 657–61.

Harwell, Amy, with Kristine Tomasik. *When Your Friend Gets Cancer*. Wheaton, IL: Harold Shaw Publishers, 1987.

Hastings, A. C., James Fadiman, and J. S. Gordon, eds. *Health for the Whole Person*. Boulder: Westview Press, 1980.

Hayes, Helen, and K. Hatch. *My Life in Three Acts*. New York: Harcourt Brace Jovanovich, 1990.

Heinrich, R. L., C. C. Schag, and P. A. Ganz. "Living with Cancer: The Cancer Inventory of Problem Situations." *Journal of Clinical Psychology* 40 (July 1984): 972–80.

Hilakivi-Clarke, L., J. Rowland, R. Clarke, and M. E. Lippman. "Psychological Factors in Development and Progression of Breast Cancer." *Breast Cancer Research and Treatment* 29 (1993): 141–60.

Hillier, Richard. "Terminal Care—The Doctor's Anxieties." *Cancer Care* 5 (1988): 9–10.

Hilton, Cheryl. "New Drug Offers Relief from Chemotherapy Nausea." *University Currents* (University of Cincinnati, May 21, 1993): 5.

Hinton, John. "Bearing Cancer." *British Journal of Medical Psychology* 46 (1973): 105–13.

———. "The Influence of Previous Personality Reactions to Having Cancer." *Omega: Journal of Death and Dying* 6 (1975): 95–111.

———. "Sharing and Withholding Awareness of Dying between Husband and Wife." *Journal of Psychosomatic Research* 25 (1981): 337–43.

Hirshaut, Yashar, and P. I. Pressman. *Breast Cancer: The Complete Guide*. New York: Bantam, 1992.

Hirst, Sandra. "The Significance of Breast Pain." *Nursing Times* 80 (January 25, 1984): 34–35.

Holland, J. C., and L. O. Cullen. "New Insights and Attitudes," in A. I. Holleb, ed., *American Cancer Society Cancer Book*. Garden City, NY: Doubleday, 1986, pp. 3–14.

Holleb, A. I., ed. *The American Cancer Society Cancer Book*. Garden City, NY: Doubleday, 1986.

Holm, Lars-Erik, E. Nordevang, E. Ikkala, L. Hallstrom, and E. Callmer. "Dietary Intervention as Adjuvant Therapy in Breast Cancer Patients—A Feasibility Study." *Breast Cancer Research and Treatment* 16 (1990): 103–9.

Holmes, F. A., and A. B. Deisseroth. "Genetic and Molecular Approaches to the Use of Autologous Stem Cells to Enhance the Therapeutic Index of Chemotherapy for Breast Cancer." *Cancer Bulletin* 45 (1993): 146–152.

Hortobagyi, G. N., and S. E. Singletary. "Spectrum of Breast Cancer." *Cancer Bulletin* 45 (1993): 471–72.

Humphrey, L. J. "Subcutaneous Mastectomy Is Not a Prophylaxis against Carcinoma of the Breast: Opinion or Knowledge?" *American Journal of Surgery* 145 (1983): 311–12.

Huntington, M. "Weight Gain in Patients Receiving Adjuvant Chemotherapy for Carcinoma of the Breast." *Cancer* 56 (1985): 472–74.

Ilfeld, F. W. "Understanding Marital Stressors: The Importance of Coping Style." *Journal of Nervous and Mental Disease* 168 (1980): 375–81.

Inglis, Brian, and Ruth West, eds. *The Alternative Health Guide*. New York: Knopf, 1983.

Ireland, Jill. *Life Wish*. Boston: Little, Brown, 1987.

Isley, C. "The Fatal Choice: Cancer Quackery." *RN Magazine* (September 1974): 55–59.

Jacobs, E. R., J. C. Holland, T. Chaglassian, et al. "Reconstructive Breast Surgery after Mastectomy: A Comparative Study of Psychosocial Aspects." *Proceedings, Thirteenth International Cancer Conference* 167 (1982), Abstract 938.

James, N. D. "Bone Marrow Transplantation," in D. Carney and K. Sikora, eds., *Genes and Cancer*. New York: John Wiley, 1990, pp. 329–37.

Jamison, K., D. K. Wellisch, K. L. Katz, and R. O. Pasnau. "Phantom Breast Syndrome." *Archives of Surgery* 114 (1979): 93–95.

Jamison, K. R., D. K. Wellisch, and R. O. Pasnau. "Psychological Aspects of Mastectomy: I. The Woman's Perspective." *American Journal of Psychiatry* 135 (1978): 432–35.

Jansen, C., P. Hamilton, S. Dibble, and M. J. Dodd. "Family Problems during Cancer Chemotherapy." *Oncology Nursing Forum* 20 (May 1993): 689–96.

Johnson, J. L., and P. A. Norby. "We Can Weekend: A Program for Cancer Families." *Cancer Nursing* 4 (1981): 23–28.

Kalish, R. A. "Dying and Preparing for Death: A View for Families," in H. Feifel, ed., *New Meanings of Death*. New York: McGraw-Hill, 1977, pp. 215–32.

Kaplan, B. H., and J. C. Cassel. "Social Support and Health." *Medical Care* 15 (1977): 47–57.

Kaplan, D. M., Aaron Smith, Rose Grobstein, and S. E. Fischman. "Family Mediation of Stress," in R. H. Moos, ed., *Coping with Physical Illness*. New York: Plenum, 1977, pp. 82–96.

Katz, J. L., Herbert Weiner, T. F. Gallagher, and Leon Hellman. "Stress, Distress and Ego Defenses: Psychoendocrine Response to Impending Breast Tumor Biopsy." *Archives of General Psychiatry* 23 (1970): 131–42.

Kaufman, M. *Homeopathy in America*. Baltimore: Johns Hopkins Press, 1971.

Kaye, Ronnie. *Spinning Straw into Gold: Your Emotional Recovery from Breast Cancer*. New York: Simon & Schuster, 1991.

Kelley, O. E. "Make Today Count," in H. Feifel, ed., *New Meanings of Death*. New York: McGraw-Hill, 1977, pp. 181–93.

Kennedy, S., J. K. Kiecolt-Glaser, and R. Glaser. "Immunological Consequences of Acute and Chronic Stressors: Mediating-Role of Interpersonal Relationships." *British Journal of Medical Psychology* 61 (1988): 77–85.

Kent, Saul. "Coping with Sexual Identity Crises after Mastectomy." *Geriatrics* 30 (1975): 145–46.

Keough, Carol, et al., eds. *The Complete Book of Cancer Prevention*. Emmaus, PA: Rodale Press, 1988.

Kesselring, Annmarie, A. M. Lindsey, M. J. Dodd, and N. C. Lovejoy. "Social Network and Support Perceived by Swiss Cancer Patients." *Cancer Nursing* 9 (1986): 156–63.

Kiecolt-Glaser, J. K., R. Glaser, et al. "Modulation of Cellular Immunity in Medical Students." *Journal of Behavioral Medicine* 9 (1986): 5–21.

Kiecolt-Glaser, J. K., and R. Glaser. "Stress and Immune Function in Humans," in P. Ader, D. L. Felton, and N. Cohen, eds., *Psychoneuroimmunology*, 2d ed. New York: Academic Press, 1991.

Kiecolt-Glaser, J. K., L. Fisher, P. Ogrocki, et al. "Marital Quality, Marital Disruption, and Immune Function." *Psychosomatic Medicine* 49 (1987): 13–34.

Kievman, Beverly, with Susie Blackmun. *For Better or For Worse: A Couple's Guide to Dealing with Chronic Illness*. Chicago: Contemporary Books, 1989.

Kim, E. E., D. A. Podoloff, L. A. Moulopoulos, et al. "Magnetic Resonance Imaging, Positron Emission Tomography, and Radioimmunoscintography of Breast Cancer." *Cancer Bulletin* 45 (1993): 500–505.

King, M. C., S. Rowell, and S. M. Love. "Inherited Breast and Ovarian Cancer— What Are the Risks? What Are the Choices?" *Journal of the American Medical Association* 269 (1993): 1975–80.

Klagsbrun, S. C. "Communications in the Treatment of Cancer." *American Journal of Nursing* 71 (May 1971): 944–48.

Klein, R. F., Alfred Dean, and M. D. Bogdonoff. "The Impact of Illness upon the Spouse." *Journal of Chronic Disease* 20 (1967): 241–48.

Klein, Roberta. "A Crisis to Grow On." *Cancer* 28 (1971): 1660–65.

Klopfer, Bruno. "Psychological Variables in Human Cancer." *Journal of Projective Techniques* 21 (1957): 331–40.

Knobf, M. T., and Richard Stahl. "Reconstructive Surgery in Primary Breast Cancer Treatment." *Seminars in Oncology Nursing* 7 (August 1991): 200–206.

Krause, Kaisa. "Contracting Cancer and Coping with It: Patients' Experiences." *Cancer Nursing* 14 (1991): 240–45.

Kriss, Regina. "Effectiveness of Group Therapy for Problems of Self-Perception, Body Image and Sexuality." Dissertation, California Graduate School of Marital and Family Therapy, Stanford University, 1982.

Kübler-Ross, Elisabeth. *Death: The Final Stage of Growth*. Englewood Cliffs, NJ: Prentice-Hall, 1975.

———. *On Children and Death*. New York: Macmillan, 1983.

———. *On Death and Dying*. New York: Macmillan, 1969.

———. *Questions and Answers on Death and Dying.* New York: Macmillan, 1974.

Kushner, Rose. *Alternatives: New Developments in the War on Breast Cancer.* New York: Warner Books, 1985.

———. *Breast Cancer: A Personal History and an Investigative Report.* New York: Harcourt Brace Jovanovich, 1975.

Laing, R. D., H. Phillipson, and A. D. Lee. *Interpersonal Perception: A Theory and a Method of Research.* London: Tavistock, 1966.

Lamb, M. A., and N. F. Woods. "Sexuality and the Cancer Patient." *Cancer Nursing* 4 (April 1981): 137–43.

Laszlo, John. *Understanding Cancer.* New York: Harper & Row, 1987.

Lazarus, R. S. *Patterns of Adjustment.* 3rd ed. New York: McGraw-Hill, 1976.

———. *Psychological Stress and the Coping Process.* New York: McGraw-Hill, 1966.

Lazarus, R. S., and Susan Folkman. *Stress, Appraisal and Coping.* New York: Springer, 1984.

Lee, Harper. *To Kill a Mockingbird.* New York: Warner Books, 1960.

Leiber, L., M. M. Plumb, M. L. Gerstenzang, and J. D. Holland. "The Communication of Affection between Cancer Patients and Their Spouses." *Psychosomatic Medicine* 38 (1976): 379–89.

Lerner, Harriet G. *The Dance of Anger.* New York: Harper & Row, 1985.

———. *The Dance of Intimacy.* New York: Harper & Row, 1989.

LeShan, Eda. *Learning to Say Goodby: When a Parent Dies.* New York: Macmillan, 1976.

LeShan, Lawrence. *Cancer as a Turning Point.* Rev. ed. New York: Penguin, 1994.

———. *Cancer as a Turning Point: A Handbook for People with Cancer, Their Families and Health Professionals.* New York: E. P. Dutton, 1989.

———. *You Can Fight for Your Life.* New York: M. Evans, 1980.

Levy, S. M. "Death and Dying," in T. G. Burish and L. A. Bradley, eds., *Coping with Chronic Disease: Research and Applications.* New York: Academic Press, 1983.

Lewin, Margaret. "Principles of Cancer Chemotherapy," in A. I. Holleb, ed., *The American Cancer Society Cancer Book.* Garden City, NY: Doubleday, 1986, pp. 126–39.

Lewis, F. M. "The Impact of Cancer on the Family: A Critical Analysis of the Research Literature." *Patient Education and Counseling* 8 (1986): 269–89.

———. "Strengthening Family Supports: Cancer and the Family." *Cancer* 65 (1990): 752–59.

Lewis, F. M., N. F. Woods, L. Bensley, and E. Hough. "Family Functioning in Chronic Illness: The Spouse's Perspective." *Social Science Medicine* 29 (1989): 1261–69.

Lichtman, R. R., et al. "Relations with Children after Breast Cancer: The Mother-Daughter Relationship at Risk." *Journal of Psychosocial Oncology* 2 (1984): 1–19.

Lichtman, Rosemary. "Close Relationships after Breast Cancer." Doctoral Dissertation, University of California, 1982. Dissertation Abstracts International, 43,3411B.

Lichtman, R. R., S. E. Taylor, and J. V. Wood. "Social Support and Marital Adjustment after Breast Cancer." *Journal of Psychosocial Oncology* 5 (1987): 47–74.

Lindsey, A. M., J. S. Norbeck, V. L. Carrieri, and E. Perry. "Social Support and

Health Outcomes in Post-Mastectomy Women: A Review." *Cancer Nursing* 4 (1981): 377–84.

Lipowski, Z. J. "Physical Illness, the Individual and the Coping Process." *International Journal of Psychiatry in Medicine* 1 (1970–1971): 91–102.

Littlejohn, S. W. *Theories of Human Communication*, 2d ed. Belmont, CA: Wadsworth, 1983.

Ljungdahl, Lars. "Laugh If This Is a Joke." *Journal of the American Medical Association* 261 (1989): 558.

Lonetto, Richard, *Children's Conceptions of Death*. New York: Springer, 1980.

Love, R. R. "Genetics and Human Cancer: Family History and Common Cancers." *Wisconsin Medical Journal* 86 (1987): 20–21.

———. "Tamoxifen Therapy in Primary Breast Cancer: Biology, Efficacy, and Side Effects." *Journal of Clinical Oncology* 7 (1989): 803–15.

Love, Susan, with Karen Lindsey. *Dr. Susan Love's Breast Book*. Reading, MA: Addison-Wesley, 1990.

Lovejoy, N. C. "Family Responses to Cancer Hospitalization." *Oncology Nursing Forum* 13 (March/April 1986): 33–37.

Loveys, B. J., and K. Klaich. "Breast Cancer: Demands of Illness." *Oncology Nursing Forum* 18 (1991): 75–80.

Lynch, H. T., and J. F. Lynch. "Breast Cancer Genetics in an Oncology Clinic: 328 Consecutive Patients." *Cancer Genetics and Cytogenetics* 22 (1986): 369–71.

Lynch, H. T., W. A. Albano, J. J. Heieck, et al. "Genetics, Biomarkers and Control of Breast Cancer: A Review." *Cancer Genetics and Cytogenetics* 13 (1986): 43–92.

Lynch, J., P. Fain, D. Golgar, et al. "Familial Breast Cancer and Its Recognition in an Oncology Clinic." *Cancer* 47 (1981): 2730–39.

MacDonald, Sue. "Finding Strength in Cancer." *Cincinnati Enquirer* (March 28, 1990): 1–3, Sec. B.

MacKay, R. C., E. J. Carver, and J. R. Hughes. "The Professional's Use of Empathy and Client Care Outcomes," in R. C. MacKay et al., eds., *Empathy in the Helping Relationship*. New York: Springer, 1990, pp. 120–32.

MacVicar, M. G., and Pat Archbold. "A Framework for Family Assessment in Chronic Illness." *Nursing Forum* 15 (1976): 180–94.

Maguire, G. P., E. G. Lee, D. J. Bevington, C. S. Kuchemann, R. J. Crabtree, and C. E. Cornell. "Psychiatric Problems in the First Year after Mastectomy." *British Medical Journal* 1 (April 1978): 963–65.

Maguire, Peter. "Breast Conservation vs. Mastectomy: Psychological Considerations." *Seminar in Surgical Oncology* 5 (1989): 137–44.

———. "The Psychological and Social Consequences of Breast Cancer." *Nursing Mirror* 140 (1975): 54–57.

———. "The Psychological and Social Sequelae of Mastectomy," in J. G. Howells, ed., *Modern Perspectives in Psychiatric Aspects of Surgery*. New York: Brunner/Mazel, 1976.

———. "The Psychological Impact of Cancer." *British Journal of Hospital Medicine* 34 (August 1985): 100–109.

———. "The Repercussions of Mastectomy on the Family." *International Journal of Family Psychiatry* 1 (1981): 485–503.

Maguire, Peter, A. Tait, and M. Brooke. "A Conspiracy of Pretense." *Nursing Mirror* 150 (January 10, 1980): 17–19.

Maguire, P., A. Tait, M. Brooke, C. Thomas, and R. Sellwood. "Effect of Counseling on Psychiatric Morbidity Associated with Mastectomy." *British Medical Journal* 281 (November 29, 1980): 1454–56.

Maguire, P., A. Tait, M. Brooke, and R. Sellwood. "Emotional Aspects of Mastectomy: Planning a Caring Programme." *Nursing Mirror* 150 (1980): 35–37.

Mailick, Mildred. "The Impact of Severe Illness on the Individual and Family: An Overview." *Social Work in Health Care* 5 (Winter 1979): 117–28.

Mandler, G. "Stress and Thought Processes," in L. Goldberger and S. Breznitz, eds., *Handbook of Stress.* New York: Free Press/Macmillan, 1984.

Matje, Sister Diane. "Stress and Cancer: A Review of the Literature." *Cancer Nursing* 7 (1984): 399–404.

Maxwell, M. B. "The Use of Social Networks to Help Cancer Patients Maximize Support." *Cancer Nursing* 5 (August 1982): 275–81.

May, Harold J. "Integration of Sexual Counseling and Family Therapy with Surgical Treatment of Breast Cancer." *Family Relations* 30 (1981): 291–95.

McAllister, R. M., S. T. Horowitz, and R. V. Gilden. *Cancer.* New York: Basic Books, 1993.

McBridge, A. B. *The Secret of a Good Life with Your Teenager.* New York: Times Books, 1987.

McCubbin, H. I. "Integrating Coping Behavior in Family Stress Theory." *Journal of Marriage and the Family* 41 (1979): 237–44.

McCubbin, H. I., and C. R. Figley, eds. *Stress and the Family, Vol. II: Coping with Catastrophe.* New York: Brunner/Mazel, 1983.

McCubbin, H. I., and J. M. Patterson. "Family Transitions: Adaptation to Stress," in H. I. McCubbin and R. Figley, eds., *Stress and the Family, Vol. I: Coping with Normative Transitions.* New York: Brunner/Mazel, 1983, pp. 5–25.

McCubbin, H. I., A. E. Cauble, and Joan Patterson. *Family Stress, Coping and Social Support.* Springfield, IL: Charles C. Thomas, 1983.

McCubbin, H. I., B. Dahl, G. Lester, et al. "Coping Repertoires of Families to Prolonged War-Induced Separation." *Journal of Marriage and the Family* 38 (1976): 461–72.

Metzger, L. F., T. Rogers, and L. J. Bauman. "Effects of Age and Marital Status on Emotional Distress after a Mastectomy." *Journal of Psychosocial Oncology* 1 (Fall 1983): 17–33.

Meyerowitz, Beth. "The Psychological Correlates of Breast Cancer and Its Treatment." *Psychological Bulletin* 87 (1980): 108–31.

Meyerowitz, B. E. "The Impact of Mastectomy on the Lives of Women." *Professional Psychology* 12 (1981): 118–27.

Meyerowitz, B. E., F. C. Sparks, and I. K. Spears. "Adjuvant Chemotherapy for Breast Carcinoma, Psychosocial Implications." *Cancer* 43 (1979): 1613–18.

Meyerowitz, B. E., R. Heinrich, and C. Schag. "A Competency-Based Approach to Coping with Cancer," in L. S. Bradley and T. G. Burish, eds., *Coping with Chronic Disease: Research and Application.* New York: Academic Press, 1983, pp. 137–58.

Meyerowitz, B. E., S. M. Levy, and T. G. Burish. "Cancer, Nutrition and Eating Behavior: Introduction and Overview," in B. Meyerowitz, S. Levy, and T.

Burish, eds., *Cancer, Nutrition and Eating Behavior: A Behavioral Perspective.* Hillsdale, NJ: Lawrence Earlbaum, 1985, pp. 1–7.

Miller, M. W., and C. Nygren. "Living with Cancer—Coping Behaviors." *Cancer Nursing* 1 (1978): 297–302.

Miller, S., E. Nunnally, and D. B. Wackman. *Couple Communication I. Talking Together.* Sydney: Family Life Movement of Australia, 1980.

Moetzinger, C. A., and L. G. Dauber. "The Management of the Patient with Breast Cancer." *Cancer Nursing* 5 (1982): 287–92.

Moffit, P. F., N. D. Spence, and R. D. Goldney. "Mental Health in Marriage: The Roles of Need for Affiliation, Sensitivity to Rejection, and Other Factors." *Journal of Clinical Psychology* 42 (1986): 68–76.

Montagu, Ashley. *Touching: The Human Significance of Skin.* New York: Harper & Row, 1971.

Moos, R. H. "Psychological Techniques in the Assessment of Adaptive Behavior," in G. V. Coelho, D. A. Hamburg, and J. E. Adams, eds., *Coping and Adaptation.* New York: Basic Books, 1974, pp. 334–99.

Moos, R. H., and J. A. Schaefer. "The Crisis of Physical Illness: An Overview and Conceptual Approach," in R. H. Moos and J. A. Schaefer, eds., *Coping with Physical Illness 2: New Perspectives.* New York: Plenum, 1984, pp. 3–21.

Moos, R. H., and V. D. Tsu. "The Crisis of Physical Illness: An Overview," in R. H. Moos, ed., *Coping with Physical Illness.* New York: Plenum, 1977.

Morgan, Brian L. G. *Nutrition Prescription: Strategies for Preventing and Treating 50 Common Diseases.* New York: Crown, 1987.

Morris, Tina, H. S. Greer, and P. White. "Psychological and Social Adjustment to Mastectomy: A Two-Year Follow-Up Study." *Cancer* 40 (1977): 2381–87.

Moss, Ralph, and Leslie Strong. "A Real Choice." *Ladies Home Journal* (November 1984): 101–8.

Moss, Ralph W. *The Cancer Syndrome.* New York: Grove Press, 1980.

Murcia, Andy, and Bob Stewart. *Man to Man: When the Woman You Love Has Breast Cancer.* New York: St. Martin's Press, 1989.

Murphy, D. C., and Mendelson, L. A. "Communication and Adjustment in Marriage: Investigating the Relationship." *Family Process* 12 (1973): 317–26.

Napier, Augustus Y. *The Fragile Bond.* New York: Harper & Row, 1988.

Nerenz, D. R., and H. Leventhal. "Self-Regulation Theory in Chronic Illness," in T. G. Burish and L. A. Bradley, eds., *Coping with Chronic Disease.* New York: Academic Press, 1983.

Nessim, Susan, and Judith Ellis. *Cancervive: The Challenge of Life after Cancer.* Boston: Houghton Mifflin, 1991.

Neuling, S. J., and H. R. Winefield. "Social Support and Recovery after Surgery for Breast Cancer: Frequency and Correlates of Supportive Behaviors by Family, Friends and Surgeon." *Social Science and Medicine* 27 (1988): 385–92.

Nielsen, Beverly, C. Miaskowski, and S. L. Dibble. "Pain with Mammography: Fact or Fiction?" *Oncology Nursing Forum* 20 (May 1993): 639–42.

Nimocks, M.J.A., L. Webb, and J. R. Connell. "Communication and the Terminally Ill: A Theoretical Model." *Death Studies* 11 (1987): 323–44.

Nolen, W. A. *Crisis Time!* New York: Dodd, Mead & Co., 1984.

———. *Healing: A Doctor in Search of a Miracle.* New York: Random House, 1974.

————. *A Surgeon's Book of Hope*. New York: Coward, McCann & Geoghegan, 1980.

Northouse, Laurel L. "The Impact of Cancer on the Family: An Overview." *International Journal of Psychiatry in Medicine* 14 (1984): 215–42.

————. "Mastectomy Patients and the Fear of Cancer Recurrence." *Cancer Nursing* 4 (June 1981): 213–20.

————. "Social Support in Patients' and Husbands' Adjustment to Breast Cancer." *Nursing Research* 37 (March/April 1988): 91–95.

Northouse, Laurel L., Ann Cracchiolo-Caraway, and C. P. Appel. "Psychologic Consequences of Breast Cancer on Partner and Family." *Seminars in Oncology Nursing* 7 (August 1991): 216–23.

Northouse, L. L., and M. A. Swain. "Adjustment of Patients and Husbands to the Initial Impact of Breast Cancer." *Nursing Research* 36 (July/August 1987): 221–25.

Northouse, P. G., and L. L. Northouse. "Communication and Cancer: Issues Confronting Patients, Health Professionals, and Family Members." *Journal of Psychosocial Oncology* 5 (1987): 17–46.

Novotny, Elizabeth, J. M. Hyland, L. Coyne, J. W. Travis, and H. Pruyser. "Factors Affecting Adjustment to Cancer." *Bulletin of the Menninger Clinic* 48 (July 1984): 318–28.

Nuehring, E. M., and W. E. Barr. "Mastectomy: Impact on Patients and Families." *Health and Social Work* 5 (1980): 51–58.

Oberst, M. T., and R. H. James. "Going Home: Patient and Spouse Adjustment following Cancer Surgery." *Topics in Clinical Nursing* (1985): 46–57.

O'Hare, P. A., D. Malone, E. Lusk, and R. McCorkle. "Unmet Needs of Black Patients with Cancer Posthospitalization: A Descriptive Study." *Oncology Nursing Forum* 20 (May 1993): 659–64.

Olsen, E. H. "The Impact of Serious Illness on the Family System." *Postgraduate Medicine* 47 (1970): 169–74.

Olson, D. H., H. I. McCubbin, H. Barnes, A. Larsen, M. Muxen, and M. Wilson. *Families: What Makes Them Work*. Beverly Hills, CA: Sage, 1983.

O'Neill, M. P. "Psychological Aspects of Cancer Recovery." *Cancer* 36 (1975): 271–73.

Ostchega, J., and K. Jacob. "Providing Safe Conduct: Helping Your Patient Cope with Cancer." *Nursing* 4 (1984): 43–48.

Panos, M. B., and Jane Heimlich. *Homeopathic Medicine at Home*. Los Angeles: Tarcher, 1980.

Parker, J. H., and R. B. Parker. *Three Weeks in Spring*. Boston: Houghton Mifflin, 1978.

Parker, S. H., J. D. Lovin, W. D. Jobe, B. J. Burke, K. D. Hopper, and W. F. Yakes. "Nonpalpable Breast Lesions: Stereotactic Automated Large-Core Biopsies." *Radiology* 180 (1991): 403–7.

Parkes, C. M. "The Emotional Impact of Cancer on Patients and Their Families." *Journal of Laryngology and Otology* 89 (1975): 1271–79.

Parkes, Colin M. *Studies of Grief in Adult Life*. Madison, CT: International Universities Press, 1986.

Pauley, J. "Breast Care Test." *PBS Special*, October 15, 1993.

Pearlin, L., and C. Schooler. "The Structure of Coping." *Journal of Health and Social Behavior* 19 (1978): 2–21.

Pearlin, L. I., and J. S. Johnson. "Marital Status, Life-Strains and Depression." *American Sociological Review* 42 (1977): 704–15.

Pearsall, Paul. "Emotional Reactions to Having Cancer." *American Journal of Roentgenology* 114 (1972): 591–99.

———. *Superimmunity.* New York: McGraw-Hill, 1987.

Pederson, L. M. "The Impact of Breast Cancer on Interpersonal Relationships." Paper delivered at World Communication Association, Norwich, England, 1987.

Pederson, L. M., and B. G. Valanis. "The Effects of Breast Cancer on the Family: A Review of the Literature." *Journal of Psychosocial Oncology* 6 (1988): 95–118.

Pelletier, K. R. *Holistic Medicine: From Stress to Optimum Health.* New York: Delacorte Press, 1979.

Peters-Golden, Holly. "Breast Cancer: Varied Perceptions of Social Support in the Illness Experience." *Social Science Medicine* 16 (1982): 483–91.

Photopulos, Georgia, and B. Photopulos. "What to Say to Someone Who's Really Sick." *Looking Forward* 6 (Cincinnati: Good Samaritan Hospital, Fall 1993): 6.

Physicians' Desk Reference. Oradell, NJ: Medical Economics Data, 1994.

Polivy, Janet. "Psychological Effects of Mastectomy on a Woman's Feminine Self-Concept." *Journal of Nervous and Mental Disease* 164 (1977): 77–87.

Poss, Sylvia. "How the Terminal Patient Accepts Dying," in R. H. Moos and J. A. Schaefer, eds., *Coping with Physical Illness 2: New Perspectives.* New York: Plenum, 1984, pp. 391–403.

Preece, P., M. Baum, and R. Mansel. "Importance of Mastalgia in Operable Breast Cancer." *British Medical Journal* 284 (1982): 1299–1300.

Quigley, Pat, and Marilyn Shroyer. *Making It through the Night: How Couples Can Survive a Crisis Together.* Berkeley, CA: Conari Press, 1992.

Raber, M. N., and S. P. Tomasovic. "Spectrum of Breast Cancer." *Cancer Bulletin* 45 (1993): 471.

Rando, Theresa A. *Grieving: How to Go On Living When Someone You Love Dies.* Lexington, MA: D. C. Heath, 1988.

Recht, A., J. L. Connelly, S. J. Schnitt, et al. "Conservative Surgery and Primary Radiation Therapy for Early Breast Cancer: Results, Controversies and Unresolved Problems." *Seminars in Oncology* 13 (1986): 434–49.

Redd, W. H., and M. A. Andrykowski. "Behavioral Intervention in Cancer Treatment: Controlling Aversion Reactions to Chemotherapy." *Journal of Consulting Clinical Psychology* 50 (1982): 1018–29.

Redd, W. H., T. G. Burish, and M. A. Andrykowski. "Aversive Conditioning and Cancer Chemotherapy," in T. Burish, S. Levy, and B. Meyerowitz, eds., *Cancer, Nutrition and Eating Behavior.* Hillsdale, NJ: Lawrence Earlbaum, 1985, pp. 117–32.

Register, Cheri. *Living with Chronic Illness: Days of Patience and Passion.* New York: Free Press, 1987.

Renneker, Richard, and Max Cutler. "Psychological Problems of Adjustment to Cancer of the Breast." *Journal of the American Medical Association* 148 (1952): 833–38.

Richards, Dick. *The Topic of Cancer: When the Killing Has to Stop.* New York: Pergamon Press, 1982.

Rollin, Betty. *First You Cry.* Philadelphia: J. B. Lippincott, 1976.

Rose, D. P., J. M. Connolly, R. T. Chlebowski, et al. "The Effects of a Low-Fat Dietary Intervention and Tamoxifen Adjuvant Therapy on the Serum Estrogen and Sex Hormone—Binding Globulin Concentrations of Postmenopausal Breast Cancer Patients." *Breast Cancer Research and Treatment* 27 (1993): 253–62.

Rosenbaum, E. H. *Living with Cancer.* New York: Praeger, 1975.

Rosenberg, S. A. "Immunotherapy and Gene Therapy of Cancer." *Cancer Research—Supplement* 51 (September 15, 1991): 5074S–79S.

Rosenberg, S. A., and J. M. Barry. *The Transformed Cell: Unlocking the Mysteries of Cancer.* New York: G. P. Putnam's Sons, 1992.

Roud, P. C. *Making Miracles: An Exploration into the Dynamics of Self.* New York: Warner Books, 1990.

Royak-Schaler, Renee, and B. L. Benderly. *Challenging the Breast Cancer Legacy.* New York: Harper Collins, 1992.

Rubin, T. I., with Eleanor Rubin. *Compassion and Self-Hate: An Alternative to Despair.* New York: David McKay, 1975.

Rutter, Michael. "Stress, Coping and Development: Some Issues and Some Questions." *Journal of Child Psychology and Psychiatric Medicine* 22 (1981): 323–56.

Sabo, D., J. Brown, and C. Smith. "The Male Role and Mastectomy: Support Groups and Men's Adjustment." *Journal of Psychosocial Oncology* 4 (1986): 19–31.

Sahin, A. A., and N. Sneige. "Pathologic Assessment of Prognostic Factors in Patients with Operable Breast Cancer." *Cancer Bulletin* 45 (1993): 495–99.

Sands, R. G. "Crisis Intervention and Social Work Practice in Hospitals." *Health and Social Work* 8 (Fall 1983): 253–61.

Sanger, C. K., and M. Reznikoff. "A Comparison of the Psychological Effects of Breast-Saving Procedures with the Modified Radical Mastectomy." *Cancer* 48 (1981): 2341–46.

Scanlon, E. F., and Philip Strax. "Breast Cancer," in A. I. Holleb, ed., *The American Cancer Society Cancer Book.* Garden City, NY: Doubleday, 1986, pp. 297–340.

Schag, C. C., R. L. Heinrich, and P. A. Ganz. "Cancer Inventory of Problem Situations: An Instrument for Assessing Cancer Patients' Rehabilitation Needs." *Journal of Psychosocial Oncology* 1 (Winter 1983): 11–23.

Schain, W. S. "Sexual Functioning, Self-Esteem and Cancer Care." *Frontiers of Radiation Therapy and Oncology* 14 (1980): 12–19.

Schain, W. S., D. K. Wellisch, R. O. Pasnau, and J. Landsverk. "The Sooner the Better: A Study of Psychological Factors in Women Undergoing Immediate vs. Delayed Breast Reconstruction." *American Journal of Psychiatry* 142 (1985): 40–46.

Schatzkin, A., D. Y. Jones, R. N. Hoover, P. R. Taylor, et al. "Alcohol Consumption and Breast Cancer in the Epidemiologic Follow-Up Study of the First National Health and Nutrition Examination Survey." *New England Journal of Medicine* 316 (1987): 1169–73.

Schatzkin, A., P. Greenwald, D. P. Byar, et al. "The Dietary Fat–Breast Cancer Hypothesis Is Alive." *Journal of the American Medical Association* 261 (1988): 3284–87.

Schier, M. J. "Clinical Trials Expanding for Breast Cancer." *Cancer Bulletin* 45 (1993): 109.

Schoenung, Patricia. "Raising Self-Esteem Crucial after Mastectomy." *Prime Times* (November 1991): 9 (Cincinnati, Deaconess Hospital).

Schover, L. R. "The Impact of Breast Cancer on Sexuality, Body Image, and Intimate Relationships." *Ca—A Cancer Journal for Clinicians* 41 (March/April 1991): 112–20.

Scoresby, A. L. *The Marriage Dialogue.* Reading, MA: Addison-Wesley, 1977.

Scott, D. M. "Quality of Life following the Diagnosis of Breast Cancer." *Topics in Clinical Nursing* 4 (1983): 20–37.

Seidman, H., S. D. Stellman, M. H. Mushinski. "A Different Perspective on Breast Cancer Risk Factors: Some Implications of the Nonattributable Risk." *Cancer* 32 (1982): 301–13.

Seltzer, V. L. *Every Woman's Guide to Breast Cancers: Prevention, Treatment, Recovery.* New York: Penguin, 1988.

Shook, R. L. *Survivors Living with Cancer: Portraits of Twelve Inspiring People.* New York: Harper & Row, 1983.

Siegel, Bernie S. *Love, Medicine and Miracles.* New York: Harper & Row, 1986.

———. *Peace, Love and Healing.* New York: Harper & Row, 1989.

Silberfarb, P. M., L. H. Maurer, and C. S. Crouthamel. "Psychiatric Themes in the Rehabilitation of Mastectomy Patients." *International Journal of Psychiatry in Medicine* 8 (1977–1978): 159–67.

———. "Psychosocial Aspects of Neoplastic Disease: I. Functional Status of Breast Cancer Patients during Different Treatment Regimens." *American Journal of Psychiatry* 137 (April 1980): 450–55.

Sillars, Alan L., T. S. Jones, and M. A. Murphy. "Communication and Understanding in Marriage." *Human Communication Research* 10 (1984): 317–50.

Simonton, O. Carl, S. Matthews-Simonton, James Creighton. *Getting Well Again.* Los Angeles: J. P. Tarcher, 1978.

Simonton, Stephanie, with R. L. Shook. *The Healing Family: The Simonton Approach for Families Facing Illness.* New York: Bantam Books, 1984.

Singletary, S. E., M. H. Schusterman, and M. D. McNeese. "Breast Conservation vs. Breast Reconstruction." *Cancer Bulletin* 45 (1993): 512–16.

Smuts, J. S. *Holism and Evolution.* London: Macmillan, 1927.

Sobel, David, ed. *Ways of Health, Holistic Approaches to Ancient and Contemporary Medicine.* New York: Harcourt Brace Jovanovich, 1979.

Spear, Ruth. "Breast Cancer: New Research, New Options." *New York* (January 16, 1984): 24–33.

Spiegel, David. *Living beyond Limits.* New York: Random House, 1993.

Spiegel, David, J. Bloom, H. Kraemer, et al. "Effect of Psychosocial Treatment on Survival of Patients with Metastatic Breast Cancer." *Lancet* 2 (1989): 888–91.

Staerkel, G. A. "Fine-Needle Aspiration: Technique and Application in the Evaluation of Malignancies." *Cancer Bulletin* 45 (1993): 8–12.

Stefanek, M. E., and Patti Wilcox. "First Degree Relatives of Breast Cancer Patients:

Screening Practices and Provision of Risk Information." *Cancer Detection and Prevention* 15 (October 1991): 379–85.

Steinberg, D., L. Juliano, and L. Wise. "Psychological Effects of Lumpectomy versus Mastectomy for Breast Cancer." *American Journal of Psychology* 142 (1985): 34–39.

Steinberg, Joyce, and P. J. Goodwin. "Alcohol and Breast Cancer Risk—Putting the Controversy into Perspective." *Breast Cancer Research and Treatment* 19 (1991): 221–31.

Stetz, K. M., F. M. Lewis, and J. Primomo. "Family Coping Strategies and Chronic Illness in the Mother." *Family Relations* 35 (1986): 515–22.

Stevens, L. A., M. H. McGrath, R. D. Druss, S. J. Kister, F. E. Grump, and K. A. Forde. "The Psychological Impact of Immediate Breast Reconstruction for Women with Early Breast Cancer." *Plastic and Reconstructive Surgery* 73 (April 1984): 619–26.

Stinnett, Nick, and John De Frain. *Secrets of Strong Families.* Boston: Little, Brown, 1985.

Stolar, G. E. "Coping with Mastectomy: Issues for Social Work." *Health and Social Work* 7 (1982): 26–34.

Stommel, M., and M. Kingry. "Support Patterns for Spouse-Caregivers." *Cancer Nursing* 14 (August 1991): 200–205.

Sullivan, C. F., and K. K. Reardon. "Social Support Satisfaction and Health Locus of Control: Discriminators of Breast Cancer Patients' Styles of Coping," in M. L. McLaughlin, ed., *Communication Yearbook 9.* Beverly Hills: Sage, 1986, pp. 707–22.

Sullivan, Irene. "Cancer: Curriculum for Well Siblings of Pediatric Cancer Patients," in A. Blitzer et al., eds., *Communicating with Cancer Patients and Their Families.* Philadelphia: Charles Press, 1990, pp. 90–114.

Taylor, S., R. Lichtman, and J. Wood. "Attributions, Beliefs about Control and Adjustment to Breast Cancer." *Journal of Personality and Social Psychology* 46 (1984): 489–502.

Thiadens, S.R.J. *Lymphedema: An Information Booklet,* 3d edition. San Francisco: National Lymphedema Network, 1993.

Thomas, Patricia. "The Muddle over Screening Breast Cancer." *Medical World News* (May 9, 1988): 34–38.

Thorne, S. E. "Helpful and Unhelpful Communications in Cancer Care: The Patient Perspective." *Oncology Nursing Forum* 15 (1989): 167–72.

Thorne, Sally. "The Family Experience." *Cancer Nursing* 8 (1985): 285–91.

Trillin, A. S. "Of Dragons and Garden Peas: A Cancer Patient Talks to Doctors," in R. H. Moos and J. A. Schaefer, eds., *Coping with Physical Illness 2: New Perspectives.* New York: Plenum, 1984.

Tse, N. Y., C. K. Hoh, R. A. Hawkins, et al. "The Application of Positron Emission Tomographic Imaging with Fluorodeoxyglucose to the Evaluation of Breast Disease." *Annals of Surgery* 216 (1992): 27–34.

Vachon, M.L.S. "A Comparison of the Impact of Breast Cancer, Personality, Social Support and Adaptation," in S. E. Hobfall, ed., *Stress, Social Support and Women.* Washington, DC: Hemisphere, 1986.

———. "Psychotherapy and the Person with Cancer: An Analysis of One Nurse's Experience." *Oncology Nursing Forum* 12 (July/August 1985): 33–40.

Vachon, M.L.S., A. Formo, K. Freedman, W.A.L. Lyall, J. Rogers, and S.J.J. Freeman. "Stress Reactions to Bereavement." *Essence* 1 (1976): 15–21.

Valanis, B. G., and C. H. Rumpler. "Helping Women to Choose Breast Cancer
Treatment Alternatives." *Cancer Nursing* 8 (June 1985): 167–75.

Veer, P., F. Kok, R. Herman, and F. Sturmans. "Alcohol Dose: Frequency and Age
at First Exposure in Relation to the Risk of Breast Cancer." *International
Journal of Epidemiology* 18 (1989): 511–17.

Veninga, Robert L. *A Gift of Hope: How We Survive Our Tragedies.* Boston: Little,
Brown, 1985.

Verderber, R. F., and K. S. Verderber. *Inter-Act,* 6th ed. Belmont, CA: Wadsworth,
1992.

Vess, J. D., J. R. Moreland, and A. I. Schwebel. "An Empirical Assessment of the
Effects of Cancer on Family Role Functioning." *Journal of Psychosocial Oncology* 3 (1985): 1–16.

Vettese, JoAnn. "Family Stress and Mediation in Cancer," in P. Ahmed, ed., *Living
and Dying with Cancer.* New York: Elsevier, 1981, pp. 273–84.

Vinokur, A. D., B. A. Threatt, R. D. Caplan, and B. L. Zimmerman. "Physical and
Psychological Functioning and Adjustment to Breast Cancer: Long-term Follow-Up of a Screening Population." *Cancer* 63 (1989): 394–405.

Viorst, Judith. *Necessary Losses.* New York: Ballantine Books, 1987.

Vogel, C. L. "Treatment of Metastatic Breast Cancer." *Seminars in Oncology Nursing* 7 (August 1991): 194–99.

Vogel, V. G., and A. C. Yeomans. "Evaluation of Risk and Preventive Approaches
to Breast Cancer." *Cancer Bulletin* 45 (1993): 489–94.

Wabrek, A. J., and C. J. Wabrek. "Mastectomy: Sexual Implications." *Primary Care*
3 (1976): 803–10.

Wainstock, J. M. "Breast Cancer: Psychosocial Consequences for the Patient." *Seminars in Oncology Nursing* 7 (August 1991): 207–15.

Wallis, Claudia. "A Puzzling Plague: What Is It about the American Way of Life
That Causes Breast Cancer?" *Time* (January 14, 1991): 48–52.

Ward, Sandra, Susan Heidrich, and William Wolberg. "Factors Women Take into
Account When Deciding upon Type of Surgery for Breast Cancer." *Cancer
Nursing* 12 (1989): 344–51.

Wass, Hannelore, and C. A. Corr. *Helping Children Cope with Death: Guidelines and
Resources,* 2d ed. New York: Hemisphere, 1984, 1982. McGraw-Hill International Book Co.

Watson, Maggie. S. Greer, L. Rowden, et al. "Relationships between Emotional
Control, Adjustment to Cancer and Depression and Anxiety in Breast Cancer
Patients." *Psychological Medicine* 21 (1991): 51–57.

Weinstein, Bernard. "Cancer Prevention: Recent Progress and Future Opportunities." *Cancer Research—Supplement* (September 15, 1991): 5080S–85S.

————. "The Syndrome of Understanding the Cancer Patient: Caregiver's Plight,"
in R. H. Moos and J. A. Schaefer, eds., *Coping with Physical Illness 2: New
Perspectives.* New York: Plenum, 1984, pp. 345–58.

Weisman, A. D., and H. J. Sobel. "Coping with Cancer through Self-Instruction: A
Hypothesis." *Journal of Human Stress* 5 (March 1979): 3–8.

Weisman, A. D., and J. W. Worden. "The Existential Plight in Cancer: Significance of the First 100 Days." *International Journal of Psychiatry in Medicine* 7 (1976–1977): 1–15.

Welch, Deborah. "Anticipatory Grief Reactions in Family Members of Adult Cancer Patients." *Issues in Mental Health Nursing* 4 (1982): 149–58.

———. "Planning Nursing Interventions for Family Members of Adult Cancer Patients." *Cancer Nursing* 4 (October 1981): 365–70.

Wellisch, D. K. "Family Relationships of the Mastectomy Patient: Interactions with the Spouse and Children." *Israel Journal of Medical Science* 17 (1981): 993–96.

———. "Intervention with the Cancer Patient," in C. K. Prokop and L. A. Bradley, eds., *Medical Psychology: Contributions to Behavioral Medicine.* New York: Academic Press, 1981, pp. 224–40.

Wellisch, D. K., E. R. Gritz, W. Schain, He-Jing Wang, and J. Siau. "Psychological Functioning of Daughters of Breast Cancer Patients." *Psychosomatics* 32 (1991): 324–36.

Wellisch, D. K., F. I. Fawzy, J. Landsverk, et al. "Evaluation of Psychosocial Problems of the Homebound Cancer Patient: The Relationship of Disease and the Sociodemographic Variables of Patients to Family Problems." *Journal of Psychosocial Oncology* 1 (1983): 1–15.

Wellisch, D. K., J. Landsverk, K. Guidera, et al. "Evaluation of Psychosocial Problems of the Homebound Cancer Patient: I. Methodology and Problem Frequencies." *Psychosomatic Medicine* 45 (March 1983): 11–21.

———. "The Psychologic Impact of Breast Cancer on Relationships." *Seminars in Oncology Nursing* 1 (1985): 195–99.

Wellisch, D. K., K. R. Jamison, and R. O. Pasnau. "Adolescent Acting Out When a Parent Has Cancer." *International Journal of Family Therapy* 1 (1979): 230–41.

———. "Psychosocial Aspects of Mastectomy: II. The Man's Perspective." *American Journal of Psychiatry* 135 (May 1978): 543–46.

Westlake, S. B., and F. E. Selder. "Breast Cancer: Living with Uncertainty," in A. Blitzer et al., eds., *Communicating with Cancer Patients and Their Families.* Philadelphia: Charles Press, 1990, pp. 125–33.

Wilkinson, S., P. Maguire, and A. Tait. "Life after Breast Cancer." *Nursing Times* 84 (October 5, 1988): 34–37.

Willet, W. C., M. J. Stampfer, G. A. Colditz, et al. "Moderate Alcohol Consumption and the Risk of Breast Cancer." *New England Journal of Medicine* 316 (1980): 1174–80.

Witkin, M. H. "Psychosexual Counseling of the Mastectomy Patient." *Journal of Sex and Marital Therapy* 4 (1978): 20–28.

———. "Sex Therapy and Mastectomy." *Journal of Sex and Marital Therapy* 1 (1975): 290–304.

Wolfe, J. N. "Breast Cancer Screening: A Brief Historical Review." *Breast Cancer Research and Treatment* 18 (1991): S89–S92.

Wolfrom, D. M., A. R. Rao, and C. W. Welsch. "Caffeine Inhibits Development of Benign Mammary Gland Tumors in Carcinogen-Treated Female Sprague-Dawley Rats." *Breast Cancer Research and Treatment* 19 (1991): 269–75.

Woods, N. F. "Influences on Sexual Adaptation to Mastectomy." *Journal of Obstetric and Gynecological Nursing* 4 (1975): 33–37.

Woods, N. F., and J. Earp. "Women with Cured Breast Cancer: A Study of Mastec-
    tomy Patients in North Carolina." *Nursing Research* 27 (1978): 279–85.
Worden, J. W. "Psychosocial Screening of Cancer Patients." *Journal of Psychosocial
    Oncology* 1 (Winter 1983): 1–10.
Worden, J. W., and H. J. Sobel. "Ego Strength and Psychosocial Adaptation to Can-
    cer." *Psychosomatic Medicine* 40 (December 1978): 585–92.
Wortman, C. B. "Social Support and the Cancer Patient." *Cancer* 53 (1983): 2339–
    60.
Wortman, C. B., and Christine Dunkel-Schetter. "Interpersonal Relationships and
    Cancer: A Theoretical Analysis." *Journal of Social Issues* 35 (1979): 120–55.
Wright, K., and S. Dyck. "Expressed Concerns of Adult Cancer Patients' Family
    Members." *Cancer Nursing* 7 (1974): 371–74.
Yasko, J. M., and P. Greene. "Coping with Problems Related to Cancer and Cancer
    Treatment," in A. I. Holleb, ed., *The American Cancer Society Cancer Book.*
    Garden City, NY: Doubleday, 1986, pp. 171–200.
Zanca, J. A. "Making Decisions about Breast Reconstruction." *Cancer Nursing* 11
    (Winter 1993): 2–4.
Zemore, Robert, and L. F. Shepel. "Effects of Breast Cancer and Mastectomy on
    Emotional Support and Adjustment." *Social Science and Medicine* 28 (1989):
    19–27.

Index

Acceptance, 22; of death, 164, 166; of diagnosis, 14, 18, 117, 118; of loss, 22, 78; of one's life, 165; of self, 53, 128, 166; spouses and reconstruction, 53

Achterberg, Jeanne, on imagery, 64

Adenocarcinomas, 29. *See also* Invasive or infiltrating ductal carcinoma

Adjustment: to breast cancer, 13, 25; effect of marital quality, 79; on expressing feelings, 110; of family members, 134; influence of age and other factors, 13–14; influence of health care professionals, 101; most difficult, 78; prior adjustments, 26; spousal/partner reassurance, 150; suggestions for helping, 89; support, 131

Adjuvant chemotherapy, 33, 38, 42; in reducing recurrence, 37. *See also* Chemotherapy

Adjuvant hormone therapy, 42

Adolescents: and anger, 20, 86; behavioral changes, 86; conflict, 86; coping with, 87; effects of death and grief, 171–72; need of support; 172; psychological stresses, 86–87

Affection, need for, 185–86

Age: and breast cancer risk, 9; and treatment choices, 16

AIDS, 68. *See also* Controversial treatments; Immuno-augmentative therapy

Alcohol: and breast cancer, 64; and children, 89; and coping, 117, 119, 157

Alliances, in families, 124

Alopecia, 39. *See also* Hair loss

Alternative/Complementary treatments, 39, 56, 60–69; reasons for interest in, 57

American Cancer Society: on detection guidelines, 6, 7; on implants and mammograms, 49–50; for information about, 96; on nutrition, 63; on safe radiation levels, 8; for sources of information, 113; on supplies, 154; on support groups, 138–39. *See also* Detection methods

American College of Radiology, on implants and mammograms, 49

American Society of Aesthetic Plastic Surgery, 52

American Society of Plastic and Reconstructive Surgeons (ASPRS): on implant ruptures and removal of implants, 51–52; on implants and mammograms, 49; telephone number, 51

Analgesic drug therapy, 19

Androgens, 41. *See also* Hormones

Anesthesia, 32; in reconstruction, 47–48

Anesthetist, 94

Anger: in adolescents, 20; and communication, 153; in coping with death, 164; in daughters, 83, 87–88; as positive reaction, 18; and post-traumatic stress, 151, 156; as reaction to diagnosis, 17, 18, 21, 22; in sons, 89

Anti-cancer drugs, 38

Anticipatory reaction: to chemotherapy, 38; to death, 76

Anti-nausea drugs, 39

Antioncogene, 27

Anxiety: and breast lumpiness, 7; of children, 84, 114; of decision-making, 16; of family, 133; and fear of recurrence, 22, 26; of physicians, 98; of prosthesis, 78; of recovery, 149; and sexual adjustment, 78, 112; of spouses/partners, 75, 76; of treatment and side effects, 40, 123; of waiting for diagnosis and surgery, 5

Areola, 45; grafting, 46; nipple sharing, 46; tattoo, 45–46

Aspiration, of pseudolumps, 29

ASPRS (American Society of Plastic and Reconstructive Surgeons), 51, 56

Assertiveness, 6, 176, 194

Attitude, 89; healing, 110; positive, 159

Autogolous bone marrow transplant, 26, 42. *See also* Bone marrow rescue; Bone marrow transplant

Autoimmune (rheumatic) disorders: and silicone implants, 50; symptoms of, 50

Autosomal dominant syndrome, 34. *See also* Preventive surgery; Prophylactic surgery

Avoidance: as coping method, 81; of others, 74; of spouses, 74–75

Awareness, of breast cancer symptoms, 6

Axilla, 36

Axillary dissection, 33, 36. *See also* Lymph nodes

Axillary lymph nodes, 33

Axillary metastases, 36

Axioms of holistic medicine, 68. *See also* Holism

B-A-Fiter formula, 65, 66

Bankruptcy, 147

Bargaining, in coping with death, 164

Baseline mammogram, 2, 29. *See also* Mammogram

Bayh, Marvella, 167, 194. *See also* Growth, personal and family

Bennett, Dr. Howard, *The Best of Medical Humor*, 67. *See also* Humor and laughter; Laughter

Benson, Herbert, on relaxation, 60

Bilateral surgery, 5, 35, 55, 77. *See also* Double mastectomy

Bill of 10 Rights, for patients and family members, 166. *See also* Kaye, Ronnie

Biofeedback, and pain, 19, 60

Biopsy, 4–6; excisional biopsy, 31–32; fear of, 11; fine-needle biopsy, 31; incisional biopsy, 31–32; of pseudolumps, 29, 40; stereotactic breast biopsy (mammotest), 32. *See also* Detection methods

BIPRN (Breast Implant Patient Relation Network), 52

Birth control pills, and breast cancer: risk, 10; guilt, 20

Black, Shirley Temple, 143. *See also* Personal care

Blood counts, 38, 39, 40

BMT. *See* Bone marrow transplant

Body image, 21–22; and chemotherapy, 39; effect of spousal rejection on, 24, 73; and reconstruction, 47

Body imbalance, 47, 53; and survival, 154. *See also* Post-traumatic stress disorder

Bombeck, Erma, 194

Bone marrow rescue, 19; process, 41–42. *See also* Autologous bone marrow transplant, Bone marrow transplant

Bone marrow transplant (BMT), 28, 41. *See also* Bone marrow rescue

Breast augmentation, 46

Breast cancer: classifications by cell type, 29–30; incidence in men, 12; incidence in women, 10; negative effects, 21–22, 193; predictions for new cases, 11–12; rate of growth, 5, 28; risk factors, 4, 9–10; treatment approaches, 28 (*see also* Treatment options)

Breast conservation, 16. *See also* Lumpectomy

Breast Implant Patient Relations Network (BIPRN), 52

Breast implants: coping with rupture, 51; detection of, 49–50; fixation of, 44; guidelines for handling problems, 50–52; insertion of, 47; removal of, 44; risks of rupture, 48–49; saline-filled, 44; silicone gel–filled, 43–44

Breast pain, 3, 98; with capsular contraction, 48; cyclical and menstrual cycle, 19; nonbreast pain, 19; noncyclical or target-zone, 3, 19; phantom breast pain, 77, 155. *See also* Holistic treatment methods; Mastaglia

Breast reconstruction, 18, 33; as a choice, 48, 54; historical perpective, 43–44; women's reactions to, 47, 51–54. *See also* Reconstructive surgery

Breast reduction, 5

Breast self-examination (BSE), 2, 3, 7, 10; failure to practice, 10; procedure for, 8. *See also* BSE; Detection methods; Mammogram

Breast size, and treatment selection, 16. *See also* Treatment options, conditions for selection

Breast symmetry, 35; with reconstructive surgery, 54

Breast symptoms of cancer, 3, 6, 7

Breast tissue: change in, 2, 7 (*see also* Lumpy breasts); and radiation, 36

Breastfeeding, 6

Breasts as symbols of femininity, 12, 54

Brinker, Nancy: on coping, 155–56; on exercise, 64; on lymphedema, 154–55; *The Race Is Run One Step at a Time*, 64

BSE (breast self-examination), 2, 7, 8, 10. *See also* Breast self-examination

Caffeine, and breast cancer, 64

Calcifications, 5, 29, 30. *See also* Lesions; Microcalcifications

Cancer Care Inc., 123, 138

Cancer cells, 5, 28, 31, 41; growth rate of, 5, 28; metastasis of, 28 *See also* Love, Dr. Susan M.

Cancer Counseling and Research Center, Fort Worth, 60

Cancer risk: alcohol consumption, 64; caffeine, 64; diet, 64; family history, 4; genetic factors, 28; preventive surgery, 34; weight, 63

Cancer Share, 23, 56

Cancers of the breast, by cell types: infiltrating comedocarcinoma, 30; inflammatory breast carcinoma, 30; invasive ductal carcinoma, 29; invasive lobular carcinoma, 30; medullary carcinoma, 29–30; mucinous carcinoma, 30; noninvasive breast carcinoma in situ, 30; Paget's disease, 30; tubular ductal carcinoma, 30. *See also* Carcinomas of the breast

Cancervive, 150. *See also* Nessim, Susan

Capsular contracture, 44; and breast reconstruction, 48

Carcinogen, 28

Carcinomas of the breast, 3, 28; by cell type, 29–30. *See also* Cancers of the breast

CAT scan (computerized axial tomography), 4, 9; cost of, 9; detection of metastasis, 9; and radiation, 9. *See also* CT scan; Detection methods

Cells: behavior of, 27–28; future genetic alteration of, 28. *See also* Love, Dr. Susan M.

Check-ups, 2, 4; importance of, 10, 152

CHEER (Center for Health Enhancement, Education and Research), 58. *See also* Cousins, Norman

Chemotherapy, 3, 5, 18–19; adjuvant chemotherapy, 38; and bone marrow rescue, 41; effects of, 22, 38–40; effect on cancer cells, 38; how administered, 38; as a major treatment, 42, 61; and stress, 26; weight gain, 73. *See also* Bone marrow rescue

Childbearing, effect of breast cancer on, 24, 25

Childcare, 25

Children's reactions: by age and developmental stage, 84–89; anger, 83, 88; fear, 84–85; guilt, 20; helping them cope, 84–87, 184; reactions to death, 171–72; reactions to parent's recovery, 151; symptoms of stress, 85–89, 115

Cholesterol, 66

Chromosomes, 27

Clinical breast examinations, 6, 7, 8, 10

Collagen vascular disease, criteria for treatment option, 16, 57, 58. *See also* Cousins, Norman

Communication, 80, 107; on benefits of good communication, 106–7; with children, 56, 85, 114–15, 179; and conflict, 83; and death, 168, 170, 172–73; with friends, 104–6, 180; in good marriages, 82; and growth, 160; during illness, 83; improving communication, 107–12; with other family members 106, 179; with professional caregivers, 11, 91, 106, 121; and sexuality, 81; with spouses/partners, 71–72, 104–5, 112–14, 132–33, 185

Communication difficulties, 72; with children, 114; with family and friends, 135–36; family avoidance, 74; with health professionals, 98; mixed messages, 74; reasons for, 81;

83; with sexual issues, 81; between spouses, 73, 104–6, 112–14. *See also* Secrecy

Communication training seminars, for health care providers, 75

Community support resources, 138. *See also under names of specific organizations*

Computerized Nutrition, Health and Activity Profile, 64. *See also* Pelletier, K. R.

Conflicts, 80, 83, 87, 99, 108, 124; of children, 84; with daughters, 83; with family members, 90, 153

Conspiracy of silence, 74. *See also* Secrecy

Constraints: environmental, 26, 123; personal, 122–23

Control, 19, 69; on loss of, 136; on relinquishing, 183

Controlled substances, 19. *See also* Narcotic drugs

Controversial treatments, 68. *See also* Immuno-augmentative therapy (IAT); Laetrile

Copers, good: characteristics of, 126–27; examples of, 90, 103, 128–29, 167–69

Coping, 14, 117–29; of children, 171; and communication, 103; with crises, 14–15, 17–18; with death, 163–64; defined, 118; emotional, 25; rational, 25; with recovery, 149

Coping resources, 21, 119, 166; collective resources, 123; community and professional resources, 115, 122, 127; competency resources, 121; individual, 123; material resources, 121–22; physical resources, 120; psychological resources, 120–21, 127, 129, 141, 166; social support, 122; spiritual resources, 161. *See also* Hansen, Barbara; Harwell, Amy

Coping strategies, 80, 81, 118–19; with death, 164; with dying, 164; holistic coping methods, 57–69; Lerner's patterns of coping, 124; problem-solving coping, 56; with recovery, 150–51; self-protective methods, 119 (*see also* Coping); of successful families, 123; therapists' suggestions for coping, 127. *See also* Kübler-Ross, Elisabeth; Theories

Cornerstone Group, on communication seminars, 99

Cosmetic, Toiletry, and Fragrance Association, 142

Counseling, 56; on sexual problems, 78

Cousins, Norman, 57–59, 66, 68; *Anatomy of an Illness*, 58, 68; on growth, 162. *See also* Humor and laughter; Laughter

Cremation, 157, 164

Crisis events: defined, 14, 158; effects on family, 14, 26, 118; "pile-up" of difficulties, 120; threats of, 120

Crisis intervention, 78

Cronkite, Walter, on Marvella Bayh, 167

CT scans (CAT scans), 9

Cysts, 29; age and, 29; aspiration of, 29; incidence of malignancy, 29; and menopause, 29; milk cysts, 6

Daughters of women with breast cancer, 71–72, 83, 87

Death, 93, 98, 193; benefits of communication, 165; childrens' fears of, 89; communication tasks, 173; coping with, 157, 163; effects on bereaved children, 85, 171 (*see also* Children's reactions); effects on bereaved spouse, 157, 169–70, 187 (*see also* Evans, Dame Edith); effects on communication, 109, 172–73; and empathy, 109; examples of, 167–69 (*see also* Kievman, Beverly; Bayh, Marvella); fears of women, 73, 104; preparation for, 166, 169, 181, 186–87; reactions of dying person, 157, 166, 168–69 (*see also* Harwell, Amy; Kaye, Ronnie); stages of, 164; strengthening inner resources, 170; transcendental death, 165–66. *See also* Coping; Coping Strategies; Kübler-Ross, Elisabeth

Decision-making, 13; with help of nurses, 96, 118; with help of spouses/partners 183–84; listening, 17, 45, 48, 54–55; about preventive surgery, 34; woman's involvement in, 15–16

Defense mechanisms, 119. *See also names of specific behaviors*

Deformity, 34–35, 47. *See also* Mobility of arm and shoulder

Denial, 6, 11; of death, 164; effect of prolonged denial, 76, 90, 109; as maladaptive, 81, 110; as self-protective coping, 6, 118

Deoxyribonucleic acid (DNA), 27, 38

Dependency: fear of, 73; and guilt, 20

Depression, 6, 14; and breast reconstruction, 47; in children, 86; in daughters, 87–88; and death, 164; delayed depression, 23; and expressing feelings, 110; of family members, 76; in lack of treatment choice, 16; and relaxation, 58; as a survivor, 151; and withdrawal, 112, 117, 138

Describing feelings: and adjustment, 110; and children, 86

Detection methods, 2, 8; awareness of body changes, 4, 6; biopsy, 31; breast self-examination, 6, 175; CAT scan, 9; checking out other problems, 4; clinical examination, 5, 6, 7, 175; delayed reconstructive surgery, 65; importance of early detection, 6, 11–12, 88; by intuition, 4; mammography, 2, 6, 42, 175–76; MRI, 9; ultrasound, 8–9. *See also* Lumps

Developmental stages: adolescent, 86–87; schoolage child, 84–86; teenaged and older daughters, 87–89; teenaged and older sons, 89; young child, 85

Diagnosis, 14, 76, 134, 149, 176; impact on family, 84. *See also* Acceptance; Adjustment; Women's reactions

Diet: and chemotherapy, 22 (*see* Chemotherapy, effects of); as complementary treatment, 66; physicians

and, 22; as prevention, 64; and pro-
moter agents, 28; as risk factor, 10.
See also Dreher, Henry; Morgan,
Brian L.G.
Disability, arm and shoulder immobil-
ity, 177
Disfigurement: fear of, 73, 76, 79; reactions of women to, 33, 47, 52
Displacement, 81; as self-protective
coping method, 15, 79. *See also* Defense mechanisms
Distant metastases, 12, 31. *See also* Metastases
Divorce: and breast cancer, 75, 81,
117; and children, 85, 109; after recovery, 151
DNA (deoxyribonucleic acid), 27, 38
Doctor/patient relationships: communication about treatment, 36, 99–100;
communication barriers, 98–99; conflict within families, 98–99; disagree-
ments with, 71; on doctor's failure to
convey hope, 98; on ending treatment, 93, 152–53; expectations of
doctors, 94–95, 99; importance of
good communication, 94, 99; insensitivity of, 94–95; questions to ask,
176; responsibilities of patient and
family to, 100; selecting doctors, 55,
177, 184–85; stresses on professionals, 98; supportiveness of doctors, 93,
100; therapeutic effects of good partnership, 57, 68. *See also* Physicians
Double mastectomy, 5, 53. *See also* Bilateral surgery
Dreher, Henry, 64. *See also* Prevention
Drug abuse, and adjustment, 13–14.
See also Substance abuse
Drugs: analgesic, 19; anti-cancer, 38;
anti-inflammatory, 19; cell cycle nonspecific, 38; cell-specific, 38; narcotic,
19; nonprescription, 19
Dying: effects on bereaved, 169–72; effects on communication, 172–73;
fear of, 22, 76, 87; needs of dying
person, 166; needs of other members, 169–70; preparation for, 166–
69; reactions to, 164; suggestions for

"good death" experience, 173; tasks
of bereaved, 168 (*see also* Kievman,
Beverly). *See also* Death
Dysplasia, 1, 31

Eckland (four views) mammogram, 49;
on finding accredited mammography
equipment, 49. *See also* Modified
compression technique
Ego-strength, 150
Emotional balance, effects of body
changes, 15
Emotional coping, 14, 18, 21, 25–26,
76, 183; choosing treatment, 16;
preparation for treatment, 56
Emotional needs of patients and families, 42
Empathy, 101, 106; defined, 108; examples of, 108–10; how to develop,
108–9; importance of, 80, 108–9;
specific need for, 109–10. *See also*
Death; Dying; Grieving
Employment, 118; and post-traumatic
stress, 150
Endorphins, 19. *See also* Natural
opiates
Enkalphins, 19. *See also* Natural
opiates
Estrogen: and breast cancer risk, 10;
and hormone therapy, 40, 41
Estrogen-receptor test, 40. *See also*
Hormones
Evans, Dame Edith, 165; effects of
spouse's death on, 169
Excisional biopsy, 31, 32. *See also* Biopsy
Expressing feelings: of anger, 110; of
children, 115; learned behavior, 81;
of overwhelming emotions, 133; of
patients, 98; in recovery, 150, 178;
on sensitive issues, 113; on sexuality,
79
External prosthesis, 52, 53

FACT (Facing a Cancer Trauma: Psychological Support for Women), 138
Faith and prayer: as a coping strategy,
15; loss of, 88; strengthening, 89

Families: characteristics of "low-stress" and "high-stress" families, 123; family relationships, 123; structure of, 84; successful families, 120. *See also* Coping strategies, of successful families

Family history, 175; and risk factors, 9; and treatment choice, 16

Family members: adjustment and being supportive, 134; needs of, 42, 97, 138; responsibilities to health care professionals, 100; on taking care of own needs, 135; what they value in nurses, 97

Fasting, and holism, 57

Fat intake, 63. *See also* Diet

Fatigue: and emotional trauma, 26; and marital relationship, 79; and radiation, 36

FDA (Food and Drug Administration), 44; guidelines for ruptured implants, 50; handling problems with implants, 50–51; on risk of implants, 49, 50; toll-free number, 51

Fears, of children: of getting cancer, 88; of mother dying, 89

Fears, of spouses: of hurting wife, 79, 112; of wife dying, 76

Fears of women: of cancer screening, 10–11; of disfigurement, 73; of dying, 22; of effect on family, 19, 73; Five D's, 19; and guilt, 20; of loss of attractiveness, 73; of pain, 19, 73; and preventive surgery, 34; of recurrence, 22, 73; of sexual relationship, 23

Felder, Leonard: on financial challenges of illness, 147; on guilt, 20 (*see* Guilt); *When a Loved One Is Ill*, 20, 147

Felson, Benjamin, 67; *Humor in Medicine . . . and Other Topics*, 67

Femininity, and reconstructive surgery, 47

Fibroadenomas, 6, 29; age and menstruation, 29

Fibrocystic disease, 3, 11, 29. *See also* Lumps; Pseudolumps

Fibrosis, 47

Fibrous membrane, 44; and capsular contraction, 48

Financial resources, 25, 121–22, 145; financial advisors, 147. *See also* Coping resources

Fine-needle aspiration biopsy, 31. *See also* Biopsy

Five D's, 19; *See also* Fears

Food and Drug Administration (FDA), advisory panel of, 44; guidelines for, 44; toll-free number, 51

Food toxins, 27

Forbes, Bryan, 165; on life of Dame Edith Evans, 165

Ford, Gerald, 143

Freeman, Lucy, 20; *Guilt: Letting Go* (with H. L. Strean), 20

Friends: on attitudes of, 136; suggestions for, 135–37; and supportiveness, 135; on what to do and say, 136

FSC (Family Success Consortium, Ohio), 138

Genes, 27–28, 69; oncogenes (normal genes transformed into tumors), 27; regulator genes (normal or growth-supporting protooncogenes), 27; tumor-suppressor (or antioncogenes), 27. *See also* Risk factors; *names of specific genes*

Genetic alterations, 28

Genetic research, 42

Graft-taking in bone marrow rescue, 41

Gravelle, Karen, 171–72. *See also* Adolescents; Death, effects on bereaved children

Gray, Lynn, 158, outcome of growth, 161

Grieving, 18; of adolescents, 171; of bereaved spouse, 169–70; and empathy, 110; on expressing feelings, 133; and families, 76; for losses, 55, 56, 65; and physical changes, 118; on stages of grief, 164–65; of young children, 171. *See also* Death; Gravelle, Karen; Kübler-Ross, Elisabeth

Group support: for sexuality, 78

Growth: beginning the process, 160–
61; challenge for, 73, 150; children,
160; commitment to, 160; defined,
158; importance of communication,
160; opportunities for, 89, 181;
outcomes of, 161–62; personal and
family, 158, 160; steps toward, 21,
66, 160. *See also* Quality of life
Growth-supporting genes (protoocoge-
nes), 27
Guidelines. *See* Survival guidelines
Guilt, and breast cancer, 15, 20, 88,
119. *See also* Felder, Leonard; Freeman, Lucy
Gynecologist, 1, 3

Hair loss, 22, 39; chemotherapy and,
22, 141; coping with, 141
Halstead procedure, 34
Hanneman, Samuel, 67. *See also* Home-
opathy
Hansen, Barbara: on acceptance of
death, 166; on growth, 161; on in-
ner resources, 170; *Picking Up the
Pieces*, 161, 170
Harwell, Amy: on friends, 152; suggestions for friends, 189–91; *When Your
Friend Gets Cancer* (with Kristine
Tomasik), 152, 189
Hayes, Helen, 165
Health care, 57
Hepatitis, 68
Holism: areas of concern, 68; defined,
57; four axioms of, 68; historical per-
spective, 57. *See also* Alternative/
complementary treatments; Holistic
treatment methods
Holistic treatment methods, 19, 54, 56,
62; benefits of, 68; dangers of, 68–
69; goals of, 69. *See also* Alternative/
complementary treatments
Homeopathic physicians, 67; goals of,
67. *See also* Alternative/complemen-
tary treatments; Holism
Homeopathy, 54, 67
Hope, 59, 90, 127, 164, 194; false
hope, 60
Hormone-sensitive tumor, 25

Hormones: hormonal changes, 11, 29;
hormonal imbalance, 79; hormonal
problems, 3; hormone-responsive
breast cancer, 40; and osteoporosis,
10, 26; as a risk factor, 10. *See also*
Breast pain
Hospice, 75, 157
Hospitalization, 76
Housekeeping tasks, 25, 80
Hugo, Norman, 47
Humor and laughter, 5, 21; physicians
and humor, 67; putting into our
lives, 66–67; as self-treatment, 58;
therapeutic effects of, 66. *See also*
Cousins, Norman; Laughter
Hypnosis, 19
Hysterectomy, 3, 55, 71

IAT (immuno-augmentative therapy),
68. *See also* Controversial treatments
I Can Cope, 138
Imagery: as a coping method, 62; for
pain, 19. *See also* Visualization
Imaging, 39
Immune disease, 54; guidelines for handling, 50; symptoms of, 50
Immune system: and bone marrow rescue, 41; and cancer, 31; and exercise,
64; and holism, 69; and positive
emotions, 59; and relaxation, 58, 60;
strengthening of, 65. *See also* B-A-
Fiter formula
Immunizer-program, 65. *See also* Pearsall, Paul
Immuno-augmentative therapy (IAT),
68. *See also* IAT; Controversial treatments
Implants: on ASPRS position, 51; capsular contraction, 44; coping with
rupture, 48; FDA guidelines for handling problems with implants, 51, 54;
fixation of, 44; on frequency of ruptures, 51; guidelines for detection,
49; hinderance in detection of breast
cancer, 49; implant removal and replacement, 51; insertion of, 47; polyurethane coating, 44; removal of, 44;
risk of rupture, 48, 51; saline-filled,

44, 50–51; silicone gel-filled, 44, 50–51; on surgical fee, 51; tissue expander, 44

In situ (noninvasive) cancer cells, 1, 30. *See* Noninvasive breast carcinoma in situ

Incisional biopsy, 31–32. *See also* Biopsy

Independence, 130

Infiltrating comedocarcinoma, 30. *See also* Tumors

Inflammatory breast carcinoma, 30. *See also* Tumors

Information: for making treatment decisions, 16; obtaining and absorbing, 17, 56; reasons for difficulty, 17

Initiators in cells, 28. *See also* Cells: behavior of

Inner resources, 65, 129, 166, 178, 180, 194; steps for using, 170; ways of strengthening, 170. *See also* Coping resources; Hansen, Barbara; Kaye, Ronnie

Insurance coverage, 4, 18, 121–22; claims, 25; on dealing with reconstructive surgery, 146; high cost, 147; for implant removal and replacement, 51; on information sources, 145, 147; on keeping records, 143, 145; for mammograms, 11; and PTSD, 156; on risk pools, 146. *See also* Nessim, Susan

Interpersonal relationships, 69; children's relationships, 84–89; communication about, 104; on couples, 71–73, 75–77; difficulty discussing sensitive issues, 106; fulfilling affection and intimacy needs, 77–81, 186; misperceptions of one another, 80–81; how misunderstandings occur, 105–6; other family members, 90, 114–15, 171–72; recovery stresses, 151–52; strains of death, 163–68; strains on single women, 24

Intervention approaches, 75; family-centered program, 122; for reducing stress, 75, 81; for sexual functioning, 78, 81

Invasive or infiltrating ductal carcinoma (adenocarcinoma), 29–30. *See also* Cancers of the breast

Invasive or infiltrating lobular carcinoma, 30. *See also* Cancers of the breast

Inverted nipples, 8. *See also* Nipple changes

Ireland, Jill, 150; *Life Wish*, 150; on coping, 156, 167

Iridium implants, 121

Jillian, Ann: on reconstruction, 53; on surgical scar, 76, 77, 183

Job responsibilities, of spouses, 84

Kaye, Ronnie, 131; on Bill of 10 Rights, 166; on confronting death, 158; on crying, 133; on making needs known, 132, 180; on personal growth, 158

Kievman, Beverly: on children's reactions, 115; on coping, 127–28; on financial and practical matters, 147, 168; *For Better or For Worse* (with S. Blackmun), 113, 147, 168; on sensitive issues, 113–14

Kübler-Ross, Elisabeth, 162; on children and death, 171; on coping with death, 164; criticism of theory, 164–65; *On Death and Dying*, 164; on philosophy of death, 169, 173

Kushner, Rose, 34, 156, 180

Lactation, 7

Laetrile, 68. *See also* Controversial treatments

Laing, R. D., 105

Laughter, 5, 21, 58, 194. *See also* Humor and laughter

Laying-on-of-hands (therapeutic touch), 62–63

Lazarus, R. S., 127

LDMF procedure, 45. *See also* Myocutaneous flap

Lee, Harper, *To Kill a Mockingbird*, 108

Lerner, Harriet G.: on changing reactions and coping, 125–26; *The Dance of Intimacy*, 123; examples of coping, 124–25; on guilt, 20 (*see* Guilt); on managing anxiety, 115, 123, 125; patterns of coping, 124; on rebuilding a relationship, 151–52

LeShan, Lawrence, 68, 81, 85; on communication, 103; on improving quality of life, 158; on professional help, 106; on self-healing, 159; suggestions for, 160–61; on transcendental death, 165; on transforming failure, 159

Lesions, 12, 31, 39; implants and detection of, 49; nonpalpable lesions, 30. *See also* Dysplasia; Neoplasms

Leukemias, 28–29

Life-cycle stages, and coping, 14, 120

Life-strains, and coping, 14, 120, 129

Life-style, 58, 64, 66; and growth, 156, 158, 162

Listening, 17, 100–101, 108–9; effectiveness, 111–12, 189, 194. *See also* Communication skills

Lobular and ductal carcinoma in situ, 30. *See also* Noninvasive breast carcinoma in situ

Local treatment, 31

Loeff, Phyllis, on information and growth, 161

"Look Good, Feel Better" program, 139

Love, Dr. Susan M., 7; on alternative therapies, 69; on BSE, 8; on cancerous growth rate, 28; on nondrug treatments and immune system, 19; on pregnancy, 25; on risks of cancer, 9; on therapeutic touch, 63; on troublesome lumps, 29; on ultrasound, 9, 49

Luce, Clare Boothe, 195

Lumpectomy, 15; compared to mastectomy, 16, 32, 121; criteria for performing, 33; with radiation, 16; reaction to, 33. *See also* Partial mastectomy

Lumpectomy with radiation, 5, 16; compared to mastectomy, 16

Lumps, in the breast: benign, 3; cysts, 29; fibroadenomas, 29; finding of, 1, 2, 4, 6; malignant, 1, 2, 3, 27, 175; pseudo lumps, 29; troublesome lumps (benign and malignant), 29. *See also under specific names*

Lymph nodes, 5, 28; and axillary dissection, 33, 76; removal of, 33–35. *See also* Axillary dissection

Lymphatic system, 28, 31

Lymphedema, 35, 154; dangers and precautions, 154–55

Lymphomas, 28. *See also* Tumors

Lumpy breasts, 6; characteristics of dominant lumps, 29; confusion caused by, 6

Magnetic resonance imaging (MRI), 9

Malaria, 67. *See also* Homeopathy; Hanneman, Samuel

Malignancy, 3, 28, 30, 32

Mammogram, 1–7; age and, 7–8, 29; avoidance of, 10–11, 15; as baseline, 2, 29; calcified areas, 29; as detection, 28, 29–30; and implants, 49, 50; limitations of, 7; and pain, 11; possible radiation risks, 8; selecting accredited equipment, 7–8

Mammography, 3, 7, 9, 42, 49; insurance coverage, 11; proper practice of, 10

Mammotest, 32. *See also* Stereotactic breast biopsy

Marital-sexual relationship: and communication on issues, 78, 112–13; in low-stress families, 123; prior relational quality, 78; reactions to stresses, 75, 79–80; satisfaction with, 81; spousal/partner reactions, 79–81; women's feelings of femininity, 78–81

Marriage: characteristics of strong marriage, 80; quality of relationship, 79; rebuilding impaired marriage, 151

Mastalgia, 19. *See also* Breast pain

Mastectomy, 1–3, 23, 30, 33, 43, 45; modified radical, 16–33; modified radical with radiation, 16; modified radical with reconstruction, 16; partial mastectomy, 32, 33 (*see also* Lumpectomy; Quadrantectomy; Segmental mastectomy; Wide excision); possible complications from, 35; radical, 34

M. D. Anderson Hospital and Tumor Institute, 13

Meaning of life, 158, 166, 194

Medicaid, 147

Medical costs, 145, 147; preparatory measures, 147–48

Medical forms, 145

Medication, 18

Meditation: defined, 60; and pain, 19, 54, 57, 127; and Siegel, 61. *See also* Holistic treatment methods

Medullary carcinoma, 29–30. *See also* Tumors

Memorial Sloan-Kettering Cancer Center in New York, 142

Menopause, 25, 80; ages, 30; and cysts, 29–30; and hormone therapy, 40

Menstruation: and chemotherapy, 25, 39; family history, 10; and fibroadenomas, 6, 29

Metastases, 12, 31; risk of, 42

Metastasis, 28, 31, 63; and Tamoxifen, 41

Microcalcifications, 5. *See also* Calcifications; Lesions

Milk cysts, 6. *See also* Cysts

Mobility of arm and shoulder, 34, 35. *See also* Disability

Modified compression technique, 49–50

Modified radical mastectomy, 16, 33, 34; with reconstruction, 16

Mood changes (or swings), 21, 73; and chemotherapy, 39; spouse's acceptance of, 132; spouse's reaction, 107; and tension, 80

Morgan, Brian L. G., 64

Mortality rates: and mammograms, 40; for men, 12; predictions for 1994, 12; for women, 11–12. *See also* Breast cancer, predictions for new cases

Mothers, of women with breast cancer: conflict with, 90; reactions of, 90

Motivation, and treatment options, 16

Motor nerve, injury of, 35. *See also* Disability; Lymphedema

MRI (magnetic resonance imaging), 9. *See also* Detectionmethods

Mucinous carcinoma, 30. *See also* Cancers of the breast

Murcia, Andy: *Man to Man: When the Woman You Love Has Breast Cancer* (with Bob Stewart), 77; on providing support, 183; on viewing of scar, 76–77

Mutilation: male attitude, 77; women's feelings of, 47, 79

Myocutaneous flap (or TRAM flap), 45; advantages of, 45

Myths about breast cancer, 19, 153

Napier, Augustus Y.: *The Fragile Bond*, 105; on marriage and communication, 105

Narcotic drugs, 19

National Cancer Institute, 8, 10; on exercise, 64; on fat and protein, 63; on partial mastectomy, 33; toll-free number, 33, 49

National Institute of Health, on effectiveness of lumpectomy, 33

Natural killer (NK) cells, 58–59

Natural opiates, 19. *See also* Endorphins; Enkalphins

Nausea: and chemotherapy, 22, 38–39; and emotional trauma, 26; and hormonal imbalance, 79

Neoadjuvant systemic therapy, 38, 42. *See also* Chemotherapy

Neoplasms, 31. *See also* Dysplasia; Lesions

Nessim, Susan: *Cancervive: The Challenge of Life After Cancer* (with Judith Ellis), 122, 147, 150; on insurance, 122, 146; on physicians, 152; on stigma and myths, 153; on survival, 149–50

New normalcy, 119, 147, 149, 180

Newly married women, and breast cancer, 137. *See also* Friends; Single women

Nipple changes, 30; dimpling, 8; discharge, 8; inversion, 8; nipple epidermis, 30 (*see also* Paget's disease); retraction, 29 (*see also* invasive or infiltrating ductal carcinoma)

Nipple and areola reconstruction, 45; decision about, 46

Nolen, Dr. William A., 63; *Crisis Time!*, 105; on marriage and communication, 105

Noncyclical pain, 5. *See also* Breast pain

Noninvasive breast carcinoma in situ. *See also* Lobular and ductal carcinoma in situ; Cancers of the breast

Nonmedical therapies, 19, 56. *See also* Alternative/Complementary treatments; Holistic treatment methods

Nonprescription drugs, 19. *See also* Drugs

Non-steroidal, anti-inflammatory drugs, 19. *See also* Drugs

Nonverbal communication, 74, 107, 132, 180; communicating affection, 112; of health care professionals, 98

Nurses, 94; examples of supportive nurses, 96–97, 100; how they can help the family, 99; insensitivity of, 94; kinds of information nurses can give, 96; patient and family expectations of, 95–96; pressures on them, 100; support to family, 96–98. *See also* Interpersonal relationships, Physicians

Nutrition: fat intake, 63–64, 88, 134; and holism, 57

Oncogenes, 27. *See also* Genes

Oncologist, 16, 39, 59, 94, 114. *See also* Oncology radiologist

Oncology radiologist, 16, 94. *See also* Oncologist

Oophorectomy, 40

Openness in communication, 106, 132

Osteoporosis, 10

p53 (tumor suppressor gene), 28. *See also* Genes

Pac-men, 62

Paget's disease, 30. *See also* Cancers of the breast; Nipple changes

Pain: fear of, 19; and mammograms, 11; tolerance, 11. *See also* Breast pain

Palpable mass, 5

Parker, Joan H.: on sexual adjustment, 78; *Three Weeks in Spring* (with R. B. Parker), 78

Partial mastectomy, 32, 33. *See also* Lumpectomy; Quadrantectomy; Segmental mastectomy; Wide excision

Pathologist, 32, 33

Patterns of coping, 124. *See also* Lerner, Harriet G.

Pearsall, Paul, 64; on B-A-Fiter formula, 65; on laughter, 66; *Superimmunity*, 66. *See also* B-A-Fiter formula; Humor and laughter; Immune system

Pelletier, K. R.: on nutrition and health, 64. *See also* Computerized Nutrition, Health and Activity Profile

Personal care, 25, 138; benefits of, 141–42; coping, 141–42; "Look Good, Feel Better" seminars for, 142–43; spousal assistance, 134. *See also* Black, Shirley Temple; Brinker, Nancy; Murcia, Andy

Phantom breast sensation, 77, 155. *See also* Breast pain

Phlebitis, 35

Physical contact, patient's need for, 77

Physical exercise: for arm mobility, 35; for immune system, 58, 64; and lymphedema, 64, 154; for pain, 19; for stress and well-being, 57, 88, 127; therapists' suggestion for, 127

Physical therapy, 19

Physicians, 93; attitudes and philosophy of, 127; communication with, 35, 41, 55, 61, 98–100, 106–7; emotional support, 93, 99; expectations of 94–96; and holistic treatment, 68; and homeopathy, 67; and humor, 67; and implant problems, 51; insensitiv-

ity of, 93–95; questions to ask, 176; release after treatment, 152–53; selection of, 177, 184–85. *See also* Doctor/patient relationships; Nurses
Polyurethene, as coating for implants, 44
Post-traumatic stress disorder (PTSD), 147, 149; problems of, 156
Practical matters (legal, financial), 145–46, 167–68
Prayer, 54, 61, 62, 63
Predictions. *See* Breast cancer, predictions for new cases
Pregnancy, 6, 7; and risk factors, 10, 24, 25
Prevention: to decrease risk, 63; good eating habits, 65; lowered fat intake, 64. *See also* Diet; Dreher, Henry; Morgan, Brian L. G.
Preventive surgery, 34
Problem-solving (rational) coping techniques, 14, 25–26, 118–19; advantages, 119. *See also* Coping strategies
Progesterone: and hormone therpy, 40, 41
Prognosis, 30, 59. *See also names of cancers of the breast*
Projection, as self-protective strategy, 15
Promoters in cells, 28. *See also* Cells, behavior of
Prophylactic surgery, 34
Prosthesis, 22, 52–53, 78, 136, 154
Protooncogenes, 27. *See also* Genes
Pseudolumps, 6, 29. *See also* Lumps; Fibrocystic disease
Psychic healing, 54, 62–63
Psychological makeup, and coping, 5
Psychological well-being, and marital quality, 81
Psychosocial problems, 13, 26; counseling for, 78
Psychotherapist, helpfulness of, 18, 94, 103, 131
Psychotherapy, 25, 104
PTSD (post-traumatic stress disorder), 147, 156; anger and resentment, 153; fear of recurrence, 155; main-

taining self-esteem, 150; physical effects, 154; relationships, 150–53; stigma, 153

Quackery, 68
Quadrantectomy, 32, 35. *See also* Partial mastectomy
Quality of life, 13, 26, 37, 42, 60, 69, 158, 162. *See also* Growth
Questioning: hesitancy about, 17; open-ended questions, 110–11
Questionnaire responses, 71, 79, 88
Questions to ask, 177, 185

Radiation: compared to chemotherapy, 38; fear of, 11; as major treatment, 42; and mammograms, 7–8; possible side effects and risks, 36; uses for, 33, 35–36; and visualization, 61–62
Radiation therapy, 19. *See also* Radiotherapy
Radical mastectomy, 34. *See also* Mastectomy
Radioisotopes, 35
Radiologist, 8, 11, 32
Radiotherapy, 26, 37. *See also* Radiation therapy
Rando, T. A., 169
Rational coping, 14. *See also* Problem-solving coping techniques
Reach to Recovery, 18, 56, 104, 114, 134, 155
Recoil, 76
Reconstructive surgery: benefits of, 22, 77, 79; history of, 43; immediate versus delayed, 46; psychological effects of, 43, 47–48; physicians on, 45, 147; risks of 48, 50; spouses' reactions to, 53–54; women's reactions to, 52–53, 77. *See also* Love, Dr. Susan M.
Recovery, 71, 131; coping with long term effects, 149–55; need for supportive friends, 152, 190; and self sufficiency, 134. *See also* Brinker, Nancy; Nessim, Susan; Survival
Recuperation, and weight gain, 73, 119, 129, 130

Recurrence, 4, 5; comparative survival rates in mastectomy and lumpectomy with radiation, 16; fear of, 22–23, 73; and post-traumatic stress, 155, 179; Tamoxifen, 41. *See also* Fears, of women

Regulator genes, 27

Rejection: fears of women, 73, 75, 78, 79 (*see* Fears, of women); of friends, 136, 152; spousal misperception of, 151

Relational distancing, 82, 105, 124; coping with, 179

Relaxation, 19; depression and, 58; relaxation response, 60; Simonton's techniques for, 61. *See also* Holistic treatment methods; Simonton, O. Carl

Resentment, 20

Resources, 14. *See also* Coping resources

Responsibility, for one's health, 6, 194

Risk factors: age, 9; in breast cancer, 8, 9–10; diet and obesity, 10, 63; family history, 7; genetic risk, 10; national origin, 10; other factors (pregnancy, menstrual history, hormones), 10; previous cancer, 10; sex, 9; social and economic status, 10

Risk pools, 146. *See also* Insurance coverage

Rosenbaum, E. H., 75, 100; on communication, 106–7, 111; *Living with Cancer*, 75, 100

Rubin, T. I., *Compassion and Self Hate: An lternative Despair* (with E. Rubin), 128

Saline implants, 44, 47, 48; on availability, 51; on FDA guidelines for ruptures, 50–51. *See also* Implants

Sarcomas, 3

Scar tissue, 48, 51

Scoresby, Lynn, *The Marriage Dialogue*, 106

Screening mammograms, 7. *See also* Detection methods

Second opinions, of physicians, 3, 184

Secrecy, 103–4, 122 (*see also* Conspiracy of silence); children's misgivings, 84; examples of, 104; reasons for, 74

Segmental mastectomy, 32. *See also* Partial mastectomy

Self-blame: on holistic practices, 69; on Simonton technique, 20. *See also* Guilt

Self-concept, 71

Self-criticism, 20. *See also* Freeman, Lucy

Self-disclosure, 101, 108

Self-esteem, 11, 14, 15, 21, 73, 126; effect of spousal reaction, 77; effects of reconstructive surgery on, 52–53; and post-traumatic stress, 150. *See also* Breasts as symbols of femininity

Self-healing, 63, 66, 68; holistic approaches, 159

Self-hypnosis, 127

Self-image, 15, 22, 47; effect of breast reconstruction, 54, 79, 88, 109, 117

Self-protective coping methods, 12, 14, 15, 119. *See also* names of specific methods

Self-worth, 53, 59, 88, 150

Sensitive issues, 79, 81, 104, 178, 186

Sex therapy, 78

Sexual attractiveness: effect on relationship, 79; fears about, 73, 117, 150

Sexual functioning: and breast reconstruction, 47; modes of treatment for problems, 78

Shook, Robert, *The Healing Family*, 127

Side effects, 26. *See also* specific treatments

Siegel, Bernie, 61, 66; *Love, Medicine and Miracles*, 61; *Peace, Love and Healing*, 61

Silent ruptures, 50. *See also* Implants

Silicone gel-filled implants, 43, 44; autommune disease, 50 (*see also* Implants); detection of lesions, 49; FDA guidelines for ruptures and risk of implants, 50–51; and risk, 49; and rupture, 48. *See also* FDA

Simonton, Stephanie: on communicating affection, 112; on communication and support, 106; on expressing feelings, 110, 111

Simonton, O. Carl, 60, 61–62, 81, 133. *See also* Simonton technique

Simonton technique: and guilt, 20; and relaxation, 60–61

Single women, 77, 137. *See also* Friends; Unmarried women

Size of breasts, and treatment options, 16

Skin: dimpling, 29; edema of, 30; grafting, 34; local stimulation of, 19 (*see also* Holistic treatment methods)

Sons of women with breast cancer, reactions to, 89. *See also* developmental stages

Spiegel, David, 68–69, 193; *Living beyond Limits*, 68, 193

Spiritual growth, 62, 167; a spiritual vision, 168–69

Spousal/partner reactions to breast cancer: avoidance and rejection, 74, 75; compassion and worry, 22, 24, 25, 40, 72; effect on wife's coping, 80; needs for support, 137; stresses on, 76, 80. *See also* Supportiveness

Spousal/partner reactions to reconstruction: approval, 53–54; disapproval, 43

Spousal/partner reactions to viewing scar, 76; explanations of reactions, 81

Stages of tumor growth, 14, 31, 38, (*see also* Adjustment); and radiation therapy, 35, 36; and survival rate, 12; and treatment options, 16

Stepfamilies, 84

Stereotactic breast biopsy, 32. *See also* Mammotest

Stigma, 22, 136; of survival, 153

Stoicism-fatalism, 15

Stress-reduction, on teaching methods and counseling, 81

Substance abuse, 13. *See also* Adjustment

Support, professional, 93–97, 131, 149; lack of support, 93–95; need for, 150

Support groups, 100, 104, 117, 130; for treatment of adverse effects on sexuality, 78; on women's reactions to, 137, 178

Supportiveness: communication and, 106; defined, 131; empathy, 149; family support, 90, 106, 187; importance of, 81, 133, 158; making needs known, 132; professional support, 131–32; programs for, 122; spousal/partner support, 21, 77, 114–15; on ways of providing support, 134; what spouses can do, 126; woman's responsibility in 129–30. *See also* Spousal/partner reactions

Supportiveness, of friends: attitudes of, 151; examples of, 133–36; kinds of friends, 136; rejection by, 136; in relieving family stress, 106, 129, 130–31, 135–36; suggestions for 135–36, 137

Surgery, 19, 21, 31

Surgical scar: adjusting to, 77–78; viewing of, 21, 76–77. *See also* Murcia, Andy; Parker, Joan H.

Survival, 42; rates of, 12, 68

Survival guidelines, 175–91; for children, 187; for family members, 187–88; for friends, 189–91; for spouses/partners, 183–87; for women with breast cancer, 175–81

Systemic therapy, 31, 38, 40

Systems theory, 123

Tamoxifen, 41; side effects of, 41

Team care, 78

Theories: family systems, 82, 84, 123–24; Kübler-Ross's theory of the death process, 164–65; Laing's theory of interpersonal perception, 105; Lazarus' theory of coping, 127; Lerner's application of systems theory, 123–24

Therapeutic touch, laying-on-of-hands, 63. *See also* Love, Dr. Susan M.

Therapists, 127

Tissue expansion, 44; advantages of, 47; problems of, 45; procedure, 44–45, 47. *See also* Implants

TM (transcendental meditation), 60

Tough love approach, 78

Traditional medical treatment, 56–57; and holistic methods, 62–63, 67–68; Siegel on, 61

Tram flap procedure, 45, 53. *See also* LDMF procedure; Myocutaneous flap

Transcendental meditation (TM), 60

Transplantation of body tissue, 43

Treatment options, 31–42; bone marrow rescue, 41; breast reconstruction, 44–46; chemotherapy, 37–39; conditions for selection, 16; hormone therapy, 40–41; local and systemic, 31; nonmedical methods (*see* Alternative/Complementary treatments; Holistic treatment methods); partial mastectomy, 32–33; preventive surgery, 34; radiation, 35–36; radical mastectomy, 34–35

Tubular ductal carcinoma, 30. *See also* Cancers of the breast

Tumors: development of, 26; major cancer types, 1, 2, 28, 30; rate of growth, 5, 28. *See also* Breast cancer

Tumor-suppressor genes (p53), 27, 28

UCLA (University of California, Los Angeles), 58

Ultrasound, 8; and age, 8–9; and radiation, 9, 49. *See also* Love, Dr. Susan M.

Ultraviolet rays, 27

Unmarried women, and breast cancer, 24, 77. *See also* Single women, Widows

U.S. Department of Health and Human Services, 138

van Nuys, Dr. Jan, 13

Vigilance, 6, 106

Vincent T. Lombardi Cancer Research Center, 142

Viorst, Judith, on adolescents, 166

Virus, 28

Visual imagery, 60

Visualization: and pain, 19, 37, 39, 54; Simonton on Siegal, 61–62, 167; *See also* Holistic treatment methods; Visual imagery

Vitamins, 63. *See also* Morgan, Brian L. G.

Vulnerability: in daughters, 87; to disease, 58; and guilt, 20

Wait-and-see approach, 11, 30

Weight gain, 22, 73, 141–42; of spouse, 157

Wellness, 149; reaction to life events, 64. *See also* Pearsall, Paul; Survival

Wide excision, 32. *See also* Partial mastectomy

Widows, 137, 178

Wigs, 22, 39, 138, 141, 143

Will to live, 5, 58, 127

Withdrawal, 75, 77; in adolescents, 87 (*see also* Developmental stages); as a coping strategy, 79; reasons for, 79

Women's reactions, to breast cancer, 131, 183; effect on self-esteem and sexual identity, 131; fears of rejection, 132; depression, 132; feeling out of control, 133; needs for support, 131–32

X rays, 8, 27, 29, 32. *See also* Mammotest; Stereotactic breast biopsy

Yoga, 60. *See also* Alternative/Complementary treatments

Zen, 60. *See also* Alternative/Complementary treatments

About the Authors

LUCILLE M. PEDERSON is Associate Professor Emerita of the Department of Communication at the University of Cincinnati.

JANET M. TRIGG is Associate Professor of Nursing at the University of Cincinnati.

ISBN 0-89789-293-3

90000>

EAN

HARDCOVER BAR CODE